Handbook of Anticancer Drug Discovery and Development

Handbook of Anticancer Drug Discovery and Development

Editor: Octavia Settle

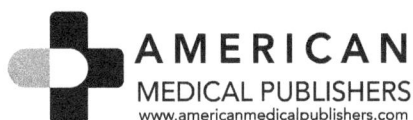

AMERICAN
MEDICAL PUBLISHERS
www.americanmedicalpublishers.com

AMERICAN
MEDICAL PUBLISHERS
www.americanmedicalpublishers.com

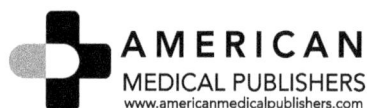

Cataloging-in-Publication Data

Handbook of anticancer drug discovery and development / edited by Octavia Settle.
   p. cm.
Includes bibliographical references and index.
ISBN 978-1-63927-880-0
1. Antineoplastic agents. 2. Drugs--Design. 3. Drug development. 4. Cancer--Chemotherapy.
5. Pharmaceutical technology. I. Settle, Octavia.
RS431.A64 H36 2023
615.798--dc23

American Medical Publishers,
41 Flatbush Avenue,
1st Floor, New York,
NY 11217, USA

ISBN 978-1-63927-880-0 (Hardback)

Contents

Preface..VII

Chapter 1   **Magnetic Graphene Oxide Nanocarrier for Targeted Delivery of Cisplatin: A Perspective for Glioblastoma Treatment**..1
Sami A. Makharza, Giuseppe Cirillo, Orazio Vittorio, Emanuele Valli, Florida Voli, Annafranca Farfalla, Manuela Curcio, Francesca Iemma, Fiore Pasquale Nicoletta, Ahmed A. El-Gendy, Gerardo F. Goya and Silke Hampel

Chapter 2   *Elaeagnus angustifolia* **Plant Extract Inhibits Epithelial-Mesenchymal Transition and Induces Apoptosis via HER2 Inactivation and JNK Pathway in HER2-Positive Breast Cancer Cells**...16
Ayesha Jabeen, Anju Sharma, Ishita Gupta, Hadeel Kheraldine, Semir Vranic, Ala-Eddin Al Moustafa and Halema F. Al Farsi

Chapter 3   **Synthesis, Anti-Cancer and Anti-Migratory Evaluation of 3,6-Dibromocarbazole and 5-Bromoindole Derivatives**..33
Krystal M. Butler-Fernández, Zulma Ramos, Adela M. Francis-Malavé, Joseph Bloom, Suranganie Dharmawardhane and Eliud Hernández

Chapter 4   **Macrocybin, a Natural Mushroom Triglyceride, Reduces Tumor Growth In Vitro and In Vivo through Caveolin-Mediated Interference with the Actin Cytoskeleton**..52
Marcos Vilariño, Josune García-Sanmartín, Laura Ochoa-Callejero, Alberto López-Rodríguez, Jaime Blanco-Urgoiti and Alfredo Martínez

Chapter 5   **3-Vinylazetidin-2-Ones: Synthesis, Antiproliferative and Tubulin Destabilizing Activity in MCF-7 and MDA-MB-231 Breast Cancer Cells**..65
Shu Wang, Azizah M. Malebari, Thomas F. Greene, Niamh M. O'Boyle, Darren Fayne, Seema M. Nathwani, Brendan Twamley, Thomas McCabe, Niall O. Keely, Daniela M. Zisterer and Mary J. Meegan

Chapter 6   **Can the Efficacy of [¹⁸F]FDG-PET/CT in Clinical Oncology be Enhanced by Screening Biomolecular Profiles?**...114
Hazel O'Neill, Vinod Malik, Ciaran Johnston, John V Reynolds and Jacintha O'Sullivan

Chapter 7   **Cytotoxic Effects of Newly Synthesized Heterocyclic Candidates Containing Nicotinonitrile and Pyrazole Moieties on Hepatocellular and Cervical Carcinomas**..........129
Amira A. El-Sayed, Abd El-Galil E. Amr, Ahmed K. EL-Ziaty and Elsayed A. Elsayed

Chapter 8   **Role of Photoactive Phytocompounds in Photodynamic Therapy of Cancer**.......................143
Kasipandi Muniyandi, Blassan George, Thangaraj Parimelazhagan and Heidi Abrahamse

Chapter 9   **Overcoming Resistance to Platinum-Based Drugs in Ovarian Cancer by Salinomycin and its Derivatives — An In Vitro Study**................164
Marcin Michalak, Michał Stefan Lach, Michał Antoszczak, Adam Huczyński and Wiktoria Maria Suchorska

Chapter 10   **In Vitro and In Vivo Anti-Breast Cancer Activities of Some Newly Synthesized 5-(thiophen-2-yl)thieno-[2,3-d]pyrimidin-4-one Candidates**....................179
Abd El-Galil E. Amr, Alhussein A. Ibrahimd, Mohamed F. El-Shehry, Hanaa M. Hosni, Ahmed A. Fayed and Elsayed A. Elsayed

Chapter 11   **Synthesis, Antiproliferative Activity and Molecular Docking Studies of Novel Doubly Modified Colchicine Amides and Sulfonamides as Anticancer Agents**....................193
Julia Krzywik, Witold Mozga, Maral Aminpour, Jan Janczak, Ewa Maj, Joanna Wietrzyk, Jack A. Tuszyński and Adam Huczyński

Permissions

List of Contributors

Index

Preface

Anticancer drugs refer to drugs that are used for treating cancerous or malignant diseases. They are classified into several categories, including antimetabolites, hormones, alkylating agents and natural products. Preclinical research, clinical research and post-clinical research are the three primary steps in the development of a novel drug. Clinical trial evaluation, in vivo confirmation, and in vitro cytotoxicity on cancer cells are the major assessment methods used while creating an anticancer drug. The evaluation of cytotoxicity towards cancer cell lines is a popular method for discovering anticancer agents. New cancer drugs can be discovered in a variety of ways including testing of animals, plants and fungi, understanding the chemical structure of a drug target, unintentional discovery, developing drugs that are similar to existing drugs, and researching the biology of cancer cells. This book unravels the recent studies on anticancer drug discovery and development. Those in search of information to further their knowledge will be greatly assisted by it.

The information contained in this book is the result of intensive hard work done by researchers in this field. All due efforts have been made to make this book serve as a complete guiding source for students and researchers. The topics in this book have been comprehensively explained to help readers understand the growing trends in the field.

I would like to thank the entire group of writers who made sincere efforts in this book and my family who supported me in my efforts of working on this book. I take this opportunity to thank all those who have been a guiding force throughout my life.

Editor

Magnetic Graphene Oxide Nanocarrier for Targeted Delivery of Cisplatin: A Perspective for Glioblastoma Treatment

Sami A. Makharza [1,2], **Giuseppe Cirillo** [1,3,*], **Orazio Vittorio** [4,5,6], **Emanuele Valli** [4,6], **Florida Voli** [4], **Annafranca Farfalla** [3], **Manuela Curcio** [3], **Francesca Iemma** [3], **Fiore Pasquale Nicoletta** [3], **Ahmed A. El-Gendy** [7], **Gerardo F. Goya** [8] and **Silke Hampel** [1]

[1]   Leibniz Institute of Solid State and Material Research Dresden, 01069 Dresden, Germany; samim@hebron.edu (S.A.M.); s.hampel@ifw-dresden.de (S.H.)
[2]   College of Pharmacy and Medical Sciences, Hebron University, Hebron 00970, Palestine
[3]   Department of Pharmacy, Health and Nutritional Sciences, University of Calabria, Rende (CS), 87036 Rende, Italy; annafranca.farfalla@gmail.com (A.F.); manuela.curcio@unical.it (M.C.); francesca.iemma@unical.it (F.I.); fiore.nicoletta@unical.it (F.P.N.)
[4]   Children's Cancer Institute, Lowy Cancer Research Centre, UNSW Sydney, Sydney 2031, Australia; OVittorio@ccia.org.au (O.V.); EValli@ccia.org.au (E.V.); FVoli@ccia.org.au (F.V.)
[5]   ARC Centre of Excellence for Convergent BioNano Science and Technology, Australian Centre for NanoMedicine, UNSW Sydney, Sydney 2052, Australia
[6]   School of Women's and Children's Health, Faculty of Medicine, UNSW Sydney, Sydney 2052, Australia
[7]   Department of Physics, University of Texas at El Paso, El Paso, TX 79968, USA; aelgendy@utep.edu
[8]   Institute of Nanoscience of Aragon (INA) & Department of Condensed Matter Physics, University of Zaragoza, 50018 Zaragoza, Spain; goya@unizar.es
*   Correspondence: giuseppe.cirillo@unical.it;

Abstract: Selective vectorization of Cisplatin (CisPt) to Glioblastoma U87 cells was exploited by the fabrication of a hybrid nanocarrier composed of magnetic γ-Fe_2O_3 nanoparticles and nanographene oxide (NGO). The magnetic component, obtained by annealing magnetite Fe_3O_4 and characterized by XRD measurements, was combined with NGO sheets prepared via a modified Hummer's method. The morphological and thermogravimetric analysis proved the effective binding of γ-Fe_2O_3 nanoparticles onto NGO layers. The magnetization measured under magnetic fields up to 7 Tesla at room temperature revealed superparamagnetic-like behavior with a maximum value of $M_S = 15$ emu/g and coercivity $H_C \approx 0$ Oe within experimental error. The nanohybrid was found to possess high affinity towards CisPt, and a rather slow fractional release profile of 80% after 250 h. Negligible toxicity was observed for empty nanoparticles, while the retainment of CisPt anticancer activity upon loading into the carrier was observed, together with the possibility to spatially control the drug delivery at a target site.

Keywords: magnetic targeting; graphene oxide; maghemite; glioblastoma; cisplatin

1. Introduction

Malignant glioma is one of the most aggressive brain tumors, and the major cause of death from central nervous system cancers (median survival times less than 15 months from diagnosis) [1–5]. Glioma treatment is still one of the most difficult challenges for oncologists [6], and current therapies involve surgical intervention to achieve tumor debulking followed by adjuvant radio- and chemo-therapy [7]. Chemotherapy approaches are of paramount importance in the case of the most devastating and lethal grade IV glioma (Glioblastoma Multiforme, GBM), because the extensive tumor infiltration into the surrounding brain parenchyma makes surgery un-effective [8]. However, the therapeutic efficiency of chemotherapy is remains unsatisfactory for two main reasons: (i) the rare brain penetration of the anticancer agents systemically administered through the blood brain barrier (BBB) [9], and (ii) the poor glioma targeting of employed chemotherapeutics [10]. The latter issue is the main obstacle in the clinical treatment of Glioma with *cis*-diamminedichloroplatinum(II) (CisPt) [11], one of the most effective anticancer agents. CisPt suffers from a nonselective distribution between normal and tumor tissues, with the insurgence of severe adverse side effects, including acute nephrotoxicity, myelosuppression, and chronic neurotoxicity in adults [12–14], and lifelong health issues when the therapy was given in children [15,16]. Therefore, it is patently clear that, for an effective Glioma treatment, there is an urgent need for powerful and targeted CisPt delivery systems in order to promote preferential accumulation in cancer cells and thereby reduce the side effects [17]. Taking advantage of the peculiar features of tumor tissues such as the leaky neovasculature and the lack of functional lymphatic drainage, a wide range of nanoparticle drug carriers have been explored for this purpose [18].

Among others, graphene nanomaterials, mainly in the form of nanographene oxide (NGO), possess superior physicochemical, thermal, optical, mechanical, and biological properties [19–21]. NGO is widely explored for drug delivery applications by virtue of the large surface area (four times higher than that of any other nanomaterials) and the high stability of its water dispersion due to the richness of oxygen containing functional groups (e.g., carboxyl, epoxide, and hydroxyl groups) [22–24]. The suitability of NGO for the preparation of CisPt delivery vehicles with high loading efficiency is related to the presence of either the sp^2-aromatic structure or the abundant oxidized sp^3-portion on the edge, top, and bottom surfaces of each sheet [25–27], allowing the drug interaction through diverse mechanisms, including π-π stacking and hydrogen bonding [28–35].

More interestingly, functionalized NGO was found to highly accumulate in U87 human glioblastoma subcutaneous tumor xenografts [36,37], confirming that such nanocarriers can be considered a valuable tool for delivering CisPt to brain cancers. The efficiency of NGO delivery vehicles can be maximized by the incorporation of magnetic materials allowing the nanocarrier to be selectively driven into tumor tissues by the application of an external magnetic field [38]. In particular, magnetic nanoparticles based on iron oxide (maghemite γ-Fe_2O_3 or magnetite Fe_3O_4) were widely used for this purpose due to their biocompatibility and superparamagnetic properties [39,40]. The resulting NGO hybrid nanodevices were proposed as effective tools for glioblastoma treatment using Doxorubicin [41] and Irinotecan [42] as cytotoxic agents. Although possessing favorable properties for magnetic drug vectorization, the different chemical stabilities of Fe_3O_4 and γ-Fe_2O_3 may affect the toxicity of the delivery vehicle [43]. The lower chemical stability of Fe_3O_4 resulted in the release of Fe^{2+} ions from the nanoparticle cores, which can catalyze the formation of reactive oxygen species (ROS) damaging cell membrane and organelles, with the insurgence of adverse long-term side effects [44]. On the other hand, γ-Fe_2O_3 was found to be a better material owing to either the magnetic features or the high chemical stability [45].

In the present study we explored the possibility to employ NGO–Iron oxide nanohybrids (γ-Fe_2O_3@NGO) as a CisPt carrier for glioblastoma treatment by intercalating γ-Fe_2O_3 nanoparticles into NGO sheets. After characterizing the physical, chemical, and morphological properties, CisPt was loaded onto the nanocarrier for several drug-to-carrier ratios and their cytotoxicity was tested on human U87 cell lines.

2. Results and Discussion

2.1. Properties of γ-Fe_2O_3@NGO Nanohybrid

As previously reported, the size of NGO is a parameter that strongly affects the drug delivery effectiveness of NGO-based systems in vitro and in vivo [46,47]. Specifically, low-sized NGOs (lateral dimension ≈100 nm) have been reported to have the best performance [46].

The average size of our graphite oxide (GO) particles, as assessed by scanning electron microscopy (SEM), revealed an average size (lateral width) of 350–400 nm. These particles were therefore subsequently sonicated until NGO with lateral width of 80–100 nm and a thickness of 6.3 nm was attained (10 NGO sheets, assuming an interlayer distance of 0.7 nm) [48] (Figure 1a–c).

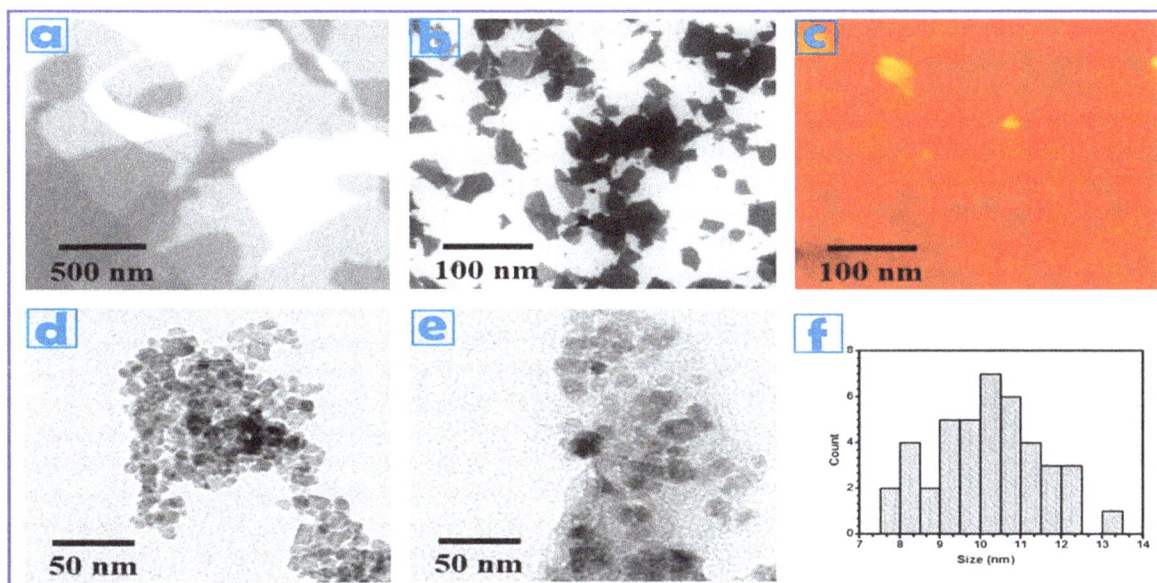

Figure 1. SEM images of (**a**) GO; and (**b**) NGO showing an average lateral width of 350–400 and 80–100 nm, respectively. (**c**) AFM image of NGO. TEM images of (**d**) γ-Fe$_2$O$_3$; and (**e**) γ-Fe$_2$O$_3$@NGO nanoparticles. (**f**) Size distribution of γ-Fe$_2$O$_3$ nanoparticles (approximately 10 nm).

The obtained NGO 100 nm were employed for the preparation of the magnetic hybrid device (γ-Fe$_2$O$_3$@NGO) as sketched in Figure 2.

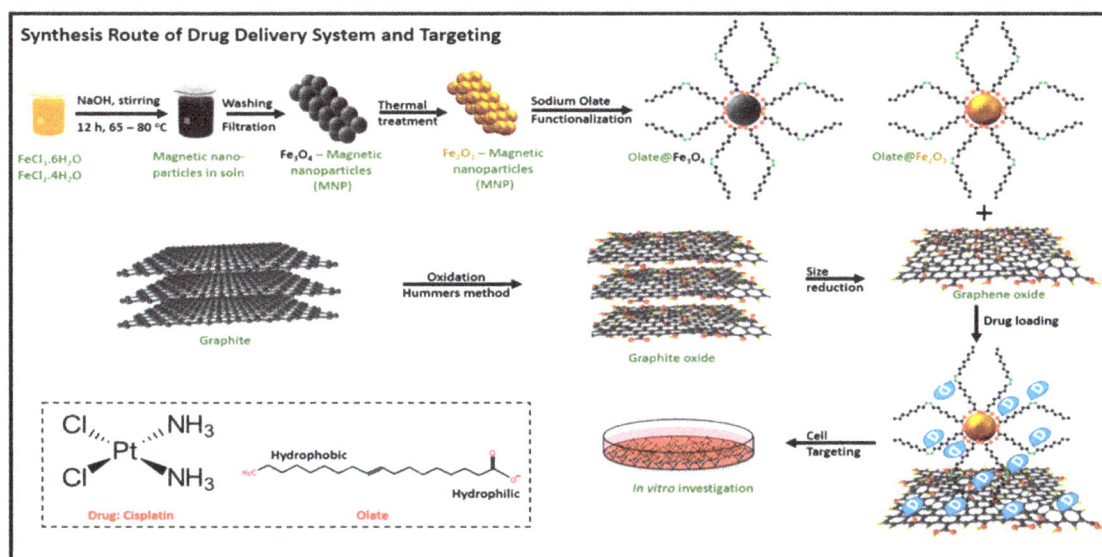

Figure 2. Schematic representation of the preparation of γ-Fe$_2$O$_3$@NGO.

Maghemite (γ-Fe$_2$O$_3$) nanoparticles were chosen to provide magnetic properties to the nanohybrids because of their high chemical stability, biocompatibility, and large magnetic moment at room temperature in its bulk form [40]. Superparamagnetism is crucial for application in biomedicine, because, despite the strong response to an external magnetic field, the absence of residual magnetic properties upon removal of the external field prevents nanoparticles from aggregation in biological environment [49–52]. γ-Fe_2O_3 nanoparticles (average size of 10 nm, see Figure 1d,f) were synthesized by annealing of magnetite Fe_3O_4 prepared by a chemical co-precipitation technique of $FeCl_3$ and $FeCl_2$ solutions [53,54], and then coated with oleic acid/sodium oleate to enhance their dispersion in water media and thus the biocompatibility features [55]. Since previously reported data proved the presence of transport systems importing fatty acids into the brain with high affinity and efficiency, it is reasonable to hypothesize that this coating strategy could be appropriate for targeting the blood brain barrier [56].

Despite the evidence of Fe_3O_4 to γ-Fe_2O_3 oxidation from the change of color of the sample (from black to reddish-brown color, see Figure 3), we investigated this phase change by XRD measurements. Figure 3 showed the XRD patterns of both compounds, and the d-spacing values emulated well the data deduced from the Joint Committee on Powder Diffraction Standards (JCPDS) cards 19-629 (Fe_3O_4) and 39-1346 (γ-Fe_2O_3).

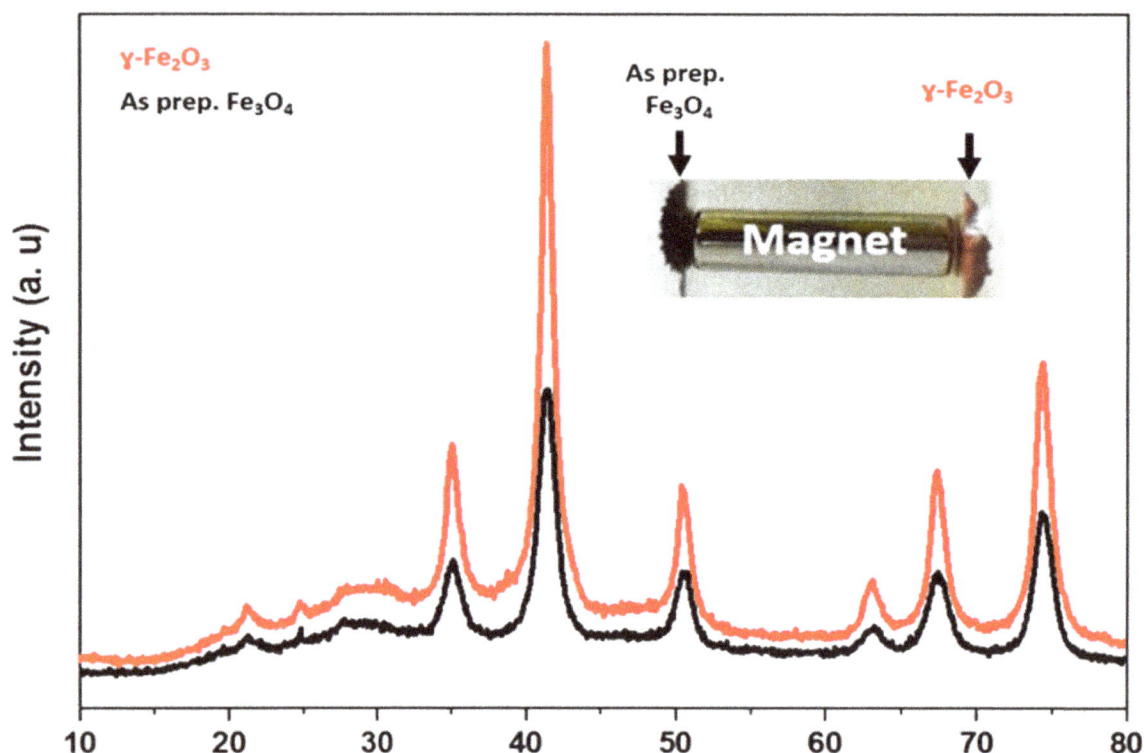

Figure 3. XRD patterns for Fe_3O_4 and γ-Fe_2O_3.

The result indicated no major differences between the two patterns, in each set of XRD patterns, the crystalline structure of magnetite and/or maghemite with indexes (hkl) ascribed to (220), (311), (400), (422), (511), and (440) were observable at the diffraction angles $2\theta = 35.1°$, $41.4.6°$, $50.4°$, $63.1°$, $67.4°$ and $74.3°$ crystal planes, respectively. This result indicated that the thermal treatment of as prepared Fe_3O_4 produced γ-Fe_2O_3 (maghemite) crystal form [57].

The magnetization vs. field M(H) curves for the annealed γ-Fe_2O_3 nanoparticles showed nearly closed hysteresis loops, with zero coercivity (Figure 4).

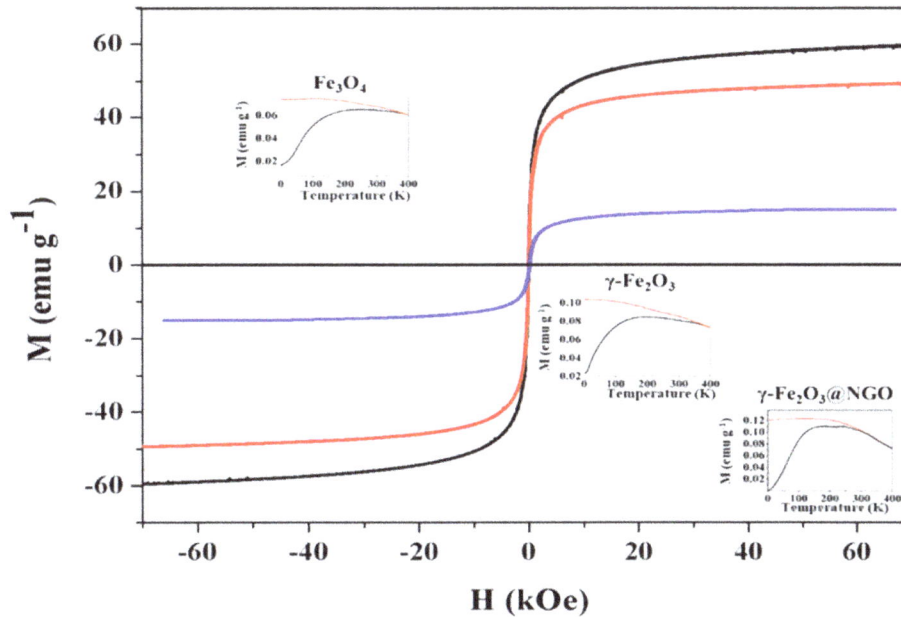

Figure 4. Hysteresis loops M(H) for Fe_3O_4 (black) and γ-Fe_2O_3 (red) and γ-Fe_2O_3@NGO (blue) nanoparticles. The insets show the Zero-field cooled (black) and field-cooled (orange) magnetization curves for Fe_3O_4, γ-Fe_2O_3, and γ-Fe_2O_3@NGO, taken with H_{FC} = 100 Oe.

The magnetization did not fully saturate within our experimentally available fields (H = 70 kOe), attaining a value of MS = 59.36 emu/g and MS = 49.25 emu/g at H = 70 kOe for Fe_3O_4 and γ-Fe_2O_3, respectively. After assembling γ-Fe_2O_3 into NGO the Ms value was 15.02 emu/g, consistent with a ≈30.5% wt. of magnetic material into NGO matrix, confirming the dispersion on magnetic nanoparticle into the hybrid platform. The coercivity values at room temperature were HC ≈ 0 for all samples. The zero field cooling (ZFC) and field cooling (FC) curves at H_{FC} = 100 Oe of Fe_3O_4, γ-Fe_2O_3 and γ-Fe_2O_3@NGO samples reflected similar features, i.e., a broad maximum in the ZFC curves originated from the distribution of blocking temperatures due to the distribution of particle sizes (see inset of Figure 4). The maxima were centered around T ≈ 194, 245, and 242 for Fe_3O_4, γ-Fe_2O_3, and γ-Fe_2O_3@NGO, respectively. These broad maxima are consistent with the blocking of the smallest nanoparticles at these temperatures, while the presence of irreversible behavior up to the highest temperature (400 K) suggests that a fraction of the largest particles are still blocked above room temperature.

The thermogravimetric analysis (TGA) curves of NGO and γ-Fe_2O_3@NGO were depicted in Figure 5.

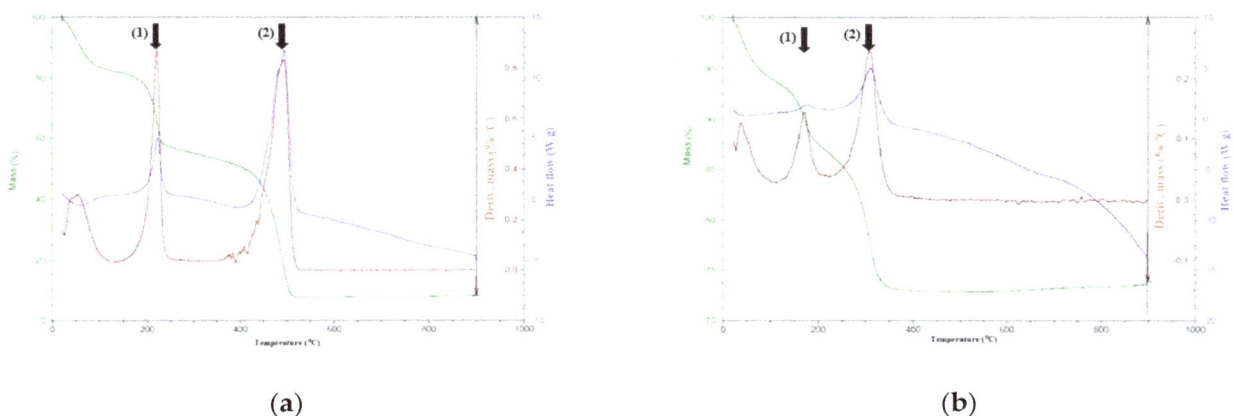

(a)

(b)

Figure 5. TGA curves for NGO (**a**) and γ-Fe_2O_3@NGO (**b**).

For the NGO sample (Figure 5a), the mass loss in the range 150–250 °C with the maximum in the derivative %M/°C graph at 215 °C (arrow (1)) was ascribed to the decomposition of decorated oxygen functionalities on the basal graphene structure, while between 400 and 525 °C (maximum at 490, see arrow (2)), a high weight loss occurs due to the discard of more thermally stable oxygen groups. On the other hand, for γ-Fe_2O_3@NGO (Figure 5b), these mass losses were found to shift to lower temperatures (maximum in the derivative %M/°C graph at 170 °C and 305 °C, respectively) as a consequence of the effective binding of γ-Fe_2O_3 nanoparticles onto NGO layers.

2.2. Evaluation of Carrier Performances

Before testing the efficiency of γ-Fe_2O_3@NGO nanohybrid as CisPt carrier, we evaluated the toxicity of the empty nanoparticles (γ-Fe_2O_3, NGO, and γ-Fe_2O_3@NGO) on human glioblastoma U87 cell lines at a concentration range of 0–25 $\mu g\ mL^{-1}$. This range of concentration was selected because of the absence of any sign of aggregation as per Dynamic light-scattering (DLS) measurements. The viability values (>96% for all samples and concentrations, see Figure 6) proved the high biocompatibility of all nanoparticle systems, confirming their suitability as drug carrier [58].

The ultimate aim of the study is to check the suitability of γ-Fe_2O_3@NGO to selectively vectorize the cytotoxic drug to the tumor site under magnetic actuation. Indeed a key requirement for this nanocarrier is the ability to retain the drug until it reaches the target site. γ-Fe_2O_3@NGO was found to possess high affinity for CisPt (Drug Loading Efficiency of 0.37 $mg\ mg^{-1}$) and the release profiles were recorded after loading the drug by a soaking procedure (drug to carrier ratio of 10% by weight).

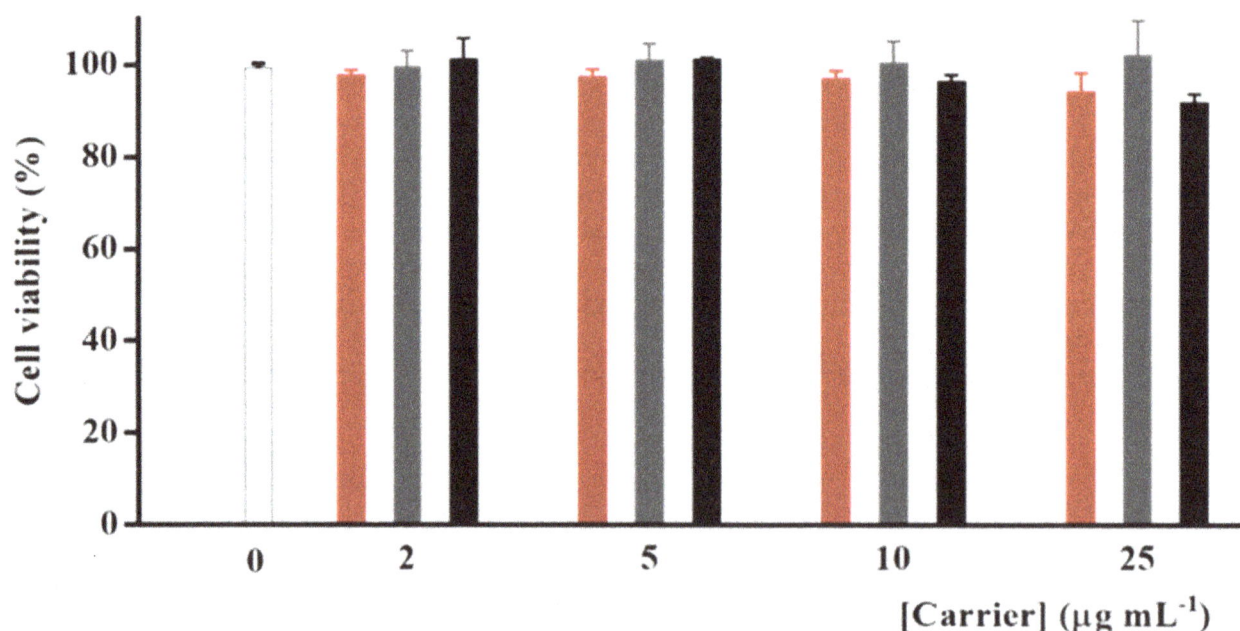

Figure 6. U87 viability after treatment with empty γ-Fe_2O_3 (**red**) and NGO (**grey**) and γ-Fe_2O_3@NGO (**black**).

The cumulative amount of drug released (M_t/M_0) was compared with those recorded when uncombined γ-Fe_2O_3 or NGO were employed as carrier (Figure 7).

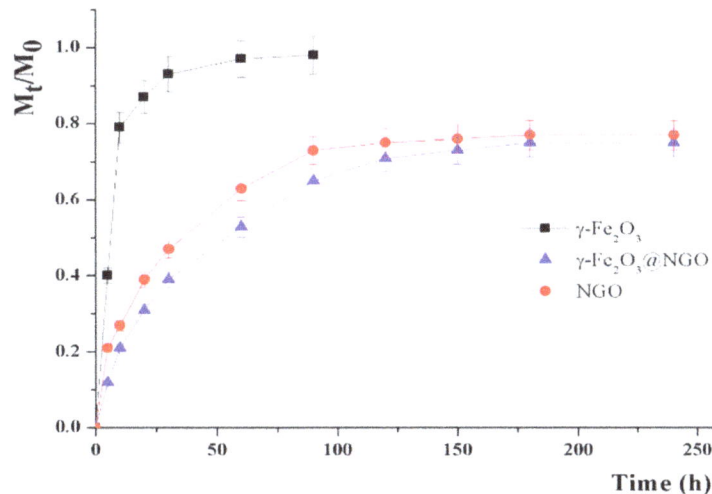

Figure 7. CisPt release profiles from γ-Fe$_2$O$_3$@NGO, γ-Fe$_2$O$_3$, and NGO.

For a more exhaustive analysis of the CisPt release profiles, a mathematical model considering the partition between the carrier and the surrounding environments and the underlying mechanism of the drug release was applied according to the literature [59]. In this model, a key parameter (α) was adopted to describe the physicochemical affinity of the drug between the carrier and solvent phases according to Equation (1):

$$\alpha = \frac{F_{max}}{1 - F_{max}} \tag{1}$$

where F_{max} represents the maximum value of relative release (M_t/M_0).

The overall drug release can be modeled according to reversible first- or second-order kinetics of Equations (2) and (3).

$$\frac{M_t}{M_0} = F_{max}\left(1 - e^{-(\frac{k_R}{F_{max}})t}\right) \tag{2}$$

$$\frac{M_t}{M_0} = \frac{F_{max}\left(e^{2(\frac{k_R}{\alpha})t} - 1\right)}{1 - 2F_{max} + e^{2(\frac{k_R}{\alpha})t}} \tag{3}$$

with k_R being the release rate constant.

The time required for reaching 50% of F_{max} ($t_{1/2}$) can be obtained by applying the following Equations (4) and (5), respectively:

$$t^1_{1/2} = \frac{F_{max}}{k_R} ln2 \tag{4}$$

$$t^2_{1/2} = \frac{\alpha}{2kR} \ln(3 - 2F_{max}) \tag{5}$$

Both models are suitable for describing the CisPt release (see R^2 in Table 1), with the presence of NGO making the release better described by reversible second-order kinetics. In the absence of NGO, a fast CisPt release was recorded (M_t/M_0 of 0.90 after 20 h), with high α value indicating a low affinity of the drug towards the carrier phase (γ-Fe$_2$O$_3$). On other hand, the strong interaction between CisPt and NGO [60–62] resulted in a more extended release over time ($F_{max} < 0.8$ even after 250 h), with the same affinity (3.54) recorded for either NGO or γ-Fe$_2$O$_3$@NGO. The presence of γ-Fe$_2$O$_3$ in γ-Fe$_2$O$_3$@NGO was found to slow the release, with reduced kinetic constant (k_R) and $t_{1/2}$ values moving from 19.01 (NGO) to 29.38 (γ-Fe$_2$O$_3$@NGO) h. This could be ascribed to the hindrance to the drug diffusion from the NGO to the solvent phase by the oleate coating of γ-Fe$_2$O$_3$ nanoparticles [55].

Table 1. R^2 values and kinetic parameters for CisPt release according to the applied mathematical model.

Mathematical Model	Parameter	γ-Fe$_2$O$_3$	NGO	γ-Fe$_2$O$_3$@NGO
$\frac{M_t}{M_0} = F_{max}\left(1 - e^{-(k_R/M_{max})t}\right)$	R^2	0.9818	0.9822	0.9909
	F_{max}	0.98	0.76	0.74
	α	49	3.17	2.85
	k_R (10^{-2})	12.71	2.76	1.85
	$t_{1/2}^1$ (h)	5.35	18.81	27.00
$\frac{M_t}{M_0} = \frac{F_{max}\left(e^{2(\frac{k_R}{\alpha})t}-1\right)}{1 - 2F_{max} + e^{2(\frac{k_R}{\alpha})t}}$	R^2	0.9340	0.9908	0.9960
	F_{max}	0.97	0.78	0.78
	α	32.33	3.54	3.54
	k_R (10^{-2})	18.28	3.42	2.25
	$t_{1/2}^2$ (h)	5.15	19.01	29.38

CisPt loaded γ-Fe$_2$O$_3$@NGO were employed in different drug-to-carrier ratios (concentration ranges of 0–25 μg mL^{-1} and 0–10 μM for carrier and drug, respectively, see Figure 8). From the data in Figure 8, it is clear that the lowest toxic concentrations of CisPt (10 μM) is unchanged after loading on the different carriers, with γ-Fe$_2$O$_3$@NGO being the most effective vehicle for killing cells.

To investigate the possibility of obtaining a selective vectorization of the drug, a proof of concept experiment was designed by incubating U87 cells with 10 μM CisPt loaded γ-Fe$_2$O$_3$@NGO for 24 h kept under the effect of a magnetic field generated by a permanent Nd-Fe-B magnet. As a result of the magnetic carrier driven spatial concentrations of the drug, a selective cell death at the region close to the magnet was reached, even at low drug concentration (10 μM), with no relevant toxicity detected on the region where the magnetic forces were negligible (Figure 9).

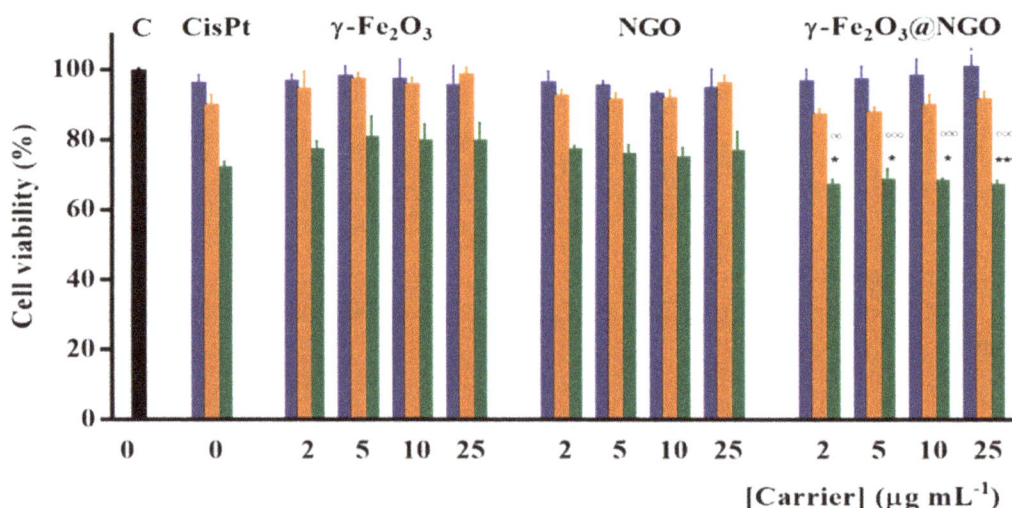

Figure 8. U87 viability after 72 h incubation with CisPt concentrations 2.5 (**blue**); 5.0 (**orange**); and 10.0 (**green**) μM in the free form and after loading on γ-Fe$_2$O$_3$; NGO; γ-Fe$_2$O$_3$@NGO. Carrier concentrations were 2.0; 5.0; 10.0; and 25.0 μg mL^{-1}. An overall p-value less than 0.05 was accepted as significant. For individual comparisons of γ-Fe$_2$O$_3$@NGO (10 μM CisPt) vs. γ-Fe$_2$O$_3$ or NGO at the same concentrations, adjusted p-values are indicate as * $p < 0.05$ vs. NGO; *** $p < 0.001$ vs. NGO; °°° $p < 0.001$ vs. γ-Fe$_2$O$_3$; °°°° $p < 0.0001$ vs. γ-Fe$_2$O$_3$. Error bars represent standard error of the mean (n = 3 independent experiments).

Overall, the obtained results are of great interest for application in cancer therapy for two main outcomes: (i) an effective magnetic vectorization of CisPt to cancer cells can be reached, since a very low amount of CisPt was released in the first 20 h ($M_t/M_0 < 0.30$) and thus negligible side toxicity can be hypothesized, and (ii) the CisPt loaded into γ-Fe$_2$O$_3$@NGO is biologically active in reducing the viability of cancerous with an efficiency comparable with that of the free drug.

Future experiments will be performed for evaluating the therapeutic performance of the designed magnetic nanohybrid, by determining the pharmacokinetics profiles with or without a magnetic field, the anticancer activity in appropriate in vivo models, and the possibility to use the system for theranostics applications.

Figure 9. Optical microscope image U87 cells incubated with 10 µM CisPt loaded γ-Fe$_2$O$_3$@NGO under the effect of a permanent magnet.

3. Materials and Methods

3.1. Synthesis of Graphite Oxide

Graphite oxide particles were prepared from graphite powder (natural, -200 mesh, 99.9995% purity, Alfa Aesar) by using a modified Hummers method [63]. Graphite powder (1.0 g) was sonicated in water for 5 min, filtrated, washed with water and dried in an oven at 40 °C for 12 h. The dried graphite was transferred to a beaker and mixed with concentrated H$_2$SO$_4$ (98%, 23 mL). The mixture was left overnight under stirring at room temperature. Thereafter, 3.0 g KMnO$_4$, as an oxidizing agent, was added gradually while keeping the reaction mixture below 10 °C, in order to decorate the surfaces of graphite by various oxygen groups (hydroxy, epoxy, carboxylic, etc.). After complete addition of KMnO$_4$, the reaction mixture was stirred for 30 min at 35 °C and 45 min at 50 °C for enhancing the degree of oxidation. 46.0 mL of distilled water was added while maintaining the temperature between 98–105 °C for 30 min 10 mL of 30% H$_2$O$_2$ was added in order to terminate the reaction. The mixture of GO was washed several times with 5% HCl and water during the suction filtration. The filtrated graphite oxide was dried in an oven at 40 °C for 5 h.

3.2. Synthesis of Nanographene Oxide

NGO particles were prepared as reported previously [46]. The resultant material of graphite oxide was cracked in distilled water with different power percent and sonication time using a horn-tipped ultrasonic probe. The material was separated to different sizes by repeated centrifuge and filtration. SEM images were obtained using a FEI, NOVA NanoSEM200 (FEI, Hillsboro, OR, USA) with an acceleration voltage of 15 kV. AFM images of well-defined NGO sizes were acquired using Digital Instruments Veeco, NanoScope IIIa, operating in the tapping mode. The images were analyzed using WSxM software designed by Nanotech Electronica (Madrid, Spain). The distribution used during this study was approximately 100 nm in lateral size and 6 nm in thickness.

3.3. Synthesis of Maghemite Nanoparticles

Maghemite γ-Fe_2O_3 nanoparticles were synthesized in a three-step procedure as follows: first, the magnetite Fe_3O_4 nanoparticles were prepared by co-precipitation method in basic medium [53]. The synthesis of Fe_3O_4 nanoparticles is shown in Equation (6):

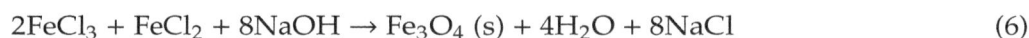

$$2FeCl_3 + FeCl_2 + 8NaOH \rightarrow Fe_3O_4 \ (s) + 4H_2O + 8NaCl \tag{6}$$

Briefly, 2.25 g of $FeCl_3 \cdot 6H_2O$ and 0.825 g of $FeCl_2 \cdot 4H_2O$ were mixed in an alkaline solution (NaOH, 1.7 g). The mixture stirred at 65–80 °C for 12 h. The resultant material was filtrated and washed many times by distilled water and ethanol.

Subsequently, magnetite Fe_3O_4 nanoparticles were employed as starting material for the synthesis of maghemite γ-Fe_2O_3. An initial amount of 1.0 g of Fe_3O_4 was placed in furnace and heated up to 450 °C in the presence of Argon and $H_{2(g)}$ for 12 h [54,57]. Thereafter, the reaction was quenched down to room temperature. The resulting material was collected, washed several times in deionized water and ethanol, dried in an oven at 65 °C for 3 h. A second annealing was applied at the same conditions in order to identify the structure of Fe_2O_3 whether it was maghemite or hematite form.

In the final step, 0.5 g of γ-Fe_2O_3 were heated to 60 °C for 15 min separately. Consequently, an excess of sodium oleate (20% wt/vol) was added under vigorous stirring for 15 min. Oleate functionalized nanoparticles were collected by magnetic decantation to remove the non-magnetic materials. The product was washed with water and acetone several times, filtrated and dried in an oven at 40 °C for 2 h.

The relevant X-ray diffraction patterns were performed by using Pert Pro MPD PW3040/60 X-ray diffractometer with Co K_α radiation ($\lambda = 0.179278$ nm) at ambient temperature.

3.4. Synthesis of γ-Fe_2O_3@NGO Nanohybrid

An amount of 0.5 g of NGO -100 nm particles was sonicated for 15 min in order to homogenize it in distilled water. The solution was heated up to 60 °C for 15 min directly; an excess of γ-$F_{e2}O_3$ system was added and stirred for 15 min. The final material was separated by magnetic decantation, washed with water and acetone, filtrated and dried in an oven at 40 °C for 2 h. TEM images were recorded on HRTEM/Tecnai F30 [300 kV] (FEI, Hillsboro, OR, USA). TGA was performed on a STA 409 PC/PG-Luxx analyzer (Netzsch, Selb, Germany). Measurements were conducted in a nitrogen atmosphere (flow of 10 mL min^{-1}), with an initial sample weight of ~10 mg in the temperature range 50–900 °C at a heating rate of 10 °C min^{-1}.

Drug loading efficiency (DLE) of γ-Fe_2O_3@NGO for CisPt was estimated by mixing drug and carrier in a 1:1 ratio (by weight) and determining the amount of unloaded CisPt by UV-Vis on a Jasco V-530 UV/Vis spectrometer (Jasco Europe s.r.l., Milan, Italy) at 301 nm [64]. DLE was calculated according to the following Equation (7):

$$DLE \left(mg \ mg^{-1} \right) = \frac{W_D}{W_C} \tag{7}$$

where W_D and W_C are the amount of loaded drug and carrier, respectively. In our condition, to ensure the same amount of drug being loaded on the three carriers (γ-Fe_2O_3@NGO, γ-Fe_2O_3, or NGO) the CisPt loading procedure was performed by mixing, in separate experiments, variable amounts of CisPt solution with the carriers and drying the products under vacuum at RT.

3.5. Magnetic Characterization

Magnetization curves were measured as function of temperature M(T) in the 4 K $\leq$ T $\leq$ 400 K temperature rage, in a SQUID magnetometer (MPMS 5000 from Quantum Design). The Zero-field-cooling (ZFC) and Field-cooling (FC) curves were measured under a field-cooling field $H_{FC} = 100$ Oe Hysteresis loops M(H) were taken at 4 K and 300 K within the -70 kOe $\leq$ H $\leq +70$ kOe field range. For all these measurements, the colloids were conditioned in cylindrical sample holders and diamagnetic signal were extracted from the total magnetization.

3.6. In Vitro Cisplatin Release

Release experiments were performed by dialysis methods using 5.0 mL phosphate buffer saline (10^{-3} M, pH 7.4) was releasing media and dialysis tubing cellulose membranes of 25 mm average flat width and 12,000 MW cutoff (Fisher Scientific, Waltham, MA, USA). 5.0 mg nanoparticles (γ-Fe$_2$O$_3$@NGO, γ-Fe$_2$O$_3$, and NGO) loaded with CisPt were inserted into the dialysis tubes and subject to dialysis. At predetermined time intervals, the amount of CisPt in the releasing media was determined by UV-Vis on a Jasco V-530 UV/Vis spectrometer (Jasco Europe s.r.l., Milan, Italy) at 301 nm [64]. The cumulative amount of drug released (F) was calculated using the following Equation (8):

$$F = \frac{M_t}{M_0} \tag{8}$$

where M_t and M_0 are the amounts of drug in solution at time t and loaded into the carrier, respectively. Sink conditions were maintained through the experiment: the maximal theoretical concentration of dissolved CisPt was 0.33 mM, with its solubility being 3.3 mM in these conditions [65].

3.7. Cell Growth Inhibition Assays

Human Glioblastoma cells (U87) were grown as a monolayer in a humidified atmosphere at 37 °C and in 5% CO$_2$ in the presence of Dulbecco's Modified Eagle Medium (DMEM) supplemented with 10% Fetal bovine serum (FBS), 1% L-glutamine, and 1% penicillin–streptomycin. Treatment effects on U87 cell growth were measured on the basis of the metabolic activity of cells using Alamar Blue assays [66]. Briefly, cells were plated in clear transparent 96-well plates at an optimized cell density of 2.5×10^3 cells per well 48 h prior to treatment. Cells were then treated with either CisPt loaded or unloaded carriers (γ-Fe$_2$O$_3$@NGO, γ-Fe$_2$O$_3$, NGO) and effects on cell growth assessed 72 h later. Treatments involved the combination of CisPt and carrier concentrations of 2.5; 5.0; 10.0 μM and 2.0; 5.0; 10.0; 25.0 μg mL^{-1}, respectively. Resazurin reduction was measured (excitation 530 nm, emission 590 nm) on a Versamax microplate reader (Molecular Devices, Sunnyvale, CA, USA).

To evaluate the magnetic vectorization ability, viability experiments were performed by treating 250×10^3 cells seeded in a 35 mm petri dish with 10 μM CisPt loaded on γ-Fe$_2$O$_3$@NGO for 24 h under the effect of a magnetic field generated by a permanent magnet (100 G).

All chemicals were purchased by from Merck/Sigma Aldrich, Taufkirchen, Germany.

3.8. Statistical Analysis

Three experiments were carried out in triplicate. Values were expressed as means ± standard error of the mean. For viability assay, statistical significance was assessed by one-way analysis of variance followed by post-hoc comparison test (Tukey's test). Significance was set at $p < 0.01$.

4. Conclusions

The possibility of CisPt delivery to specific target sites by remote actuation was reached by combining γ-Fe$_2$O$_3$ magnetic nanoparticles ensembled into a NGO nanoplatform. The correct assembly of the components was responsible for the efficiency of γ-Fe$_2$O$_3$@NGO as a drug delivery system. While NGO conferred high loading capabilities to the nanosystems, the magnetic nanoparticles provided the magnetic actuation capabilities for targeting and delivery of therapeutics.

The mathematical model of the CisPt release profiles suggested a sustained reversible second-order kinetics, which implies low amounts of CisPt released during the first seconds of the experiments. This type of release profile is of major importance if low toxicity levels are required for in vivo applications.

These findings, considered together with the retainment of CisPt toxicity upon loading and the possibility to increase the dose delivered at the target site by a magnetic actuation, make the nanocarrier developed here a valuable tool for applications in cancer therapy.

Author Contributions: Conceptualization, G.C., O.V., and S.H.; formal analysis, S.A.M., F.P.N., and A.A.E.-G.; Investigation, S.A.M., E.V., F.V., A.F., and M.C.; methodology, G.C., O.V., and A.A.E.-G.; Resources, S.H.; supervision, F.I., G.F.G., and S.H.; validation, G.C., O.V., A.A.E.-G., G.F.G., and S.H.; visualization, S.A.M., M.C., and A.A.E.-G.; writing—original draft, G.C.; writing—review and editing, F.I., F.P.N., A.A.E.-G., G.F.G., and S.H.

Acknowledgments: MIUR Excellence Department Project funds, awarded to the Department of Pharmacy and Health and Nutritional Sciences, University of Calabria (L.232/2016) is acknowledged.

References

1. Ni, D.; Zhang, J.; Bu, W.; Xing, H.; Han, F.; Xiao, Q.; Yao, Z.; Chen, F.; He, Q.; Liu, J.; et al. Dual-targeting upconversion nanoprobes across the blood-brain barrier for magnetic resonance/fluorescence imaging of intracranial glioblastoma. *ACS Nano* **2014**, *8*, 1231–1242. [CrossRef] [PubMed]

2. Huse, J.T.; Holland, E.C. Targeting brain cancer: Advances in the molecular pathology of malignant glioma and medulloblastoma. *Nat. Rev. Cancer* **2010**, *10*, 319–331. [CrossRef] [PubMed]

3. Belhadj, Z.; Ying, M.; Cao, X.; Hu, X.; Zhan, C.; Wei, X.; Gao, J.; Wang, X.; Yan, Z.; Lu, W. Design of Y-shaped targeting material for liposome-based multifunctional glioblastoma-targeted drug delivery. *J. Control. Release* **2017**, *255*, 132–141. [CrossRef]

4. Cohen, Z.R.; Ramishetti, S.; Peshes-Yaloz, N.; Goldsmith, M.; Wohl, A.; Zibly, Z.; Peer, D. Localized RNAi therapeutics of chemoresistant grade IV glioma using hyaluronan-grafted lipid-based nanoparticles. *ACS Nano* **2015**, *9*, 1581–1591. [CrossRef]

5. Dong, H.; Jin, M.; Liu, Z.; Xiong, H.; Qiu, X.; Zhang, W.; Guo, Z. In vitro and in vivo brain-targeting chemo-photothermal therapy using graphene oxide conjugated with transferrin for Gliomas. *Lasers Med. Sci.* **2016**, *31*, 1123–1131. [CrossRef]

6. Gao, H.; Qian, J.; Cao, S.; Yang, Z.; Pang, Z.; Pan, S.; Fan, L.; Xi, Z.; Jiang, X.; Zhang, Q. Precise glioma targeting of and penetration by aptamer and peptide dual-functioned nanoparticles. *Biomaterials* **2012**, *33*, 5115–5123. [CrossRef]

7. Séhédic, D.; Cikankowitz, A.; Hindré, F.; Davodeau, F.; Garcion, E. Nanomedicine to overcome radioresistance in glioblastoma stem-like cells and surviving clones. *Trends Pharmacol. Sci.* **2015**, *36*, 236–252. [CrossRef] [PubMed]

8. Cheng, Y.; Morshed, R.A.; Auffinger, B.; Tobias, A.L.; Lesniak, M.S. Multifunctional nanoparticles for brain tumor imaging and therapy. *Adv. Drug Deliv. Rev.* **2014**, *66*, 42–57. [CrossRef] [PubMed]

9. Pardridge, W.M. Brain drug development and brain drug targeting. *Pharm. Res.* **2007**, *24*, 1729–1732. [CrossRef]

10. Chowdhury, S.M.; Surhland, C.; Sanchez, Z.; Chaudhary, P.; Suresh Kumar, M.A.; Lee, S.; Peña, L.A.; Waring, M.; Sitharaman, B.; Naidu, M. Graphene nanoribbons as a drug delivery agent for lucanthone mediated therapy of glioblastoma multiforme. *Nanomed. Nanotechnol. Biol. Med.* **2015**, *11*, 109–118. [CrossRef] [PubMed]

11. Zhang, C.; Nance, E.A.; Mastorakos, P.; Chisholm, J.; Berry, S.; Eberhart, C.; Tyler, B.; Brem, H.; Suk, J.S.; Hanes, J. Convection enhanced delivery of cisplatin-loaded brain penetrating nanoparticles cures malignant glioma in rats. *J. Control. Release* **2017**, *263*, 112–119. [CrossRef]

12. Duan, X.; He, C.; Kron, S.J.; Lin, W. Nanoparticle formulations of cisplatin for cancer therapy. *Wiley Interdiscip. Rev. Nanomed. Nanobiotechnol.* **2016**, *8*, 776–791. [CrossRef]

13. Ferroni, P.; Della-Morte, D.; Palmirotta, R.; McClendon, M.; Testa, G.; Abete, P.; Rengo, F.; Rundek, T.; Guadagni, F.; Roselli, M. Platinum-based compounds and risk for cardiovascular toxicity in the elderly: Role of the antioxidants in chemoprevention. *Rejuvenation Res.* **2011**, *14*, 293–308. [CrossRef]

14. Chovanec, M.; Abu Zaid, M.; Hanna, N.; El-Kouri, N.; Einhorn, L.H.; Albany, C. Long-term toxicity of cisplatin in germ-cell tumor survivors. *Ann. Oncol.* **2017**, *28*, 2670–2679. [CrossRef] [PubMed]

15. Hartmann, J.T.; Lipp, H.P. Toxicity of platinum compounds. *Expert Opin. Pharmacother.* **2003**, *4*, 889–901. [CrossRef] [PubMed]

16. Ruggiero, A.; Trombatore, G.; Triarico, S.; Arena, R.; Ferrara, P.; Scalzone, M.; Pierri, F.; Riccardi, R. Platinum compounds in children with cancer: Toxicity and clinical management. *Anti Cancer Drugs* **2013**, *24*, 1007–1019. [CrossRef]

17. Cheng, D.; Cao, N.; Chen, J.; Yu, X.; Shuai, X. Multifunctional nanocarrier mediated co-delivery of doxorubicin and siRNA for synergistic enhancement of glioma apoptosis in rat. *Biomaterials* **2012**, *33*, 1170–1179. [CrossRef] [PubMed]

18. Cassano, D.; Santi, M.; Cappello, V.; Luin, S.; Signore, G.; Voliani, V. Biodegradable passion fruit-like nano-architectures as carriers for cisplatin prodrug. *Part. Part. Syst. Charact.* **2016**, *33*, 818–824. [CrossRef]

19. Chung, C.; Kim, Y.K.; Shin, D.; Ryoo, S.R.; Hong, B.H.; Min, D.H. Biomedical applications of graphene and graphene oxide. *Acc. Chem. Res.* **2013**, *46*, 2211–2224. [CrossRef] [PubMed]

20. Kiew, S.F.; Kiew, L.V.; Lee, H.B.; Imae, T.; Chung, L.Y. Assessing biocompatibility of graphene oxide-based nanocarriers: A review. *J. Control. Release* **2016**, *226*, 217–228. [CrossRef] [PubMed]

21. Liu, J.; Cui, L.; Losic, D. Graphene and graphene oxide as new nanocarriers for drug delivery applications. *Acta Biomater.* **2013**, *9*, 9243–9257. [CrossRef] [PubMed]

22. Rahmanian, N.; Eskandani, M.; Barar, J.; Omidi, Y. Recent trends in targeted therapy of cancer using graphene oxide-modified multifunctional nanomedicines. *J. Drug Target.* **2017**, *25*, 202–215. [CrossRef] [PubMed]

23. Deb, A.; Andrews, N.G.; Raghavan, V. Natural polymer functionalized graphene oxide for co-delivery of anticancer drugs: In-vitro and in-vivo. *Int. J. Biol. Macromol.* **2018**, *113*, 515–525. [CrossRef]

24. Arosio, D.; Casagrande, C. Advancement in integrin facilitated drug delivery. *Adv. Drug Deliv. Rev.* **2016**, *97*, 111–143. [CrossRef] [PubMed]

25. Kuila, T.; Bose, S.; Mishra, A.K.; Khanra, P.; Kim, N.H.; Lee, J.H. Chemical functionalization of graphene and its applications. *Progress Mater. Sci.* **2012**, *57*, 1061–1105. [CrossRef]

26. Fangping, O.; Huang, B.; Li, Z.; Xiao, J.; Wang, H.; Xu, H. Chemical functionalization of graphene nanoribbons by carboxyl groups on stone-wales defects. *J. Phys. Chem. C* **2008**, *112*, 12003–12007. [CrossRef]

27. Zhu, S.; Li, J.; Chen, Y.; Chen, Z.; Chen, C.; Li, Y.; Cui, Z.; Zhang, D. Grafting of graphene oxide with stimuli-responsive polymers by using ATRP for drug release. *J. Nanopart. Res.* **2012**, *14*, s11051–s12012. [CrossRef]

28. Orecchioni, M.; Cabizza, R.; Bianco, A.; Delogu, L.G. Graphene as cancer theranostic tool: Progress and future challenges. *Theranostics* **2015**, *5*, 710–723. [CrossRef]

29. Kazemi-Beydokhti, A.; Zeinali Heris, S.; Reza Jaafari, M.; Nikoofal-Sahlabadi, S.; Tafaghodi, M.; Hatamipoor, M. Microwave functionalized single-walled carbon nanotube as nanocarrier for the delivery of anticancer drug cisplatin: In vitro and in vivo evaluation. *J. Drug Deliv. Sci. Technol.* **2014**, *24*, 572–578. [CrossRef]

30. Hilder, T.A.; Hill, J.M. Modelling the encapsulation of the anticancer drug cisplatin into carbon nanotubes. *Nanotechnology* **2007**, *18*. [CrossRef]

31. Tian, L.; Pei, X.; Zeng, Y.; He, R.; Li, Z.; Wang, J.; Wan, Q.; Li, X. Functionalized nanoscale graphene oxide for high efficient drug delivery of cisplatin. *J. Nanopart. Res.* **2014**, *16*. [CrossRef]

32. Wei, Y.; Zhou, F.; Zhang, D.; Chen, Q.; Xing, D. A graphene oxide based smart drug delivery system for tumor mitochondria-targeting photodynamic therapy. *Nanoscale* **2016**, *8*, 3530–3538. [CrossRef]

33. Tran, A.V.; Shim, K.; Vo Thi, T.T.; Kook, J.K.; An, S.S.A.; Lee, S.W. Targeted and controlled drug delivery by multifunctional mesoporous silica nanoparticles with internal fluorescent conjugates and external polydopamine and graphene oxide layers. *Acta Biomater.* **2018**, *74*, 397–413. [CrossRef] [PubMed]

34. Vittorio, O.; Le Grand, M.; Makharza, S.A.; Curcio, M.; Tucci, P.; Iemma, F.; Nicoletta, F.P.; Hampel, S.; Cirillo, G. Doxorubicin synergism and resistance reversal in human neuroblastoma BE(2)C cell lines: An in vitro study with dextran-catechin nanohybrids. *Eur. J. Pharm. Biopharm.* **2018**, *122*, 176–185. [CrossRef]

35. Lerra, L.; Farfalla, A.; Sanz, B.; Cirillo, G.; Vittorio, O.; Voli, F.; Grand, M.L.; Curcio, M.; Nicoletta, F.P.; Dubrovska, A.; et al. Graphene oxide functional nanohybrids with magnetic nanoparticles for improved vectorization of doxorubicin to neuroblastoma cells. *Pharmaceutics* **2019**, *11*. [CrossRef] [PubMed]

36. Yang, K.; Zhang, S.; Zhang, G.; Sun, X.; Lee, S.T.; Liu, Z. Graphene in mice: Ultrahigh in vivo tumor uptake and efficient photothermal therapy. *Nano Lett.* **2010**, *10*, 3318–3323. [CrossRef]

37. Moore, T.L.; Podilakrishna, R.; Rao, A.; Alexis, F. Systemic administration of polymer-coated nano-graphene to deliver drugs to glioblastoma. *Part. Part. Syst. Charact.* **2014**, *31*, 886–894. [CrossRef]

38. Richard, S.; Saric, A.; Boucher, M.; Slomianny, C.; Geffroy, F.; Mériaux, S.; Lalatonne, Y.; Petit, P.X.; Motte, L. Antioxidative theranostic iron oxide nanoparticles toward brain tumors imaging and ROS production. *ACS Chem. Biol.* **2016**, *11*, 2812–2819. [CrossRef]

39. Caetano, B.L.; Guibert, C.; Fini, R.; Fresnais, J.; Pulcinelli, S.H.; Ménager, C.; Santilli, C.V. Magnetic hyperthermia-induced drug release from ureasil-PEO-γ-F_e2O_3 nanocomposites. *RSC Adv.* **2016**, *6*, 63291–63295. [CrossRef]

40. Lee, N.; Yoo, D.; Ling, D.; Cho, M.H.; Hyeon, T.; Cheon, J. Iron oxide based nanoparticles for multimodal imaging and magnetoresponsive therapy. *Chem. Rev.* **2015**, *115*, 10637–10689. [CrossRef]

41. Song, M.M.; Xu, H.L.; Liang, J.X.; Xiang, H.H.; Liu, R.; Shen, Y.X. Lactoferrin modified graphene oxide iron oxide nanocomposite for glioma-targeted drug delivery. *Mater. Sci. Eng. C* **2017**, *77*, 904–911. [CrossRef] [PubMed]

42. Huang, Y.S.; Lu, Y.J.; Chen, J.P. Magnetic graphene oxide as a carrier for targeted delivery of chemotherapy drugs in cancer therapy. *J. Magn. Magn. Mater.* **2017**, *427*, 34–40. [CrossRef]

43. Roca, A.G.; Gutiérrez, L.; Gavilán, H.; Fortes Brollo, M.E.; Veintemillas-Verdaguer, S.; Morales, M.D.P. Design strategies for shape-controlled magnetic iron oxide nanoparticles. *Adv. Drug Deliv. Rev.* **2018**. [CrossRef] [PubMed]

44. Pham, B.T.T.; Colvin, E.K.; Pham, N.T.H.; Kim, B.J.; Fuller, E.S.; Moon, E.A.; Barbey, R.; Yuen, S.; Rickman, B.H.; Bryce, N.S.; et al. Biodistribution and clearance of stable superparamagnetic maghemite iron oxide nanoparticles in mice following intraperitoneal administration. *Int. J. Mol. Sci.* **2018**, *19*. [CrossRef]

45. Kumar, N.; Kulkarni, K.; Behera, L.; Verma, V. Preparation and characterization of maghemite nanoparticles from mild steel for magnetically guided drug therapy. *J. Mater. Sci. Mater. Med.* **2017**, *28*. [CrossRef]

46. Makharza, S.; Cirillo, G.; Bachmatiuk, A.; Vittorio, O.; Mendes, R.G.; Oswald, S.; Hampel, S.; Ruemmeli, M.H. Size-dependent nanographene oxide as a platform for efficient carboplatin release. *J. Mater. Chem. B* **2013**, *1*, 6107–6114. [CrossRef]

47. Rosli, N.F.; Fojtů, M.; Fisher, A.C.; Pumera, M. Graphene oxide nanoplatelets potentiate anticancer effect of cisplatin in human lung cancer cells. *Langmuir* **2019**, *35*, 3176–3182. [CrossRef]

48. Makharza, S.; Vittorio, O.; Cirillo, G.; Oswald, S.; Hinde, E.; Kavallaris, M.; Buechner, B.; Mertig, M.; Hampel, S. Graphene oxide—Gelatin nanohybrids as functional tools for enhanced carboplatin activity in neuroblastoma cells. *Pharm. Res.* **2015**, *32*, 2132–2143. [CrossRef] [PubMed]

49. Arruebo, M.; Fernández-Pacheco, R.; Ibarra, M.R.; Santamaría, J. Magnetic nanoparticles for drug delivery. *Nano Today* **2007**, *2*, 22–32. [CrossRef]

50. Mahmoudi, M.; Sant, S.; Wang, B.; Laurent, S.; Sen, T. Superparamagnetic iron oxide nanoparticles (SPIONs): Development, surface modification and applications in chemotherapy. *Adv. Drug Deliv. Rev.* **2011**, *63*, 24–46. [CrossRef] [PubMed]

51. Mojica Pisciotti, M.L.; Lima, E., Jr.; Vasquez Mansilla, M.; Tognoli, V.E.; Troiani, H.E.; Pasa, A.A.; Creczynski-Pasa, T.B.; Silva, A.H.; Gurman, P.; Colombo, L.; et al. In vitro and in vivo experiments with iron oxide nanoparticles functionalized with DEXTRAN or polyethylene glycol for medical applications: Magnetic targeting. *J. Biomed. Mater. Res. Part B Appl. Biomater.* **2014**, *102*, 860–868. [CrossRef] [PubMed]

52. Calatayud, M.P.; Riggio, C.; Raffa, V.; Sanz, B.; Torres, T.E.; Ibarra, M.R.; Hoskins, C.; Cuschieri, A.; Wang, L.; Pinkernelle, J.; et al. Neuronal cells loaded with PEI-coated Fe_3O_4 nanoparticles for magnetically guided nerve regeneration. *J. Mater. Chem. B* **2013**, *1*, 3607–3616. [CrossRef]

53. Szalai, A.J.; Manivannan, N.; Kaptay, G. Super-paramagnetic magnetite nanoparticles obtained by different synthesis and separation methods stabilized by biocompatible coatings. *Colloids Surf. A Physicochem. Eng. Asp.* **2019**, *568*, 113–122. [CrossRef]

54. Cuenca, J.A.; Bugler, K.; Taylor, S.; Morgan, D.; Williams, P.; Bauer, J.; Porch, A. Study of the magnetite to maghemite transition using microwave permittivity and permeability measurements. *J. Phys. Condens. Matter.* **2016**, *28*. [CrossRef]

55. Mei, Z.; Dhanale, A.; Gangaharan, A.; Sardar, D.K.; Tang, L. Water dispersion of magnetic nanoparticles with selective Biofunctionality for enhanced plasmonic biosensing. *Talanta* **2016**, *151*, 23–29. [CrossRef]

56.   Mitchell, R.W.; Edmundson, C.L.; Miller, D.W.; Hatch, G.M. On the mechanism of oleate transport across human brain microvessel endothelial cells. *J. Neurochem.* **2009**, *110*, 1049–1057. [CrossRef] [PubMed]

57.   Múzquiz-Ramos, E.M.; Guerrero-Chávez, V.; Macías-Martínez, B.I.; López-Badillo, C.M.; García-Cerda, L.A. Synthesis and characterization of maghemite nanoparticles for hyperthermia applications. *Ceram. Int.* **2014**, *41*, 397–402. [CrossRef]

58.   Ryan, S.M.; Brayden, D.J. Progress in the delivery of nanoparticle constructs: Towards clinical translation. *Curr. Opin. Pharmacol.* **2014**, *18*, 120–128. [CrossRef] [PubMed]

59.   Reis, A.V.; Guilherme, M.R.; Rubira, A.F.; Muniz, E.C. Mathematical model for the prediction of the overall profile of in vitro solute release from polymer networks. *J. Colloid Interface Sci.* **2007**, *310*, 128–135. [CrossRef] [PubMed]

60.   Liu, P.; Wang, S.; Liu, X.; Ding, J.; Zhou, W. Platinated graphene oxide: A nanoplatform for efficient gene-chemo combination cancer therapy. *Eur. J. Pharm. Sci.* **2018**, *121*, 319–329. [CrossRef]

61.   Cheng, S.J.; Chiu, H.Y.; Kumar, P.V.; Hsieh, K.Y.; Yang, J.W.; Lin, Y.R.; Shen, Y.C.; Chen, G.Y. Simultaneous drug delivery and cellular imaging using graphene oxide. *Biomater. Sci.* **2018**, *6*, 813–819. [CrossRef] [PubMed]

62.   Lin, K.C.; Lin, M.W.; Hsu, M.N.; Yu-Chen, G.; Chao, Y.C.; Tuan, H.Y.; Chiang, C.S.; Hu, Y.C. Graphene oxide sensitizes cancer cells to chemotherapeutics by inducing early autophagy events, promoting nuclear trafficking and necrosis. *Theranostics* **2018**, *8*, 2477–2487. [CrossRef] [PubMed]

63.   Makharza, S.; Cirillo, G.; Bachmatiuk, A.; Ibrahim, I.; Ioannides, N.; Trzebicka, B.; Hampel, S.; Ruemmeli, M.H. Graphene oxide-based drug delivery vehicles: Functionalization, characterization, and cytotoxicity evaluation. *J. Nanopart. Res.* **2013**, *15*. [CrossRef]

64.   Czarnobaj, K.; Łukasiak, J. In vitro release of cisplatin from sol-gel processed porous silica xerogels. *Drug Deliv. J. Deliv. Target. Ther. Agents* **2004**, *11*, 341–344. [CrossRef]

65.   Hall, M.D.; Telma, K.A.; Chang, K.-E.; Lee, T.D.; Madigan, J.P.; Lloyd, J.R.; Goldlust, I.S.; Hoeschele, J.D.; Gottesman, M.M. Say No to DMSO: Dimethylsulfoxide Inactivates Cisplatin, Carboplatin, and Other Platinum Complexes. *Cancer Res.* **2014**, *74*, 3913. [CrossRef] [PubMed]

66.   Parmar, A.; Pascali, G.; Voli, F.; Lerra, L.; Yee, E.; Ahmed-Cox, A.; Kimpton, K.; Cirillo, G.; Arthur, A.; Zahra, D.; et al. In vivo [64Cu]CuCl$_2$ PET imaging reveals activity of dextran-Catechin on tumor copper homeostasis. *Theranostics* **2018**, *8*, 5645–5659. [CrossRef] [PubMed]

Elaeagnus angustifolia Plant Extract Inhibits Epithelial-Mesenchymal Transition and Induces Apoptosis via HER2 Inactivation and JNK Pathway in HER2-Positive Breast Cancer Cells

Ayesha Jabeen [1,2,†], **Anju Sharma** [1,†], **Ishita Gupta** [1,2,†], **Hadeel Kheraldine** [1,2,3], **Semir Vranic** [1], **Ala-Eddin Al Moustafa** [1,2,*] and **Halema F. Al Farsi** [1,*]

[1]   College of Medicine, QU Health, Qatar University, Doha P.O. Box 2713, Qatar; jabeen@qu.edu.qa (A.J.); anju.sharma7385@gmail.com (A.S.); ishugupta28@gmail.com (I.G.); hk1805332@student.qu.edu.qa (H.K.); svranic@qu.edu.qa (S.V.)
[2]   Biomedical Research Centre, Qatar University, Doha P.O. Box 2713, Qatar
[3]   College of Pharmacy, Qatar University, Doha P.O. Box 2713, Qatar
[*]   Correspondence: aalmoustafa@qu.edu.qa (A.-E.A.M.); halfarsi@qu.edu.qa (H.F.A.F.);

[†]   These authors contributed equally to this work.

Academic Editors: José Antonio Lupiáñez, Amalia Pérez-Jiménez and Eva E. Rufino-Palomares

Abstract: *Elaeagnus angustifolia* (*EA*) is a medicinal plant used for treating several human diseases in the Middle East. Meanwhile, the outcome of *EA* extract on HER2-positive breast cancer remains nascent. Thus, we herein investigated the effects of the aqueous *EA* extract obtained from the flowers of *EA* on two HER2-positive breast cancer cell lines, SKBR3 and ZR75-1. Our data revealed that *EA* extract inhibits cell proliferation and deregulates cell-cycle progression of these two cancer cell lines. *EA* extract also prevents the progression of epithelial-mesenchymal transition (EMT), an important event for cancer invasion and metastasis; this is accompanied by upregulations of E-cadherin and β-catenin, in addition to downregulations of vimentin and fascin, which are major markers of EMT. Thus, *EA* extract causes a drastic decrease in cell invasion ability of SKBR3 and ZR75-1 cancer cells. Additionally, we found that *EA* extract inhibits colony formation of both cell lines in comparison with their matched control. The molecular pathway analysis of HER2 and JNK1/2/3 of *EA* extract exposed cells revealed that it can block HER2 and JNK1/2/3 activities, which could be the major molecular pathway behind these events. Our findings implicate that *EA* extract may possess chemo-preventive effects against HER2-positive breast cancer via HER2 inactivation and specifically JNK1/2/3 signaling pathways.

Keywords: *Elaeagnus angustifolia*; breast cancer; EMT; chemoprevention; apoptosis

1. Introduction

Breast cancer (BC) commonly affects women worldwide, comprising 25% of cancer cases [1]. There are several risk factors, both environmental and genetic, associated with the onset of breast cancer [2]. Gene-expression-profiling studies classified breast cancer into five molecular subtypes: Luminal (A and B), HER2, basal-like, and normal-like, using hierarchical cluster analysis [3]. Among all subtypes, HER2-positive breast cancer accounts for 20–25% and is associated with aggressive phenotype, poor prognosis, and survival rate, in addition to increased recurrence [4]. Systemic management modalities for HER2-positive breast cancer include chemotherapy, radiation, and targeted anti-HER2 treatment modalities [4–7]. Although the treatment is generally effective in the early stages of therapy, nevertheless, ~90% of primary and half of metastatic breast cancer cases resistance to therapy leads to treatment failure and mortality [8]. Thus, it is important to identify novel potent therapeutic agents that can inhibit cell proliferation of HER2+ breast cancer with minimal side-effects. An alternate to conventional therapy can be found in naturally present phytochemicals in foods such as vegetables, fruits, spices, and plant roots [9,10]. Traditionally, *Elaeagnus angustifolia* (*EA*) plant has been used extensively for centuries in the treatment of various diseases due to its antioxidant, anti-inflammatory, and antimicrobial properties [11], along with bioactive compounds (flavonoids and coumarins) [12] that regulate key events associated with cancer development, such as cell-signaling pathways, including Wnt-signaling, cell proliferation, cell-cycle progression, apoptosis, and epithelial-to-mesenchymal transition (EMT) [13,14].

Elaeagnus angustifolia (*EA*), commonly known as wild olive, oleaster, silver berry, or Russian olive [11,15], is a deciduous tree belonging to the family of *Elaeagnacea* (Araliaceae) widely distributed in the Middle East, as well as Mediterranean regions [12,16]. *EA* fruit is highly nutritious and contains vitamins (vitamin C, tocopherol, thiamine B1, and carotene), sugar, proteins, and several minerals, like potassium, iron, magnesium, and calcium [17–19]; the leaves and flower extract are rich in secondary metabolites such as coumarins, phenolcarboxylic acids, flavonoids, saponins, and tannins [16,20,21]. Previous studies have shown that *EA* exhibits anticancer effects as a result of its essential oils (ethyl cinnamate, 2-phenyl-ethyl benzoate, 2-phenyl-ethyl isovalerate, nerolidole, squalene, and acetaphenone), flavonoids (quercetin), and pro anthocyanosides [22,23]. In cancer, flavonoids are shown to enhance p53 expression and cause cell-cycle arrest in the G2/M phase [24]. Moreover, they are known to inhibit Ras protein expression and regulate heat-shock proteins in various cancers, mainly in leukemia and colorectal cancer [24]. One of the key flavonoid components of *EA* is Quercetin, which is an anti-proliferative agent [24]. Furthermore, quercetin also promotes TRAIL-induced apoptosis by enhancing the expression of Bax and inhibiting Bcl-2 protein [25–27]. Additionally, ethyl acetate has been shown to significantly reduce proliferation of Hela cells in vitro [22]. Apart from this, volatile oils present in the plant have medicinal properties and are also used in perfume industries [23,28]. *EA* possesses numerous therapeutic and pharmacological properties, including antifungal, antibacterial, antimutagenic, anti-inflammation, antioxidant, and gastroprotective effects [11,29–32]. Traditionally, *EA* is also used to cure other diseases, including osteoporosis, amoebic dysentery, jaundice, asthma, flu, cough, cold, nausea, diarrhea, sore throat, fever, tetanus, and female aphrodisiac [12,15,33,34]. However, there are limited studies regarding the role of *EA* extract on cancer. In this context, our group recently demonstrated that *EA* extract can reduce the progression of human oral cancer by the inhibition of angiogenesis and cell invasion via Erk1/Erk2 signaling pathways [12].

A previous study showed that hydroalcoholic extracts of *EA* flower significantly inhibit angiogenesis, one of the known hallmarks of cancer [35]. Nevertheless, there are no studies reported on the anticancer activity of *EA* in breast cancer, especially in HER2-positive type, and its mechanism of cancer inhibition. To investigate the potent therapeutic and antitumor properties of *EA* extract in human breast cancer and its underlying mechanism, we explored the effect of aqueous extract of *EA* flower on cell proliferation and cell-cycle progression, cell invasion, and colony formation in two HER2-positive human breast cancer cell lines (SKBR3 and ZR75-1).

2. Results

In order to determine the effects of *EA* extract on HER2-positive cell lines SKBR3 and ZR75-1, cells were treated with varying concentrations of *EA* extract (25, 50, 75, 100, 150, and 200 µL/mL) for 48 h. Treatment with EA extract reduced the number of proliferating HER2-positive breast cancer cells in a dose-dependent manner (Figure 1); notably, concentrations of 100 and 200 µL/mL showed a substantial decrease in cell viability of SKBR3 and ZR75-1 by 50% and 75%, respectively.

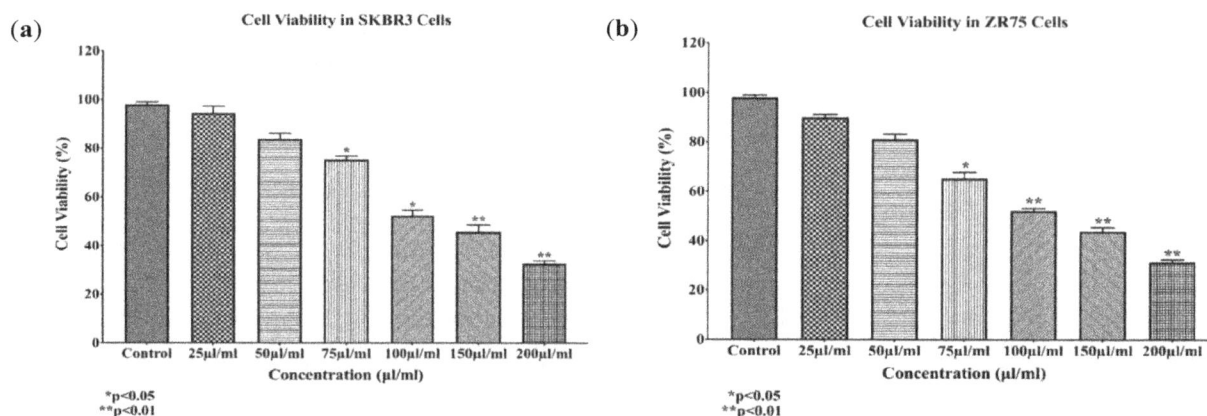

Figure 1. (a,b) The effects of different concentrations of *Elaeagnus angustifolia (EA)* plant extract on cell proliferation of HER2-positive breast cancer cell lines SKBR3 (a) and ZR75-1 (b) at 48 h. Data indicate an inverse relation between concentrations of *EA* extract and cell proliferation in both SKBR3 and ZR75-1 cell lines. Data are expressed as percent of growth ± SEM.

Meanwhile, and to examine whether the antiproliferative effect of the *EA* flower extract on SKBR3 and ZR75-1 cells is associated with cell-cycle deregulation, we analyzed cell-cycle phase distributions of *EA*-treated cells, using flow cytometric analysis. Our results showed that exposure to *EA* extract (100 and 200 µL/mL) for 48 h enhanced the G_0/G_1 phase, with a simultaneous decrease in S and G_2/M phases of both the breast cancer cell lines, thus indicating *EA*-induced cell-cycle inhibition (Figure 2). Furthermore, we observed a significant increase in the sub/G_1 phase of both cell lines, indicating that cells undergo apoptosis when treated with *EA* extract (Figure 2).

To confirm *EA*-induced apoptosis, Annexin V-FITC and 7-AAD staining by flow cytometry were performed. Therefore, the presence of apoptosis is clearly demonstrated in both cell lines (Figure 3).

Next, we examined the cell morphology of SKBR3 and ZR75-1 in addition to HNME-E6/E7 cell lines, using phase-contrast microscopy, under the effect of 100 and 200 µL/mL of *EA* extract. In the absence of treatment, SKBR3 and ZR75-1 cells displayed a round morphology and disorganized multilayered cells. In contrast, and as indicated in Figure 4a, treatment for 48 h with 100 and 200 µL/mL of *EA* plant extract led to a phenotypic conversion from round cells to epithelial-like phenotype. Clearly, cells became more flattened in appearance and showed an increase in cell-cell adhesion, in comparison with untreated cells (Figure 4a). However, at three days of treatment with 200 µL/mL of *EA* plant extract, cells started detaching from the surface of the tissue culture dish, indicating cell death in SKBR3 and ZR75-1 cells; however, this was not observed in the human normal immortalized mammary epithelial cell line (HNME-E6/E7), as shown in Figure 4b. Nevertheless, it is evident that *EA* extract inhibits cell proliferation HNME-E6/E7 cells, with a slight effect on their epithelial morphology (Figure 4b).

These results imply that moderate concentrations of 100 µL/mL of *EA* plant extract induce cell differentiation after 24 and/or 48 h, while higher concentrations (200 µL/mL of *EA* plant extract) can provoke apoptosis after 48 h of exposure.

Subsequently, and to analyze the anti-invasion effects of *EA* on HER2-positive breast cancer cells, Matrigel invasion assay was performed, using SKBR3 and ZR75-1 cells, upon *EA* treatment with 100 and 200 µL/mL concentrations; our data revealed that *EA* extract significantly inhibits cell invasion ability of both cell lines by ~70% to 88%, respectively, in comparison with control cells (Figure 5, $p < 0.05$). This suggests that *EA* plant extract can considerably downgrade cell invasion and metastasis of HER2-positive breast cancer.

On the other hand, we assessed the colony formation of SKBR3 and ZR75-1 cells, in soft agar, under the effect of *EA* plant extract at 100 and 200 µL/mL, for two weeks; we observed a significant decrease in the number of colonies for both cell lines treated with *EA* plant extract, compared with their matched control, as shown in Figure 6. SKBR3 sustained significant inhibition of colony formation by

60% ($p < 0.01$) and 80% ($p < 0.05$) when exposed to 100 and 200 µL/mL *EA* plant extract, in comparison to the control, respectively (Figure 6a). In parallel, ZR75-1 cell line also displayed a similar pattern after two weeks of treatment; the number of colonies decreased by 70% ($p < 0.05$) and 85% ($p < 0.01$) at 100 and 200 µL/mL concentrations, respectively (Figure 6b). This indicates that *EA* plant extract suppresses colony formation and probably tumor growth in vivo.

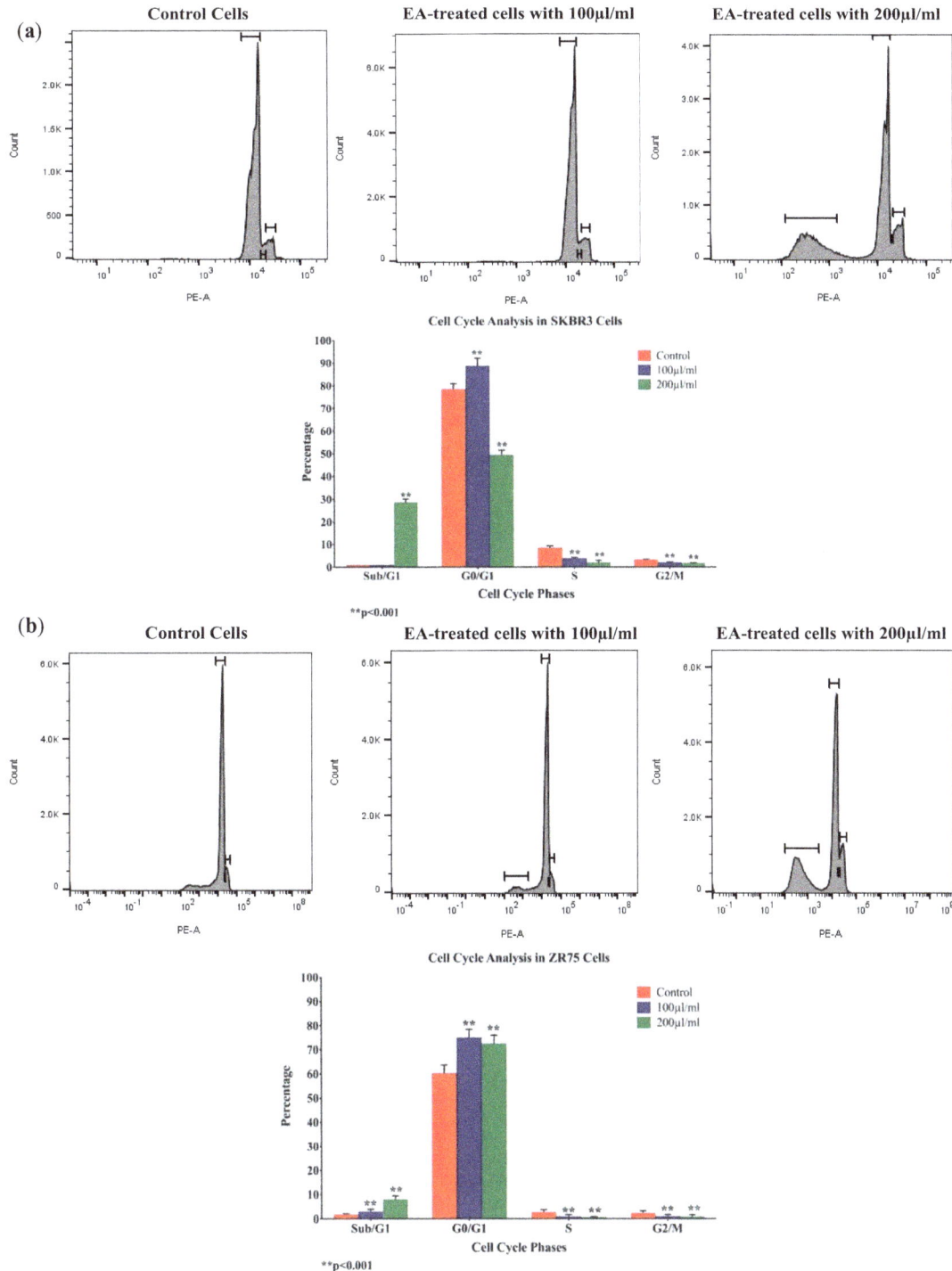

Figure 2. (a,b) Flow cytometry data analysis of SKBR3 and ZR75 cells after *EA*-treatment. Data demonstrate an increase in G_0/G_1 phase with simultaneous reduction in S and G_2/M phases in both cell lines. Meanwhile, there is a significant increase in cell apoptosis (Sub/G_1 phase) of SKBR3 cells treated with *EA*, and a small increase in cell apoptosis of treated ZR75 cells.

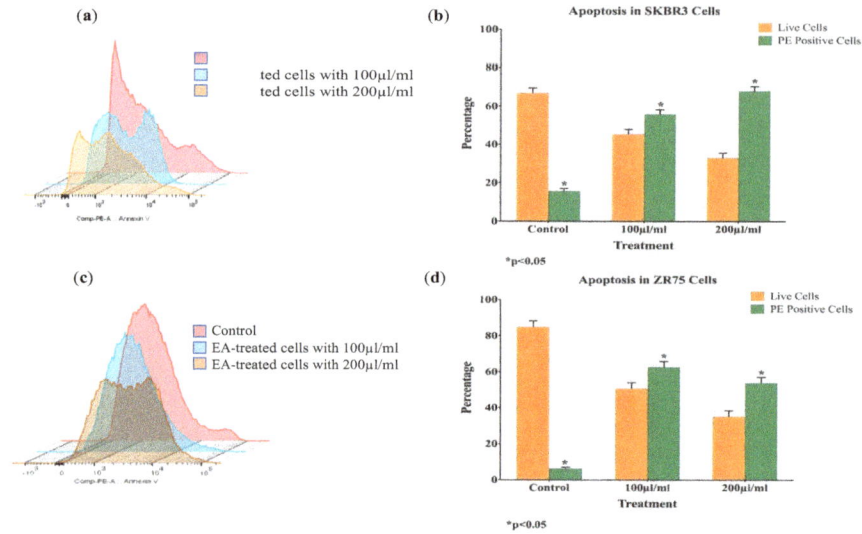

Figure 3. (**a,b**) Induction of apoptosis by *EA* extract in SKBR3 (**a**, **b**) and ZR75 (**c**, **d**) cells, as determined by Annexin V-FITC and 7-AAD apoptosis assay.

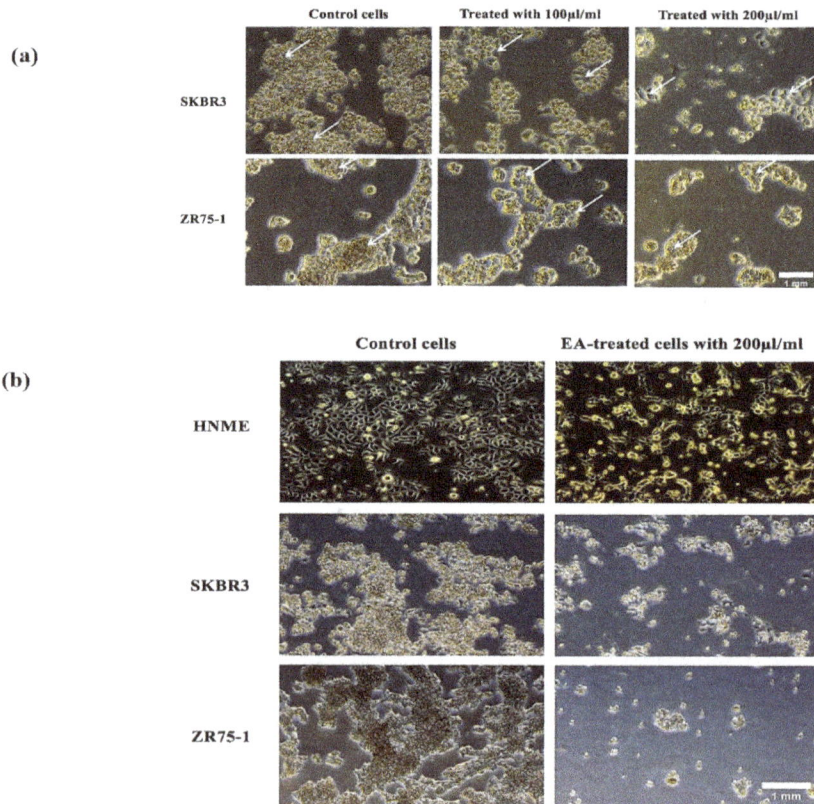

Figure 4. (**a,b**) *EA* plant extract induces morphological changes in HER2-positive cell lines, SKBR3 and ZR75-1. (**a**) We observe that treatment for 48 h with 100 and 200 μL/mL of *EA* extract induces epithelial transition and the formation of a monolayer of cells in both cell lines, in comparison with untreated (control) cells which display a round phenotype and form multilayers; arrows indicate epithelial morphology with clear cell-cell adhesion. (**b**) At three days of treatment of SKBR3, ZR75-1, and HNME-E6/E7 cell lines with 200 μL/mL of *EA* plant extract, the two cancer cell lines start detaching from the surface of the tissue culture dish, indicating cell death; this observation was not noted in the HNME-E6/E7 cells (images **a** and **b** at ×20 magnification).

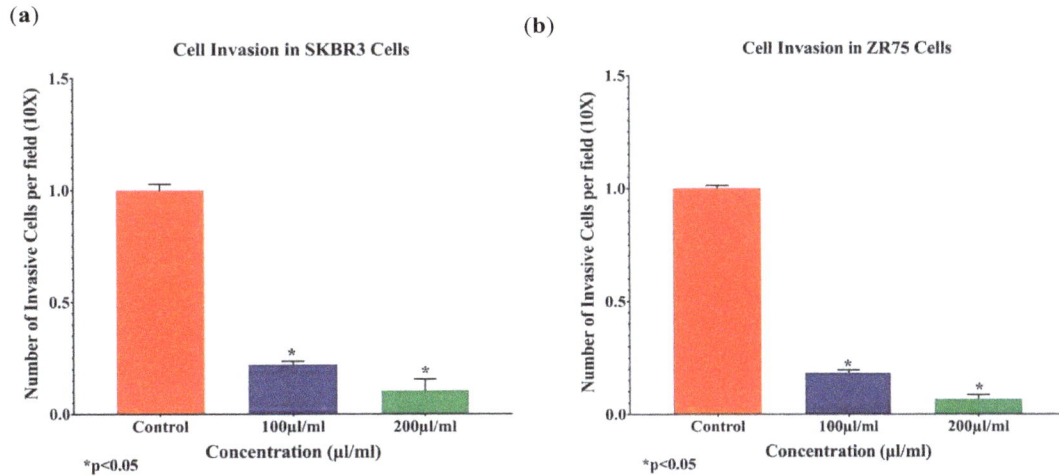

Figure 5. (**a,b**): The effects of *EA* flower extract on cell invasion of human HER2-positive breast cancer cells. *EA* extract inhibits cell invasion ability of SKBR3 (**a**) and ZR75-1 (**b**) cell lines by approximately 70% in comparison with their matched control cells (unexposed) ($p < 0.05$). Boyden chambers were used to assess cell-invasion ability of SKBR3 and ZR75-1 cell lines. Cancer cells treated for 24 h with 100 and 200 μL/mL *EA* plant extract showed a significant inhibition of cell invasion in both cell lines, when compared with their matched control ($p < 0.05$). Data are quantified by normalizing the number of invasive cells by their total number.

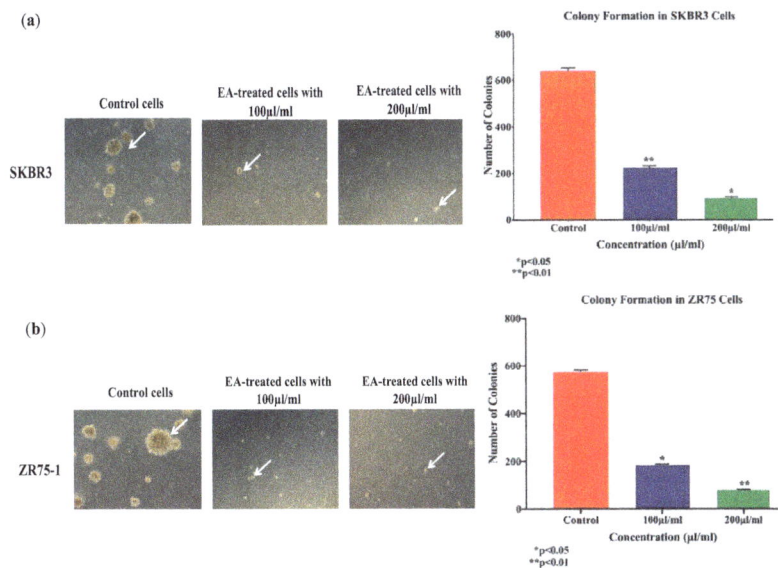

Figure 6. (**a,b**) Effect of *EA* flower extract on colony formation, in soft agar, in human HER2-positive cancer cell lines, SKBR3 (**a**) and ZR75-1 (**b**). *EA* extract inhibits colony formation of SKBR3 and ZR75-1, in comparison with their matched control cells (images of figure **a,b** at ×10 magnification). Colony formation in soft agar is a solid indicator of tumor formation in vivo. The colonies were counted manually and expressed as percentage of treatment relative to the control (mean ± SEM).

Based on the above data, we explored the expression patterns of key markers of EMT and cancer progression: E-cadherin, β-catenin, vimentin, and fascin; our data pointed out that *EA* extract enhances the expression of E-cadherin and β-catenin in SKBR3 and ZR75-1 cell lines, while the expression of vimentin and fascin are decreased in comparison to their control cells (Figures 7 and 8). In parallel, we examined the outcome of *EA* on pro-apoptotic proteins (caspase-3 and Bax) and anti-apoptotic protein (Bcl-2) with 100 and 200 μL/mL of *EA* plant extract after 24 and 48 h of exposure. We found enhanced expression of both pro-apoptotic proteins (Bax and caspase-3) in SKBR3 and ZR75-1 in *EA*-treated cells, compared to their control (Figures 7 and 8). In contrast, the expression of Bcl-2 was lost in SKBR3 and ZR75-1 (Figures 7 and 8). Our data suggest that high concentrations of *EA* induce apoptosis in HER2-positive cancer cells, which might be associated with the Bcl-2/Bax/caspase-3 signaling pathway.

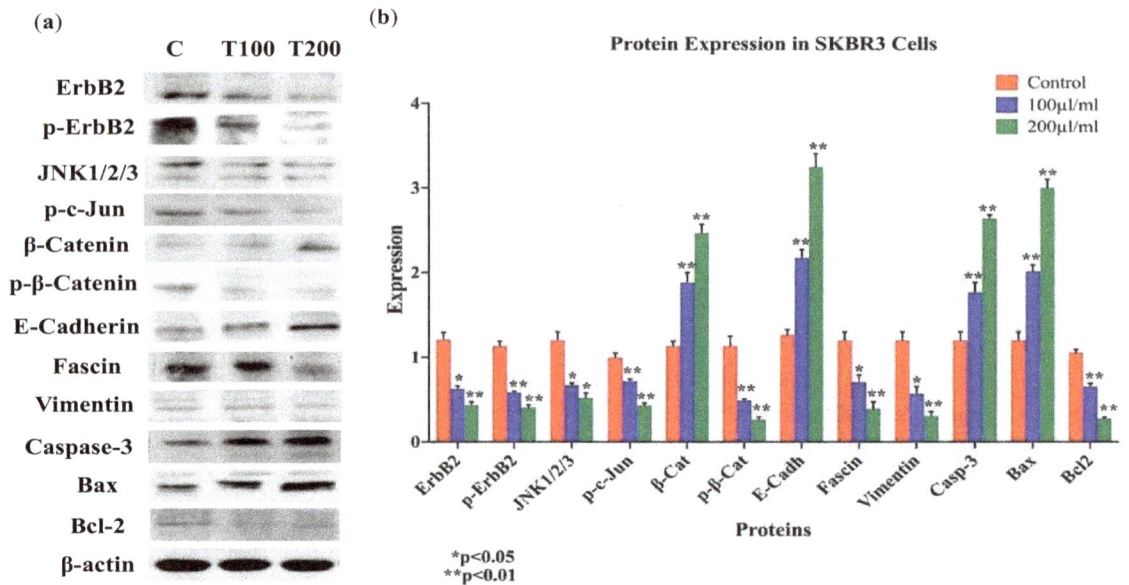

Figure 7. (**a,b**) Protein expression and molecular mechanisms of *EA* inhibitory actions in SKBR3 cell line. This plant extract induces an overexpression of E-cadherin, β-catenin, and downregulation of vimentin and fascin, while upregulating pro-apoptotic markers (Bax and Caspase-3), in comparison with their control and inhibiting anti-apoptotic markers (Bcl-2). Furthermore, *EA* plant extract inhibits the phosphorylation of ErbB2 and β-catenin, as well as the expression of JNK1/2/3. β-actin was used as a control for the proteins amount in this assay. Cells were treated with 100 and 200 μL/mL of *EA* extract for 48 h, as explained in the materials and methods and the results sections. (**a**) Blot image and (**b**) quantification of bands.

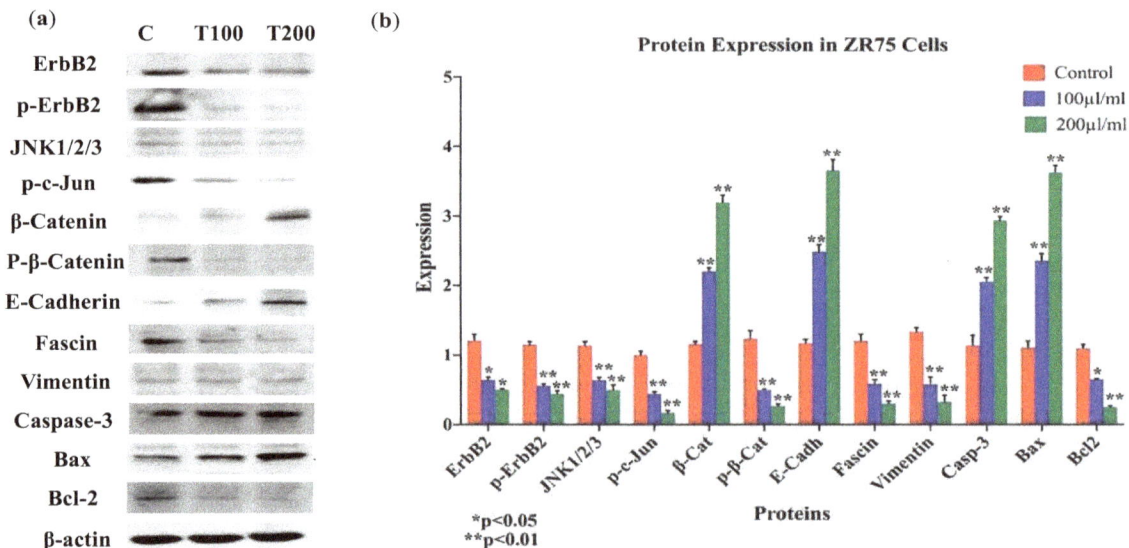

Figure 8. (**a,b**) Protein expression and molecular mechanisms of *EA* inhibitory actions in ZR75 cell line. This plant extract induces an overexpression of E-cadherin, β-catenin, and downregulation of vimentin and fascin; in addition, pro-apoptotic markers Bax and Caspase-3 are upregulated in comparison with their control, while anti-apoptotic marker Bcl-2 is inhibited. Furthermore, *EA* plant extract inhibits the phosphorylation of ErbB2 and β-catenin, as well as JNK1/2/3 expression. β-actin served as a control in this assay. Cells were treated with 100 and 200 μL/mL of *EA* extract for 48 h, as explained in the materials and Methods section. (**a**) Blot image and (**b**) quantification of bands.

Vis-à-vis the underlying molecular pathways of *EA* extract on cell proliferation, EMT progression, cell invasion, and colony formation of HER2-positive breast cancer cells, we assumed that HER2 activation, as well as c-Jun N-terminal kinase (JNK), could have major roles in regulating these events [36–39]; therefore, the expression patterns of HER2 and JNK1/2 were explored. We found that *EA* extract inhibits the phosphorylation of HER2 (with slight change in its expression level) and β-catenin, while it provokes a downregulation of JNK1/2 in SKBR3 and ZR75-1 upon treatment with *EA* plant extract after 24 and 48 h of exposure (Figures 7 and 8).

3. Discussion

In this study, we investigated the effect of *EA* extract in HER2-positive human breast cancer cell lines (SKBR3 and ZR75-1) with regard to certain parameters related to cell proliferation, cell cycle, morphological changes (round to epithelial-like transition: RELT), cell invasion, and colony formation. Additionally, we explored the molecular pathways behind these events. We report that *EA* plant extract can suppress cell proliferation, as well as dysregulate cell-cycle progression of SKBR3 and ZR75-1 cells, along with induction of RELT and inhibition of colony formation in both cell lines. *EA* plant is known for its antioxidant characteristics and has been used conventionally for the treatment of several diseases and inflammation [16,20,21]. Moreover, *EA* consists of bioactive compounds (flavonoids and neoclerodane diterpenoids), which can play a role in promoting apoptosis and cell-cycle progression, as well as inhibiting angiogenesis and EMT events, thus potentially preventing cancer development and progression [12,13,16,40]. Meanwhile, we herein demonstrate that *EA* plant extract inhibits cell proliferation and dysregulate cell-cycle and EMT progression of HER2-positive breast cancer cells.

Indeed, EMT is a crucial phenomenon in cancer progression, characterized by disruption of intracellular tight junctions and the loss of cell-cell contact and epithelial cell features, along with the gain of mesenchymal morphology [41]. On the other hand, it is well-known that cancer progression is characterized by loss of differentiation in human carcinomas, together with downregulation of E-cadherin, which is associated with the degree of tumor malignancy [33]. Moreover, previous studies on different types of human carcinomas have shown that loss of E-cadherin and β-catenin, in addition to enhanced expression of vimentin and fascin, can promote EMT, which is associated with cancer progression [41–44]. In this investigation, we analyzed the effect of *EA* on E-cadherin, β-catenin, vimentin, and fascin expression patterns in HER2-positive breast cancer cell lines. We observed two different major events that are provoked by *EA* treatment, namely induction of RELT "MET" and apoptosis. More specifically, we found that, upon *EA*-treatment for 24 and 48 h at both low and high concentrations (100 and 200 μL/mL), E-cadherin and β-catenin are upregulated, while vimentin, p-β-catenin, and fascin expressions are downregulated, which are important elements of mesenchymal-epithelial transition (MET), the opposite event of EMT, and RELT. Thus, *EA* plant extract can induce differentiation to an epithelial phenotype and consequently block cell invasion of the two HER2-positive human breast cancer cell lines. On the other hand, we found that *EA* extract inhibits colony formation of SKBR3 and ZR75-1 cell lines, which could be considered as an in vivo tumor formation.

On the other hand, regarding the molecular pathways of *EA* extract on our cell line models, we herein reported that, upon *EA*-treatment after 24 h at both low and high concentration, *EA* extract can inactivate HER2 receptor, as well as deregulate the expression patterns of JNK1/2, which can lead to increased expression of E-cadherin and β-catenin and decreased expression of vimentin and fascin, thus indicating restoration of cell-cell adhesion, especially E-cadherin/catenins complex. Furthermore, in accordance with our data, a study by Wang et al. showed overexpression of JNK to be linked with breast cancer cell migration and invasion, as well as EMT [45]. Therefore, in this present investigation, we show that *EA* plant extract can regulate the RELT/EMT event and inhibit cell invasion of the two human HER2-positive breast cancer cell lines. Moreover, these present data are concurrent with our recently published work regarding the outcome of *EA* plant extract on human oral cancer cells, where we have demonstrated that *EA* induces differentiation to an epithelial phenotype; and therefore, it causes a dramatic decrease in cell invasion and motility of human oral cancer cells, along with an upregulation of E-cadherin expression [12]. Additionally, our study of *EA* extract on oral cancer cells revealed that *EA* can inhibit the phosphorylation of Erk1/Erk2 and β-catenin, which could be behind the initiation of RELT/MET event and the overexpression of E-cadherin [12]. In the present work, we demonstrated that JNK1/2 pathway is one of the main molecular pathways of *EA* in HER2-positive human breast cancer cells.

JNK substrate proteins encompass several nuclear proteins, including transcription factors, as well as nuclear hormone receptors involved in maintaining various cellular activities comprising cell proliferation, differentiation, cell death, and cell survival [46]. JNKs phosphorylate and stimulate both, nuclear and non-nuclear proteins and form the transcription factor activator protein-1 (AP-1) by dimerization of the Jun proteins (c-Jun, JunB, and JunD) with the Fos proteins (c-Fos, FosB, Fra-1, and Fra-2); other downstream molecules include activating transcription factor 2 (ATF-2), c-Myc, p53, STAT1/3, Pax family of proteins, Elk1, NFAT, and Bcl-2 family (Bcl-2, Bcl-xl, Bad, Bim, and Bax) [47]. Of these nuclear substrates, c-jun is the most vital nuclear substrate; JNKs enhance c-jun transcription by binding and phosphorylating c-jun at Ser73 and Ser63 via Ha-Ras, c-Raf, and v-Src [48–50]. c-Jun, the downstream target of the JNK pathway, is necessary for Ras-induced carcinogenesis [51,52]. In vivo studies have indicated an oncogenic role of c-Jun in the liver [53–55], as well as intestinal cancers [54], thus indicating a pro-oncogenic role for the JNK/c-Jun axis. The activity of c-jun is essential for the Ha-Ras mediating carcinogenesis transformation. Our data indicate that *EA*-treatment reduced p-c-Jun expression, indicating an *EA*-tumor-suppressive role in cancer.

In parallel, it is evident that β-catenin signaling pathways are also involved in these events; this is based on the fact that β-catenin acts as a transcription regulator, as well as cell-cell adhesion molecule, which was elegantly reported by Kandouz et al., under the effect *Teucrium polium* on human prostate cancer cells [12,56]. Thus, it is possible that *EA* plant extract can have a similar effect on β-catenin pathways, especially since our data showed that *EA* extract inhibit β-catenin phosphorylation, consequently allowing it to translocate from the nucleus to undercoat membrane to act as a cell-cell adhesion protein leading to the inhibition of cell-invasion ability of SKBR3 and ZR75-1 cell lines. We surmise that *EA* exhibits anticancer activity due to the high levels of flavonoids, coumarins, and antioxidants [12,14,57].

Vis-à-vis the interaction between the activation of HER2 receptor and its downstream pathways, including JNK, it is well-established that HER2 overexpression causes homo- or heterodimerization, leading to phosphorylation of this receptor, which in turn triggers downstream signaling pathways responsible for important cellular functions, including cell proliferation, invasion, migration, angiogenesis, chemoresistance, and apoptosis [38,39]. We investigated the downstream target of HER2 stimuli, JNK, as JNK-dependent gene regulatory circuitry underlying cell-fate changes from epithelial to mesenchymal state. Our study demonstrates that *EA* slightly suppresses the expression of HER2 receptor, while mostly affecting its phosphorylation, as well as one of its main downstream targets JNK. More specifically, HER2 downregulation is associated with inhibition of proliferation and invasion of HER2-positive human breast cancer cells [58]; this correlates with our results of *EA*-induced decreased cell proliferation, cell invasion, and colony formation.

Regarding the outcome of high-concentration treatment of *EA* (200 μL/mL) after 48 h, we observed induction of apoptosis in *EA*-treated cells by analyzing the mitochondrial apoptosis regulators of Bcl-2 family (Bcl-2 and Bax), as well as Caspase-3 [59]. Bcl-2 homodimers have been shown to inhibit apoptosis; however, Bax homodimers initiates cell death [60]. Heterodimerization between Bax and Bcl-2 and its ratio of Bax to Bcl-2 determine the susceptibility of cells to apoptosis, whereas caspase-3 is known to act as a downstream target of Bax/Bcl-2 control and play a key role in the execution of apoptosis [60]. We herein report that *EA* can reduce the growth and provoke apoptosis of human HER2-positive breast cancer cells. This effect is associated with caspase-3 activation and reduced Bcl-2 expression. Moreover, mitochondrial Bax translocation and the expression of Bcl-2 slightly decreased upon *EA*-extract treatment, indicating that caspase-dependent pathways are involved in *EA*-induced apoptosis and Bcl2/Bax/Caspase-3-regulated cell death through JNK inactivation.

The JNK pathway is predominantly involved in the stimulation of the intrinsic apoptotic pathway facilitated by mitochondria [61]. However, the JNK pathway is also involved in TRAIL-induced apoptosis, autophagy, mitotic catastrophe, and immunogenic cell death [62–66]. Our data show upregulation of Bax and capsase-3 expression and downregulation of Bcl-2, indicating that apoptosis occurs via the extrinsic pathway as well [65]; a loss of JNK could primarily trigger extrinsic apoptosis. Moreover, Bax/Bcl-2/caspase-3 is also involved in other types of regulated cell death, including immunogenic cell death, mitotic catastrophe, and mitochondrial permeability transition (MPT)-driven necrosis [67], thus suggesting JNK inhibition to mediate Bax/Bcl-2/caspase-3 apoptosis. We herein showed loss of JNK, which is in concordance with a study by Wang et al., in breast cancer where overexpression of JNK did not cause apoptosis and correlated with poor prognosis [45]. Moreover, while activation of JNK results in loss of Bcl-2 expression [68–70], the mechanism is controversial as Bcl-2 phosphorylation enhances cell survival signaling [68,71–74], thus making the role of Bcl-2 phosphorylation in JNK-stimulated apoptosis nascent. Moreover, studies have demonstrated that JNK activation does not result in Bcl-2 phosphorylation [59,75], thus indicating that JNK might regulate another kinase or phosphatase resulting in Bcl-2 phosphorylation.

Although the roles of the Bcl-2 family of proteins in JNK-dependent apoptosis remain nascent, the results of the current study indicate that the proapoptotic Bax subfamily of Bcl-2-related proteins is not essential for JNK-dependent apoptosis. These data demonstrate a dual role of JNK in carcinogenesis which can be both oncogenic and tumor suppressive, as indicated previously. Alternatively, JNK activity can be tissue-specific and cell-type-dependent, differing based on tumor stage and status, as well as the presence of activated upstream and downstream molecules and stress signals [76–80]. Nevertheless, further work is needed to unravel the complexity of the interaction of JNK pathway and its molecules, to help pave the way for the development of anticancer therapeutic strategies. Moreover, in our laboratory, we are aiming to derive the active compounds of *EA* that can plausibly be involved in the inhibition of cancer progression.

4. Materials and Methods

4.1. Plant Collection and Extract Preparation

EA flowers were obtained during the second week of June, from Montreal, Quebec, Canada, and were dried and stored in a dark place, at room temperature, as previously described [12]. The extract was prepared by boiling 3 g of finely grounded dry *EA* flowers per 100 mL of autoclaved distilled water, at 150 °C, on a hot plate, for 20 min, with continuous stirring. The flower extract solution was then filtered, using a 0.45 μm filter unit, and stored at 4 °C until use. Dilutions were prepared in cell culture media for various applications. For each experiment, the extract was freshly prepared.

4.2. Cell Culture

Two different human HER2-positive breast cancer cell lines (SKBR3 and ZR75-1) derived from females were obtained from American Type Culture Collection (ATCC) (Rockville, MD, USA). Cell lines were grown and expanded in RPMI-1640 (Gibco, Life Technologies) supplemented with 10% fetal bovine serum (Gibco, Life Technologies, Massachusetts, MA, USA), 2 mm L-glutamine, 1% PenStrep antibiotic (Invitrogen, Life Technologies, Carlsbad, CA, USA) at 37 °C, and 5% CO_2 humidified atmosphere. Human normal mammary epithelial cells immortalized by E6/E7 of HPV type 16 (HNME-E6/E7) were used to assess plant extract toxicity [81]. Cells were maintained in Gibco® Keratinocyte-SFM (1X) media (Gibco, Life Technologies). All the experiments were carried out when cells were ~70–80% confluent.

4.3. Cell Viability Assay

HER-2-positive breast cancer cell lines, SKBR3 and ZR75-1, were seeded on clear bottom 96-well plates (10,000 cells/well) and cultured in RPMI-1640 supplemented with 10% fetal bovine serum (FBS) and 1% penicillin and streptomycin (100 μL/well).

Elaeagnus angustifolia (EA) solution was used to treat cells at different concentrations (25, 50, 75, 100, 150, and 200 μL/mL) for a period of 48 h. Control wells received 100 μL of media (control). The inhibition of cell viability was determined, using Alamar Blue Cell viability reagent (Invitrogen, Thermo Fisher Scientific, Waltham, MA, USA), according to the manufacturer's protocol. The shift in fluorescence was measured at 570 nm (excitation) and 600 nm (emission), in a fluorescent plate reader (Infinite M200, Tecan, Grödig, Austria), after 4 h of incubation with the dye. Relative cell proliferation was determined based on the fluorescence of *EA*-treated cells relative to that of control cells.

4.4. Cell Cycle and Apoptosis Assay

SKBR3 and ZR75-1 cells (1×10^6 cells/dish) were plated in 100 mm Petri dishes, with overnight incubation. The cells were then starved with serum-free RPMI-1640 medium for a period of 6–12 h to synchronize the cells into the G_0 phase of the cell cycle. Synchronized cells were then treated with *EA* extract (100 and 200 μL/mL) for 48 h. Cells were harvested, washed twice with PBS, fixed overnight in 70% ice-cold ethanol, and, subsequently, their DNA was stained with 50 μg/mL FXCycle PI/RNase staining solution (Invitrogen, Thermo Fisher Scientific) after RNase A treatment (50 μg/mL) (Thermo Fisher Scientific), at 37 °C, for 30 min, according to standard protocol [12]. Cell-cycle analysis was performed by flow-cytometry (BD Accuri C6, BD Biosciences, USA), and cells in G_0/G_1, S, G_2/M and the sub-G_0/G_1 (apoptotic) phases were quantified by using FlowJo software.

Furthermore, for apoptosis assay, the Annexin V-fluorescein isothiocyanate (FITC)/7-amino-actinomycin D (7-AAD) Apoptosis Kit-559763 (BD Biosciences, USA) was used as per the manufacturer's instructions. Briefly, cells (1×10^6 cells/dish) were seeded into 100 mm culture dishes and were maintained overnight in a medium containing 10% fetal bovine serum. The cells were collected by trypsinization and washed with phosphate buffered saline (PBS). Then, cells were resuspended in 200 μL of binding buffer. Annexin V staining was accomplished following product instructions (Clontech, Palo Alto, CA). In brief, 5 μL Annexin V-FITC and 5 μL 7-AAD were added to the samples for 15 min in the dark. However, for controls (unstained cells), they were stained with PE Annexin V (no 7-AAD) as well as with 7-AAD (no PE Annexin V). The cells were analyzed by flow cytometry (BD Accuri C6, BD Biosciences, San Jose, CA, USA). Data were presented as density plots of Annexin V-FITC and 7-AAD staining.

4.5. Cell Invasion Assay

Cell invasion assay was carried out in 24-well Biocoat Matrigel invasion chambers (pore size of 8 μm, Corning, USA) as per manufacturer's protocol. In brief, the bottom chamber was filled with RPMI-1640 medium, and the upper chamber was seeded with untreated, as well as treated, cells (5×10^4 cells), and then incubated at 37 °C. After 24 h incubation, non-invasive cells were scraped with a cotton swab, and cells that migrated to the lower surface of the membrane were fixed with methanol and stained with 0.4% crystal violet. For quantification, cells were counted under the Leica DMi1 inverted microscope (Leica Microsystems, Wetzlar, Germany) in five predetermined fields, as previously described [81]. Percentage inhibition of invasive cells was calculated with respect to untreated cells. Each experiment was carried out in triplicates.

4.6. Soft Agar Colony Formation Assay

Next, we determined the number of colonies formed prior and post-treatment, using soft agar growth assay. A total of 2×10^3 cells of SKBR3 and ZR75-1 were placed in their medium containing 0.2% agar with/without 100 and 200 μL/mL of *EA* extract (treated and control cells, respectively) and plated in a 6-well plate covered with a layer of 0.4% agar prepared in RPMI-1640 medium. Colony formation was examined every 2 days for a period of 2 weeks. Colonies in each well were counted, using the Leica SP8 UV/Visible Laser confocal microscope (Leica Microsystems, Wetzlar, Germany).

4.7. Western Blot Analysis

We analyzed the expression levels of proteins involved in the molecular pathways, such as apoptosis by Western blot analysis, as previously described by our group [81]. Briefly, SKBR3 and ZR75-1 cells (1×10^6 cells) were seeded and treated with *EA* extract (100 and 200 μL/mL) for 48 h. Cell lysates were collected, and equal amounts of protein (30 μg) were resolved on 10% polyacrylamide gels and electroblotted onto PVDF membranes. The PVDF membranes were probed with the following primary antibodies: anti-mouse E-cadherin (AbcamID#: ab1416), anti-rabbit β-catenin (CST 9562), anti-rabbit phosphorylated β-catenin (CST 4176), anti-rabbit Vimentin (Abcam: abID# 92547), anti-rabbit Fascin (AbcamID#: ab183891), anti-mouse Bax (ThermoFisher Scientific: MA5-14003), anti-mouse Bcl-2 (Abcam: abID# 692), anti-rabbit Caspase-3 (Abcam: abID# 13847), anti-mouse ErbB2 (Abcam: abID# 16901), anti-rabbit phosphorylated ErbB2 (Abcam: abID# 47262), anti-rabbit JNK1/JNK2/JNK3 (Abcam: abID# 179461), and anti-rabbit phosphorylated-c-Jun (Ser73) (Cell Signal Technologies, ID# 9164). To ensure equal loading of protein samples, the membranes were re-probed with anti-mouse β-actin (Abcam: abID# 6276).

Immunoreactivity was detected by using ECL Western blotting substrate (Pierce Biotechnology, Rockford, IL, USA), as described by the manufacturer.

In order to obtain a relative quantification of protein expressions, images acquired from Western blotting were analyzed, using ImageJ software. The intensity of the bands relative to the β-actin bands was used to calculate a relative expression of proteins in each cell line.

4.8. Statistical Analysis

The data were presented as mean ± SEM from three independent experiments performed in triplicates, and a t-test was used to compare the difference between treated and untreated cells. To evaluate significance for cell cycle, a Chi-square test was performed to compare significance between the different phases. Data were analyzed by using GraphPad Prism software (version 8.4.3), and differences with $p < 0.05$ were considered significant.

5. Conclusions

To the best of our knowledge, this is the first report, on the effect of *EA* in HER2-positive breast cancer and its underlying mechanism. Furthermore, this study brings about novel therapeutic potential by demonstrating the induced inhibition of HER2 and JNK activation by *EA* plant extract in human breast cancer cells. Our study points out that the downregulation of JNK can be one of the molecular pathways responsible of increasing E-cadherin and β-catenin and decreasing the expressions of vimentin and fascin. This is an interesting finding, since it can be potentially used as a target to inhibit cell invasion of HER2-positive breast cancer cells by reversing EMT or inducing RELT. In parallel, our data also demonstrate that high consecrations of *EA* trigger apoptosis, particularly in breast cancer cells, which is associated with Bcl-2/Bax/caspase-3 signaling pathway in HER2-positive cancer cells. We believe that *EA* might act as a candidate therapeutic agent based on its anticancer activity which can pave the way for potential more advanced therapeutic approaches in breast cancer management, especially HER2-positive cases.

Author Contributions: Conceptualization, A.-E.A.M. and H.F.A.F.; methodology, A.J., A.S., and H.K.; validation, A.J., A.S., and I.G.; resources, A.-E.A.M. and H.F.A.F.; data curation, A.J. and I.G.; writing—original draft preparation, A.S., I.G., and A.J.; writing—review and editing, I.G., S.V., and A.-E.A.M.; supervision, A.-E.A.M. and H.F.A.F.; funding acquisition, A.-E.A.M. and H.F.A.F. A.J., A.S., and I.G. contributed equally to this manuscript. All authors have read and agreed to the published version of the manuscript.

Acknowledgments: The authors would like to thank A. Kassab for her critical reading of the manuscript.

References

1. Ferlay, J.; Colombet, M.; Soerjomataram, I.; Mathers, C.; Parkin, D.M.; Piñeros, M.; Znaor, A.; Bray, F. Estimating the global cancer incidence and mortality in 2018: GLOBOCAN sources and methods. *Int. J. Cancer* **2019**, *144*, 1941–1953. [CrossRef] [PubMed]
2. Gupta, I.; Burney, I.; Al-Moundhri, M.S.; Tamimi, Y. Molecular genetics complexity impeding research progress in breast and ovarian cancers. *Mol. Clin. Oncol.* **2017**, *7*, 3–14. [CrossRef] [PubMed]
3. Perou, C.M.; Sørlie, T.; Eisen, M.B.; van de Rijn, M.; Jeffrey, S.S.; Rees, C.A.; Pollack, J.R.; Ross, D.T.; Johnsen, H.; Akslen, L.A.; et al. Molecular portraits of human breast tumours. *Nature* **2000**, *406*, 747–752. [CrossRef] [PubMed]
4. Sareyeldin, R.M.; Gupta, I.; Al-Hashimi, I.; Al-Thawadi, H.A.; Al Farsi, H.F.; Vranic, S.; Al Moustafa, A.-E. Gene Expression and miRNAs Profiling: Function and Regulation in Human Epidermal Growth Factor Receptor 2 (HER2)-Positive Breast Cancer. *Cancers* **2019**, *11*, 646. [CrossRef]
5. Giordano, S.H.; Temin, S.; Chandarlapaty, S.; Crews, J.R.; Esteva, F.J.; Kirshner, J.J.; Krop, I.E.; Levinson, J.; Lin, N.U.; Modi, S.; et al. Systemic Therapy for Patients with Advanced Human Epidermal Growth Factor Receptor 2–Positive Breast Cancer: ASCO Clinical Practice Guideline Update. *J. Clin. Oncol.* **2018**, *36*, 2736–2740. [CrossRef]
6. Ramakrishna, N.; Temin, S.; Chandarlapaty, S.; Crews, J.R.; Davidson, N.E.; Esteva, F.J.; Giordano, S.H.; Kirshner, J.J.; Krop, I.E.; Levinson, J.; et al. Recommendations on Disease Management for Patients with Advanced Human Epidermal Growth Factor Receptor 2–Positive Breast Cancer and Brain Metastases: ASCO Clinical Practice Guideline Update. *J. Clin. Oncol.* **2018**, *36*, 2804–2807. [CrossRef]
7. Vranic, S.; Beslija, S.; Gatalica, Z. Targeting HER2 expression in cancer: New drugs and new indications. *Bosn. J. Basic Med. Sci.* **2020**. [CrossRef]
8. Gonzalez-Angulo, A.M.; Morales-Vasquez, F.; Hortobagyi, G.N. Overview of Resistance to Systemic Therapy in Patients with Breast Cancer. In *Breast Cancer Chemosensitivity*; Yu, D., Hung, M.-C., Eds.; Springer: New York, NY, USA, 2007; pp. 1–22.
9. De Melo, F.H.M.; Oliveira, J.S.; Sartorelli, V.O.B.; Montor, W.R. Cancer Chemoprevention: Classic and Epigenetic Mechanisms Inhibiting Tumorigenesis. What Have We Learned So Far? *Front. Oncol.* **2018**, *8*. [CrossRef]
10. Gullett, N.P.; Amin, A.R.; Bayraktar, S.; Pezzuto, J.M.; Shin, D.M.; Khuri, F.R.; Aggarwal, B.B.; Surh, Y.-J.; Kucuk, O. Cancer Prevention with Natural Compounds. *Semin. Oncol.* **2010**, *37*, 258–281. [CrossRef]
11. Hamidpour, R.; Hamidpour, S.; Hamidpour, M.; Shahlari, M.; Sohraby, M.; Shahlari, N.; Hamidpour, R. Russian olive (Elaeagnus angustifolia L.): From a variety of traditional medicinal applications to its novel roles as active antioxidant, anti-inflammatory, anti-mutagenic and analgesic agent. *J. Tradit. Complement. Med.* **2016**, *7*, 24–29. [CrossRef]
12. Saleh, A.I.; Mohamed, I.; Mohamed, A.A.; Abdelkader, M.; Yalcin, H.C.; Aboulkassim, T.; Batist, G.; Yasmeen, A.; Al Moustafa, A.-E. Elaeagnus angustifolia Plant Extract Inhibits Angiogenesis and Downgrades Cell Invasion of Human Oral Cancer Cells via Erk1/Erk2 Inactivation. *Nutr. Cancer* **2018**, *70*, 297–305. [CrossRef] [PubMed]
13. Pudenz, M.; Roth, K.; Gerhauser, C. Impact of Soy Isoflavones on the Epigenome in Cancer Prevention. *Nutrients* **2014**, *6*, 4218–4272. [CrossRef] [PubMed]
14. Zhang, X.-J.; Jia, S.-S. Fisetin inhibits laryngeal carcinoma through regulation of AKT/NF-κB/mTOR and ERK1/2 signaling pathways. *Biomed. Pharmacother.* **2016**, *83*, 1164–1174. [CrossRef] [PubMed]

15. Amereh, Z.; Hatami, N.; Shirazi, F.H.; Gholami, S.; Hosseini, S.H.; Noubarani, M.; Kamalinejad, M.; Andalib, S.; Keyhanfar, F.; Eskandari, M.R. Cancer chemoprevention by oleaster (Elaeagnus angustifoli L.) fruit extract in a model of hepatocellular carcinoma induced by diethylnitrosamine in rats. *EXCLI J.* **2017**, *16*, 1046–1056. [PubMed]

16. Saboonchian, F.; Jamei, R.; Sarghein, S.H. Phenolic and flavonoid content of Elaeagnus angustifolia L. (leaf and flower). *Avicenna J. phytomedicine* **2014**, *4*, 231–238.

17. Boudraa, S.; Hambaba, L.; Zidani, S.; Boudraa, H. Mineral and vitamin composition of fruits of five underexploited species in Algeria: *Celtis australis* L., *Crataegus azarolus* L., *Crataegus monogyna* Jacq., *Elaeagnus angustifolia* L. and *Zizyphus lotus* L. *Fruits (Paris)* **2010**, *65*, 75–84. [CrossRef]

18. Fonia, A.; White, I.R.; White, J.M.L. Allergic contact dermatitis toElaeagnusplant (Oleaster). *Contact Dermat.* **2009**, *60*, 178–179. [CrossRef]

19. Taheri, J.B.; Anbari, F.; Maleki, Z.; Boostani, S.; Zarghi, A.; Pouralibaba, F. Efficacy of Elaeagnus angustifolia Topical Gel in the Treatment of Symptomatic Oral Lichen Planus. *J. Dent. Res. Dent. Clin. Dent. Prospect.* **2010**, *4*, 29–32.

20. Farzaei, M.H.; Bahramsoltani, R.; Abbasabadi, Z.; Rahimi, R. A comprehensive review on phytochemical and pharmacological aspects of E laeagnus angustifolia L. *J. Pharm. Pharmacol.* **2015**, *67*, 1467–1480. [CrossRef]

21. Niknam, F.; Azadi, A.; Barzegar, A.; Faridi, P.; Tanideh, N.; Zarshenas, M.M. Phytochemistry and Phytotherapeutic Aspects of Elaeagnus angustifolia L. *Curr. Drug Discov. Technol.* **2016**, *13*, 199–210. [CrossRef]

22. Torbati, M.; Asnaashari, S.; Afshar, F.H. Essential Oil from Flowers and Leaves of Elaeagnus Angustifolia (Elaeagnaceae): Composition, Radical Scavenging and General Toxicity Activities. *Adv. Pharm. Bull.* **2016**, *6*, 163–169. [CrossRef] [PubMed]

23. Ya, W.; Shang-Zhen, Z.; Chun-Meng, Z.; Tao, G.; Jian-Ping, M.; Ping, Z.; Qiu-xiu, R. Antioxidant and Antitumor Effect of Different Fractions of Ethyl Acetate Part from Elaeagnus angustifolia L. *Adv. J. Food Sci. Technol.* **2014**, *6*, 707–710. [CrossRef]

24. Kurdali, F.; Al-Shamma'A, M. Natural abundances of15N and13C in leaves of some N2-fixing and non-N2-fixing trees and shrubs in Syria. *Isot. Environ. Heal. Stud.* **2009**, *45*, 198–207. [CrossRef]

25. Murakami, A.; Ashida, H.; Terao, J. Multitargeted cancer prevention by quercetin. *Cancer Lett.* **2008**, *269*, 315–325. [CrossRef]

26. Zhang, H.; Zhang, M.; Yu, L.; Zhao, Y.; He, N.; Yang, X. Antitumor activities of quercetin and quercetin-5′,8-disulfonate in human colon and breast cancer cell lines. *Food Chem. Toxicol.* **2012**, *50*, 1589–1599. [CrossRef]

27. Duo, J.; Ying, G.G.; Wang, G.W.; Zhang, L. Quercetin inhibits human breast cancer cell proliferation and induces apoptosis via Bcl-2 and Bax regulation. *Mol. Med. Rep.* **2012**, *5*, 1453–1456. [CrossRef]

28. Kiseleva, T.I.; Chindyaeva, L.N. Biology of oleaster (Elaeagnus angustifolia L.) at the northeastern limit of its range. *Contemp. Probl. Ecol.* **2011**, *4*, 218–222. [CrossRef]

29. Faramarz, S.; Dehghan, G.; Jahanban-Esfahlan, A. Antioxidants in different parts of oleaster as a function of genotype. *BioImpacts* **2015**, *5*, 79–85. [CrossRef] [PubMed]

30. Panahi, Y.; Alishiri, G.; Bayat, N.; Hosseini, S.M.; Sahebkar, A. Efficacy of Elaeagnus Angustifolia extract in the treatment of knee osteoarthritis: A randomized controlled trial. *EXCLI J.* **2016**, *15*, 203–210. [PubMed]

31. Sahan, Y.; Dundar, A.N.; Aydın, E.; Kilci, A.; Dulger, D.; Kaplan, F.B.; Gocmen, D.; Celik, G. Characteristics of Cookies Supplemented with Oleaster (Elaeagnus angustifolia L.) Flour. I Physicochemical, Sensorial and Textural Properties. *J. Agric. Sci.* **2013**, *5*, 160. [CrossRef]

32. Tehranizadeh, Z.A.; Baratian, A.; Hosseinzadeh, H. Russian olive (Elaeagnus angustifolia) as a herbal healer. *BioImpacts* **2016**, *6*, 155–167. [CrossRef]

33. Asadiar, L.S.; Rahmani, F.; Siami, A. Assessment of genetic diversity in the Russian olive (Elaeagnus angustifolia) based on ISSR genetic markers. *Revista Ciência Agronômica* **2013**, *44*, 310–316. [CrossRef]

34. Natanzi, M.M.; Pasalar, P.; Kamalinejad, M.; Dehpour, A.R.; Tavangar, S.M.; Sharifi, R.; Ghanadian, N.; Balaei, M.R.; Gerayesh-Nejad, S. Effect of aqueous extract of Elaeagnus angustifolia fruit on experimental cutaneous wound healing in rats. *Acta medica Iran.* **2012**, *50*, 589–596.

35. Badrhadad, A.; Kh, P.; Mansouri, K. In vitro anti-angiogenic activity fractions from hydroalcoholic extract of Elaeagnus angustifolia L. flower and Nepeta crispa L. arial part. *J. Med. Plants Res.* **2012**, *6*, 4633–4639. [CrossRef]

36. Choi, Y.; Ko, Y.S.; Park, J.J.; Choi, Y.; Kim, Y.; Pyo, J.-S.; Jang, B.G.; Hwang, D.H.; Kim, W.H.; Lee, B.L. HER2-induced metastasis is mediated by AKT/JNK/EMT signaling pathway in gastric cancer. *World J. Gastroenterol.* **2016**, *22*, 9141–9153. [CrossRef]

37. Han, J.S.; Crowe, D.L. Jun amino-terminal kinase 1 activation promotes cell survival in ErbB2-positive breast cancer. *Anticancer. Res.* **2010**, *30*, 3407–3412.

38. Nahta, R. Molecular Mechanisms of Trastuzumab-Based Treatment in HER2-Overexpressing Breast Cancer. *ISRN Oncol.* **2012**, *2012*, 1–16. [CrossRef]

39. Wolf-Yadlin, A.; Kumar, N.; Zhang, Y.; Hautaniemi, S.; Zaman, M.; Kim, H.-D.; Grantcharova, V.; Lauffenburger, D.A.; White, F.M. Effects of HER2 overexpression on cell signaling networks governing proliferation and migration. *Mol. Syst. Biol.* **2006**, *2*, 54. [CrossRef]

40. Maggioni, D.; Biffi, L.; Nicolini, G.; Garavello, W. Flavonoids in oral cancer prevention and therapy. *Eur. J. Cancer Prev.* **2015**, *24*, 517–528. [CrossRef]

41. Wu, Y.; Sarkissyan, M.; Vadgama, J.V. Epithelial-Mesenchymal Transition and Breast Cancer. *J. Clin. Med.* **2016**, *5*, 13. [CrossRef]

42. Mao, X.; Duan, X.; Jiang, B. Fascin Induces Epithelial-Mesenchymal Transition of Cholangiocarcinoma Cells by Regulating Wnt/β-Catenin Signaling. *Med. Sci. Monit.* **2016**, *22*, 3479–3485. [CrossRef] [PubMed]

43. Satelli, A.; Li, S. Vimentin in cancer and its potential as a molecular target for cancer therapy. *Cell. Mol. Life Sci.* **2011**, *68*, 3033–3046. [CrossRef] [PubMed]

44. Xiao, C.; Wu, C.-H.; Hu, H.-Z. LncRNA UCA1 promotes epithelial-mesenchymal transition (EMT) of breast cancer cells via enhancing Wnt/beta-catenin signaling pathway. *Eur. Rev. Med. Pharmacol. Sci.* **2016**, *20*, 2819–2824. [PubMed]

45. Wang, J.; Kuiatse, I.; Lee, A.V.; Pan, J.; Giuliano, A.; Cui, X. Sustained c-Jun-NH2-kinase activity promotes epithelial-mesenchymal transition, invasion, and survival of breast cancer cells by regulating extracellular signal-regulated kinase activation. *Mol. Cancer Res.* **2010**, *8*, 266–277. [CrossRef]

46. Bubici, C.; Papa, S. JNK signalling in cancer: In need of new, smarter therapeutic targets. *Br. J. Pharmacol.* **2014**, *171*, 24–37. [CrossRef]

47. Bogoyevitch, M.A.; Kobe, B. Uses for JNK: The Many and Varied Substrates of the c-Jun N-Terminal Kinases. *Microbiol. Mol. Biol. Rev.* **2006**, *70*, 1061–1095. [CrossRef]

48. Leppä, S.; Saffrich, R.; Ansorge, W.; Bohmann, D. Differential regulation of c-Jun by ERK and JNK during PC12 cell differentiation. *EMBO J.* **1998**, *17*, 4404–4413. [CrossRef]

49. Li, L.; Porter, A.G.; Feng, Z. JNK-dependent Phosphorylation of c-Jun on Serine 63 Mediates Nitric Oxide-induced Apoptosis of Neuroblastoma Cells. *J. Biol. Chem.* **2004**, *279*, 4058–4065. [CrossRef]

50. Tournier, C. The 2 Faces of JNK Signaling in Cancer. *Genes Cancer* **2013**, *4*, 397–400. [CrossRef]

51. Lloyd, A.; Yancheva, N.; Wasylyk, B. Transformation suppressor activity of a Jun transcription factor lacking its activation domain. *Nature* **1991**, *352*, 635–638. [CrossRef]

52. Eferl, R.; Wagner, E.F. AP-1: A double-edged sword in tumorigenesis. *Nat. Rev. Cancer* **2003**, *3*, 859–868. [CrossRef]

53. Min, L.; Ji, Y.; Bakiri, L.; Qiu, Z.; Cen, J.; Chen, X.; Chen, L.; Scheuch, H.; Zheng, H.; Qin, L.; et al. Liver cancer initiation is controlled by AP-1 through SIRT6-dependent inhibition of survivin. *Nat. Cell Biol.* **2012**, *14*, 1203–1211. [CrossRef] [PubMed]

54. Nateri, A.S.; Spencer-Dene, B.; Behrens, A. Interaction of phosphorylated c-Jun with TCF4 regulates intestinal cancer development. *Nature* **2005**, *437*, 281–285. [CrossRef] [PubMed]

55. Maeda, S.; Karin, M. Oncogene at last—c-Jun promotes liver cancer in mice. *Cancer Cell* **2003**, *3*, 102–104. [CrossRef]

56. Kandouz, M.; Alachkar, A.; Zhang, L.; Dekhil, H.; Chehna, F.; Yasmeen, A.; Al Moustafa, A.-E. Teucrium polium plant extract inhibits cell invasion and motility of human prostate cancer cells via the restoration of the E-cadherin/catenin complex. *J. Ethnopharmacol.* **2010**, *129*, 410–415. [CrossRef] [PubMed]

57. Koirala, N.; Thuan, N.H.; Ghimire, G.P.; Van Thang, D.; Sohng, J.K. Methylation of flavonoids: Chemical structures, bioactivities, progress and perspectives for biotechnological production. *Enzym. Microb. Technol.* **2016**, *86*, 103–116. [CrossRef]

58. Roh, H.; Pippin, J.; Drebin, J.A. Down-regulation of HER2/neu expression induces apoptosis in human cancer cells that overexpress HER2/neu. *Cancer Res.* **2000**, *60*, 560–565.

59. Lei, K.; Nimnual, A.; Zong, W.-X.; Kennedy, N.J.; Flavell, R.A.; Thompson, C.B.; Bar-Sagi, D.; Davis, R.J. The Bax Subfamily of Bcl2-Related Proteins Is Essential for Apoptotic Signal Transduction by c-Jun NH2-Terminal Kinase. *Mol. Cell. Biol.* **2002**, *22*, 4929–4942. [CrossRef]

60. Gross, A.; McDonnell, J.M.; Korsmeyer, S.J. BCL-2 family members and the mitochondria in apoptosis. *Genes Dev.* **1999**, *13*, 1899–1911. [CrossRef]

61. Davis, R.J. Signal Transduction by the JNK Group of MAP Kinases. *Cell* **2000**, *103*, 239–252. [CrossRef]

62. Corazza, N.; Jakob, S.; Schaer, C.; Frese, S.; Keogh, A.; Stroka, D.; Kassahn, D.; Torgler, R.; Mueller, C.; Schneider, P.; et al. TRAIL receptor–mediated JNK activation and Bim phosphorylation critically regulate Fas-mediated liver damage and lethality. *J. Clin. Investig.* **2006**, *116*, 2493–2499. [CrossRef] [PubMed]

63. Lim, S.-C.; Jeon, H.J.; Kee, K.-H.; Lee, M.J.; Hong, R.; Han, S.I. Involvement of DR4/JNK pathway-mediated autophagy in acquired TRAIL resistance in HepG2 cells. *Int. J. Oncol.* **2016**, *49*, 1983–1990. [CrossRef] [PubMed]

64. Puduvalli, V.K.; Sampath, D.; Bruner, J.M.; Nangia, J.; Xu, R.; Kyritsis, A.P. TRAIL-induced apoptosis in gliomas is enhanced by Akt-inhibition and is independent of JNK activation. *Apoptosis* **2005**, *10*, 233–243. [CrossRef] [PubMed]

65. Recio-Boiles, A.; Ilmer, M.; Rhea, P.R.; Kettlun, C.; Heinemann, M.L.; Ruetering, J.; Vykoukal, J.; Alt, E. JNK pathway inhibition selectively primes pancreatic cancer stem cells to TRAIL-induced apoptosis without affecting the physiology of normal tissue resident stem cells. *Oncotarget* **2016**, *7*, 9890–9906. [CrossRef]

66. Reilly, E.O.; Tirincsi, A.; Logue, S.E.; Szegezdi, E. The Janus Face of Death Receptor Signaling during Tumor Immunoediting. *Front. Immunol.* **2016**, *7*. [CrossRef]

67. Galluzzi, L.; Vitale, I.; Aaronson, S.A.; Abrams, J.M.; Adam, D.; Agostinis, P.; Alnemri, E.S.; Altucci, L.; Amelio, I.; Andrews, D.W.; et al. Molecular mechanisms of cell death: Recommendations of the Nomenclature Committee on Cell Death 2018. *Cell Death Differ.* **2018**, *25*, 486–541. [CrossRef]

68. Deng, X.; Xiao, L.; Lang, W.; Gao, F.; Ruvolo, P.; May, W.S., Jr. Novel Role for JNK as a Stress-activated Bcl2 Kinase. *J. Biol. Chem.* **2001**, *276*, 23681–23688. [CrossRef]

69. Maundrell, K.; Antonsson, B.; Magnenat, E.; Camps, M.; Muda, M.; Chabert, C.; Gillieron, C.; Boschert, U.; Vial-Knecht, E.; Martinou, J.-C.; et al. Bcl-2 Undergoes Phosphorylation by c-Jun N-terminal Kinase/Stress-activated Protein Kinases in the Presence of the Constitutively Active GTP-binding Protein Rac1. *J. Biol. Chem.* **1997**, *272*, 25238–25242. [CrossRef]

70. Yamamoto, K.; Ichijo, H.; Korsmeyer, S.J. BCL-2 Is Phosphorylated and Inactivated by an ASK1/Jun N-Terminal Protein Kinase Pathway Normally Activated at G2/M. *Mol. Cell. Biol.* **1999**, *19*, 8469–8478. [CrossRef]

71. Breitschopf, K.; Haendeler, J.; Malchow, P.; Zeiher, A.M.; Dimmeler, S. Posttranslational Modification of Bcl-2 Facilitates Its Proteasome-Dependent Degradation: Molecular Characterization of the Involved Signaling Pathway. *Mol. Cell. Biol.* **2000**, *20*, 1886–1896. [CrossRef]

72. Dimmeler, S.; Breitschopf, K.; Haendeler, J.; Zeiher, A.M. Dephosphorylation Targets Bcl-2 for Ubiquitin-dependent Degradation: A Link between the Apoptosome and the Proteasome Pathway. *J. Exp. Med.* **1999**, *189*, 1815–1822. [CrossRef] [PubMed]

73. Ito, T.; Deng, X.; Carr, B.; May, W.S. Bcl-2 Phosphorylation Required for Anti-apoptosis Function. *J. Biol. Chem.* **1997**, *272*, 11671–11673. [CrossRef] [PubMed]

74. Ruvolo, P.P.; Deng, X.; May, W.S. Phosphorylation of Bcl2 and regulation of apoptosis. *Leukemia* **2001**, *15*, 515–522. [CrossRef]

75. Tournier, C.; Dong, C.; Turner, T.K.; Jones, S.N.; Flavell, R.A.; Davis, R.J. MKK7 is an essential component of the JNK signal transduction pathway activated by proinflammatory cytokines. *Genes Dev.* **2001**, *15*, 1419–1426. [CrossRef]

76. Cho, Y.-L.; Tan, H.W.S.; Saquib, Q.; Ren, Y.; Ahmad, J.; Wahab, R.; He, W.; Bay, B.; Shen, H.-M. Dual role of oxidative stress-JNK activation in autophagy and apoptosis induced by nickel oxide nanoparticles in human cancer cells. *Free. Radic. Biol. Med.* **2020**, *153*, 173–186. [CrossRef]

77. Dhanasekaran, D.N.; Reddy, E.P. JNK signaling in apoptosis. *Oncogene* **2008**, *27*, 6245–6251. [CrossRef]

78. Dou, Y.; Jiang, X.; Xie, H.; He, J.; Xiao, S.-S. The Jun N-terminal kinases signaling pathway plays a "seesaw" role in ovarian carcinoma: A molecular aspect. *J. Ovarian Res.* **2019**, *12*, 99. [CrossRef]

79. Gkouveris, I.; Nikitakis, N.G. Role of JNK signaling in oral cancer: A mini review. *Tumor Biol.* **2017**, *39*. [CrossRef]

80. Liu, J.; Lin, A. Role of JNK activation in apoptosis: A double-edged sword. *Cell Res.* **2005**, *15*, 36–42. [CrossRef] [PubMed]

81. Yasmeen, A.; Alachkar, A.; Dekhil, H.; Gambacorti-Passerini, C.; Al Moustafa, A.-E. Locking Src/Abl Tyrosine Kinase Activities Regulate Cell Differentiation and Invasion of Human Cervical Cancer Cells Expressing E6/E7 Oncoproteins of High-Risk HPV. *J. Oncol.* **2010**, *2010*, 1–10. [CrossRef] [PubMed]

Synthesis, Anti-Cancer and Anti-Migratory Evaluation of 3,6-Dibromocarbazole and 5-Bromoindole Derivatives

Krystal M. Butler-Fernández [1]**, Zulma Ramos** [1]**, Adela M. Francis-Malavé** [2]**, Joseph Bloom** [1]**, Suranganie Dharmawardhane** [3] **and Eliud Hernández** [1,*]

[1] Department of Pharmaceutical Sciences, University of Puerto Rico, School of Pharmacy, San Juan 00936, Puerto Rico
[2] Department of Biology, College of Natural Sciences, University of Puerto Rico, San Juan 00931, Puerto Rico
[3] Department of Biochemistry, University of Puerto Rico, School of Medicine, San Juan 00936, Puerto Rico
* Correspondence: eliud.hernandez@upr.edu;

Academic Editor: Qiao-Hong Chen

Abstract: In this study, a new series of N-alkyl-3,6-dibromocarbazole and N-alkyl-5-bromoindole derivatives have been synthesized and evaluated in vitro as anti-cancer and anti-migration agents. Cytotoxic and anti-migratory effects of these compounds were evaluated in MCF-7 and MDA-MB-231 breast cancer cell lines and an insight on the structure-activity relationship was developed. Preliminary investigations of their anti-cancer activity demonstrated that several compounds have moderate antiproliferative effects on cancer cell lines with GI_{50} values in the range of 4.7–32.2 μM. Moreover, carbazole derivatives **10, 14, 15, 23,** and **24** inhibit migration activity of metastatic cell line MDA-MB-231 in the range of 18–20%. The effect of compounds **10, 14,** and **15** in extension of invadopodia and filopodia was evaluated by fluorescence microscopy and results demonstrated a reduction in actin-based cell extensions by compounds **10** and **15**.

Keywords: 3,6-dibromocarbazole; 5-bromoindole; carbazole; actin; breast cancer; migration

1. Introduction

In women, breast cancer is the leading cause of death, mainly due to metastasis [1]. If breast cancer is detected and treated prior to metastasis, the patient has a higher probability of being cured of their disease. Cancer cell invasion involves cell migration through the extracellular matrix (ECM) and the accompanying degradation of the ECM [2]. Several proteins play a key role in this process, by the extension of structures known as invadopodia. Invadopodia are actin-rich protrusive structures with associated matrix degradation activity and are believed to be important for tumor cells to penetrate the basement membrane of epithelia and blood vessels [3]. In cell migration, the reorganization of the actin cytoskeleton produces the force necessary for cell migration [4]. The Rho GTPases, Rac, and Cdc42 are key molecular switches activated by a myriad of cell surface receptors to promote breast cancer cell migration/invasion, proliferation, and survival [5]. Unlike Ras, Rac and Cdc42 are not mutated in breast cancer, but activated via the deregulation of expression and/or activity of their upstream regulators, guanine nucleotide exchange factors (GEFs) [6]. The WASP family proteins are key regulators of the actin cytoskeleton and cell migration through induction of membrane protrusions at the leading edge [7]. In cancer cells, when N-WASP interacts and activates the Arp2/3 complex, it catalyzes actin polymerization and assembly into filopodia and invadopodia [7,8]. To initiate this process, the Rho GTPase Cdc42, in its GTP-activated form, binds and activates N-WASP by inducing a conformational change that liberates the autoinhibited structure, thereby interacting with Arp2/3 complex, and regulating the protrusive formation in membrane structures promoting extracellular matrix (ECM) degradation [8]. Therefore, inhibition of these processes decreases cell motility and invasion, and may greatly improve the potential therapeutic applications of such inhibitors against cancer metastasis.

Natural and synthetic carbazole derivatives comprise a wide variety of biologically active agents with diverse pharmacological activities, including antitumoral, antioxidant, anti-inflammatory, antibacterial, anticonvulsant, antipsychotic, antidiabetic, and larvicidal properties [9–28]. Carbazoles are tricyclic aromatic compounds with a benzene ring fused to the 2,3-positions of an indole ring [29]. The antitumor properties of carbazole derivatives have been correlated to their polycyclic, planar aromatic structure, and large π-conjugated backbone that noncovalently bind with DNA base pairs, hydrophobic pockets, and forms electrostatic interactions to intercalate into DNA [9,30]. In particular, among a wide variety of carbazoles, a series of N-alkyl-3,6-disubstituted carbazole derivatives has been discovered and evaluated for their potential as neuroprotective agents [31], antimalarial [32], antitumoral [33,34], anti-apoptotic [35], and antibacterial activities [36]. Selected examples of bioactive N-alkyl-3,6-disubstituted carbazole derivatives are represented in Figure 1.

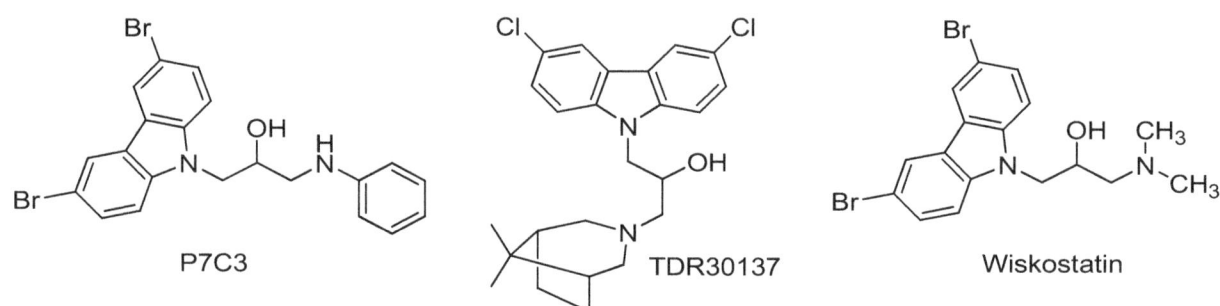

Figure 1. Structure of representative N-alkyl-3,6-dihalogencarbazole derivatives.

The compound P7C3 (Figure 1) was discovered from a library of 200,000 drug-like molecules, and showed proneurogenic and neuroprotective properties, stabilized mitochondrial membrane potential, and inhibits neuronal apoptosis [37]. Several derivatives of P7C3 have been synthesized with modifications at the linker chain. Replacement of the hydroxyl group with a fluorine atom, and an additional methylene group between the hydroxyl group and the aniline, increases activity [37]. The aromatic ring was replaced with heteroaromatic groups, but activity was found to be less effective. The commercially available TDR30137 (Figure 1) was discovered and characterized as an inhibitor of P. *falciparum* K1 (Pf-K1) in human red blood cells with an IC_{50} of 57 nM [32]. However, TDR30137 was not active in in vivo studies with the *Plasmodium berghei* mouse model. In structure-activity relationship (SAR) studies, the importance of 3,6-halogen substitution, hydroxyl group, and the tertiary amine correlated with improved activity on Pf-K1 strains [32]. A carbazole derivative named Wiskostatin (Figure 1) was identified to bind within a pocket in the GBD regulatory module that maintains N-WASP in an inactive, autoinhibited conformation [38]. In a pyrene-actin polymerization assay, using purified proteins, it was demonstrated that Wiskostatin inhibited full-length N-WASP activation of the Arp2/3 complex at $IC_{50} = 10 \mu M$ [38]. The specific binding site of Wiskostatin was determined to be within the GBD of the autoinhibited conformation of N-WASP after performing the experiment with activated Cdc42-GTP. Unfortunately, a recent report described that Wiskostatin inhibited other cellular functions that are not believed to be N-WASP dependent [39]. These studies revealed that Wiskostatin caused an irreversible decrease in cellular ATP levels, and that it does not function as a selective inhibitor of N-WASP dependent functions in intact cells, and caused an overall change in the energy status of cells; thus, inhibiting normal transport processes [39]. Herein, we designed and synthesized a new series of N-alkyl-3,6-dibromocarbazole and 5-bromoindole derivatives, tested for their antiproliferative and antimigratory activities in MCF-7 and MDA-MB-231 breast cancer cell lines, and analyzed the effect of the most active migration inhibitor on actin dynamics and actin cytoskeleton rearrangement.

2. Results and Discussion

The aim of this study is to design and synthesize a new series of *N*-alkyl-3,6-dibromocarbazole and *N*-alkyl-5-bromoindole derivatives and analyze their cytotoxic effect and potential to inhibit actin cytoskeleton rearrangement and cancer cell migration. The structural elements of Wiskostatin and derivatives identified as pharmacophoric unit are a 3,6-dihalogen carbazole and a dialkylamino-2-propanol chain. Our strategy was to design and synthesize a new series of compounds with a 3,6-dibromocarbazole or 5-bromoindole ring connected, via a three-carbon atom aliphatic chain, to an amide group. The influence of different N-alkyl or aromatic substituents at the amide group was examined.

We screened all compounds to determine their cytotoxic effect against MCF-7 and MDA-MB-231 breast cancer cells using the Sulforhodamine B (SRB) assay [40] (Figure 2). In addition, anti-migratory activity was determined using the wound healing assay (scratch method) [41] on the metastatic MDA-MB-231 cancer cells. In this assay, the relative migration of MDA-MB-231 breast cancer cells in the presence of carbazole or indole derivatives at a concentration of 10 µM (or at concentrations that do not affect cell viability) was compared to the migration in the presence of vehicle (0.02% DMSO). Representative photomicrographs of the migration inhibition of compounds **10**, **14**, **15**, and Wiskostatin are represented in Figure 3. Results show that in the vehicle-treated control experiment, wound healing is progressing considerably, and after 24 h, the wound is completely healed. When cells are incubated with compounds **10**, **14**, and **15** after 24 h, the wound healing is inhibited. However, Wiskostatin did not elicit an inhibitory effect on wound healing when incubated with MDA-MB-231 cells after 24 h at a concentration of 2 µM. Actin and Arp2/3 regulation by active WASP induce de novo actin polymerization and assembly to generate the F-actin structures filopodia and invadopodia used for cell migration [42]. Therefore, to investigate the effect of compounds **10**, **14**, **15**, and Wiskostatin on actin dynamics, we performed immunofluorescence microscopy to detect polymerized actin on MDA-MB-231 cancer cells (Figure 4). The structure and biological activities of new compounds are summarized in Tables 1 and 2.

2.1. N-Alkyl-3,6-Dibromocarbazole Derivatives

The synthetic method to construct the 3,6-dibromocarbazole derivatives library is described in Scheme 1 (see the Supplementary Materials for representative ^{1}H and ^{13}C NMR spectral data). The *N*-alkyl-3,6-dibromocarbazole derivatives were generated in a three-step synthesis using 3,6-dibromocarbazole **1** as origin of the carbazole derivatives core. Compound **1** was reacted with ethyl 4-bromobutyrate to introduce the aliphatic side chain by nucleophilic substitution (Scheme 1), followed by hydrolysis to afford the corresponding 3,6-diromocarbazole-4-butyric acid **2**. For the generation of 3,6-dibromocarbazole-4-butyramide derivatives **3**, compound **2** was therefore used as starting material, which reacted with different amines via an amide coupling reaction using N-(3-Dimethylaminopropyl)-N'-ethylcarbonate (EDAC) with Hydroxybenzotriazole (HOBt) as an additive dissolved in methylene chloride (CH$_2$Cl$_2$).

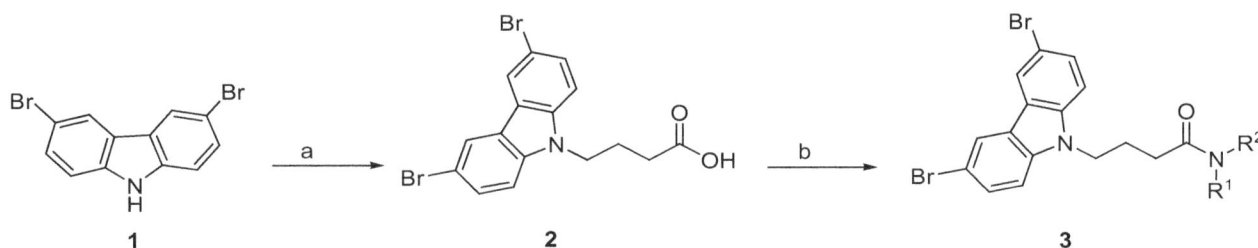

Scheme 1. General synthetic procedure of 3,6-dibromocarbazole-4-butyramide derivatives **3**. Reagents and conditions: (**a**) (i) Ethyl 4-bromobutyrate, K$_2$CO$_3$, DMF, 80 °C, 2h; (ii) KOH, DMF/water, 80 °C, 2-6 h, 86%; (**b**) HOBt, EDAC, CH$_2$Cl$_2$, Et$_3$N, rt, amine: R-NH$_2$ or HNR^{1}R^2, 2-8 h.

The in vitro anti-proliferative and anti-migratory activities of compounds **4–27**, and Wiskostatin are represented in Table 1. From the twenty-four compound derivatives of 3,6-dibromocarbazole, it can be observed that in the MCF-7 (ER+) cancer cell line, compounds **6–10, 14, 16–21,** and **32** showed good to moderate antiproliferative activity with a GI_{50} in the range of 6.8–32.2 μM. In the MDA-MB-231 cell line, compounds **6–10, 14, 16, 18, 20–21,** and **23** inhibited cell proliferation with a GI_{50} in the range of 4.7–23 μM. The remaining compounds in that series had a GI_{50} above 50 μM in both breast cancer cell lines. Compound **8** with a 2-piperazinyl ethyl butyramide chain showed very good anticancer activity against both cancer cell lines MCF-7 and MDA-MB-231 with GI_{50} values of 8 and 4.7 μM, respectively. Also, compound **18** with a piperazinyl amide showed significant anticancer activity against both cancer cell lines with GI_{50} values of 7.5 and 6.7 μM, respectively. Similarly, compound **21**, another piperazinyl amide derivative, showed very good in vitro anticancer activity against both cancer cell lines with GI_{50} values of 6.5 and 8 μM, respectively. Shortening the aliphatic chain between the N-atom of the amide group and the morpholine from C3 (**9**), over C2 (**4**), to C0 (**12**) led to a complete loss of antiproliferative activity on both cancer cell lines. On the other hand, introduction of an aromatic ring or aromatic heterocycle (**22–27**, Table 1) in the amide group led to lack of antiproliferative activity with GI_{50} above 50 μM on both cancer cell lines. Thus, in general, compounds with a piperazinyl butyramide group attached to the N-atom of the carbazole appear to be more cytotoxic than compounds with other butyramide group in this series of compounds. In addition, three compounds—**8, 18,** and **21**—were found to be more cytotoxic against both cancer cell lines MCF-7 and MDA-MB-231 than Wiskostatin, which in this assay showed GI_{50} values of 9.7 and 8.3 μM, respectively (Table 1, Figure 2).

To further assess the anti-migratory activity of carbazole derivatives in vitro, we examined its inhibitory effects on the migration of the metastatic breast cancer cell line MDA-MB-231 using the wound-healing assay at concentrations that do not affect cell viability. We chose the MDA-MB-231 breast cancer cells over MCF-7 due to its enhanced metastatic and migratory properties, with concomitant Rac and Cdc42 expression, compared to the non-metastatic and poorly migrating MCF-7 cells. The relative migration of treated cells with 3,6-dibromocarbazole derivatives compared with control (MDA-MB-231 cells) are summarized in Table 1.

Table 1. Cell growth inhibition and anti-migration activity of 3,6-dibromocarbazole derivatives.

Comp.	R =	GI_{50} (μM)[a]		Migration (%)[b,c]
		MCF-7	MDA-MB-231	
4		>50	>50	99 ± 6.03
5		>50	>50	99 ± 5.98
6		16.8	16	94 ± 3.93
7		6.8	10	99 ± 0.03 (at 2 μM)
8		8	4.7	97 ± 4.90 (at 1 μM)
9		13.4	15.4	99 ± 1.58 (at 3.1 μM)
10		8.1	10.5	87 ± 4.65 (at 2.1 μM)

Table 1. *Cont.*

Comp.	R =	GI$_{50}$ (μM)[a] MCF-7	MDA-MB-231	Migration (%)[b,c]
11	piperidine-ethyl carbamate	>50	>50	99 ± 0.02
12	morpholine	>50	>50	97 ± 6.41
13	thiomorpholine	>50	25	99 ± 0.03
14	piperidine-CN	11.8	16.7	81 ± 8.96
15	piperazine-N-Ph	>50	>50	80 ± 5.87
16	piperazine-N-acetyl (CH$_3$)	18.2	23	82 ± 7.52
17	piperazine-N-Boc	17.5	>50	99 ± 2.09
18	piperazine-NH	7.5	6.7	99 ± 0.02
19	piperazine-ethyl-morpholine	12.4	>50	99 ± 0.97
20	piperazine-acetamide-isopropyl (CH$_3$, CH$_3$)	9.1	13.4	99 ± 0.05 (at 2.7 μM)
21	piperazine-ethyl-N(CH$_3$)$_2$	6.5	8	99 ± 0.48 (at 1.6 μM)
22	NH-phenyl-morpholine	>50	>50	97 ± 4.19
23	NH-trimethoxyphenyl (OCH$_3$, OCH$_3$, OCH$_3$)	>50	19	90 ± 6.60
24	NH-quinoline	32.2	>50	82 ± 5.19
25	NH-indole	>50	>50	96 ± 4.69
26	NH-benzimidazole	>50	>50	99 ± 6.52
27	NH-phenyl-O-CH$_3$	>50	>50	99 ± 0.05
Wiskostatin		9.7	8.3	95 ± 6.79 (at 2 μM)

[a] GI$_{50}$ = compound concentration required to inhibit MDA-MB-231 proliferation by 50% after 48 h treatment. Values are expressed as the mean of triplicate experiments, and standard deviation (SD) is <10%. [b] After 24 h, MDA-MB-231 cellular migration was determined by measuring the distance traveled from the edge of the scratch toward the center of the scratch, relative to control. [c] Percent relative migration values at 10 μM (or at concentrations that do not affect cell viability). Results are presented as means ± SD of three independent experiments.

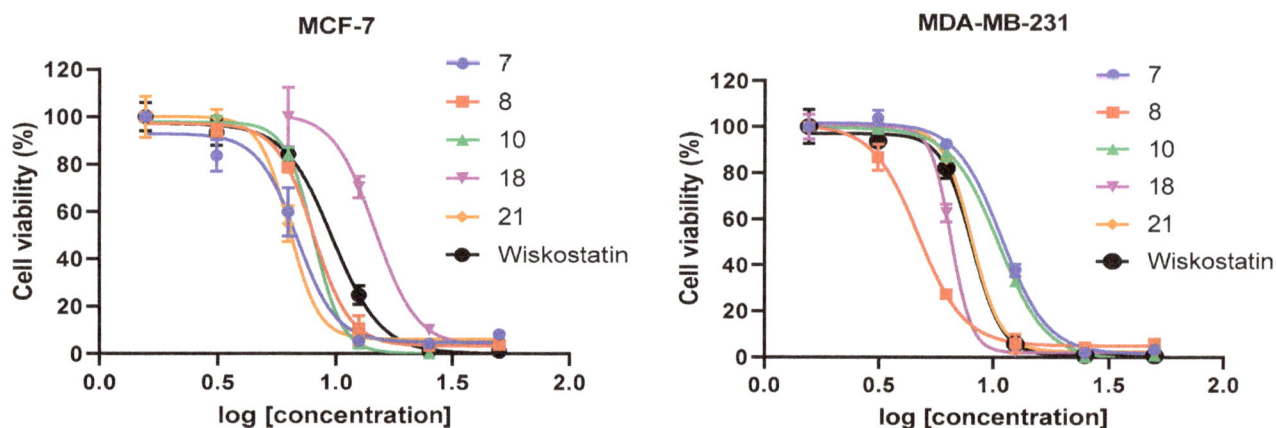

Figure 2. Log-dose response curve for compounds **7**, **8**, **10**, **18**, **21**, and Wiskostatin on MCF-7 and MDA-MB-231 breast cancer cell lines. Each data point represents the mean of three replicates and error bars represent ± SD. Each GI_{50} value was calculated based on sigmoidal curve fitting to the respective data set.

Among the twenty-four compounds tested for their anti-migratory effect, five compounds (**10**, **14**, **15**, **23**, **24**) inhibited migration in the range of 10–20%. While compounds **7**, **8**, **18**, and **21** were among the most cytotoxic compounds tested against MDA-MB-231 and MCF-7 cancer cell lines, they did not show significant anti-migratory effect. In contrast, compounds **14–16** and **24** inhibited migration in the range of 18–20%, compared to Wiskostatin that inhibit 5% of migration at 2 µM. Compound **14**, a carbazole derivative with a piperidine-4-carbonitrile amide group that showed moderate anti-proliferative activity on both MCF-7 and MDA-MB-231 cell lines, inhibit 19% of migration. Both compounds **15** and **16**, with phenyl- and acetyl-piperazine amide group, respectively, showed comparable anti-migratory activity with 20% and 18%, respectively. The anti-proliferative effect of **16** on both cancer cell lines was moderate, compared to **15**, which lacks cytotoxic activity. On the other hand, the 3-aminoquinoline amide **24**, showed anti-migratory activity of 18% with GI_{50} above 50 µM on MDA-MB-231 cell line. When comparing Wiskostatin and carbazole derivatives from Table 1, compound **10** exhibited anti-proliferative activity with GI_{50} values comparable with Wiskostatin on both cancer cell lines. However, compound **10** showed higher anti-migratory potency with 13% at 2.1 µM, compared with 5% anti-migratory effect of Wiskostatin at 2 µM on MDA-MB-231 breast cancer cells. Therefore, compound **10** exhibits similar cytotoxicity with improved anti-migratory potential compared to Wiskostatin.

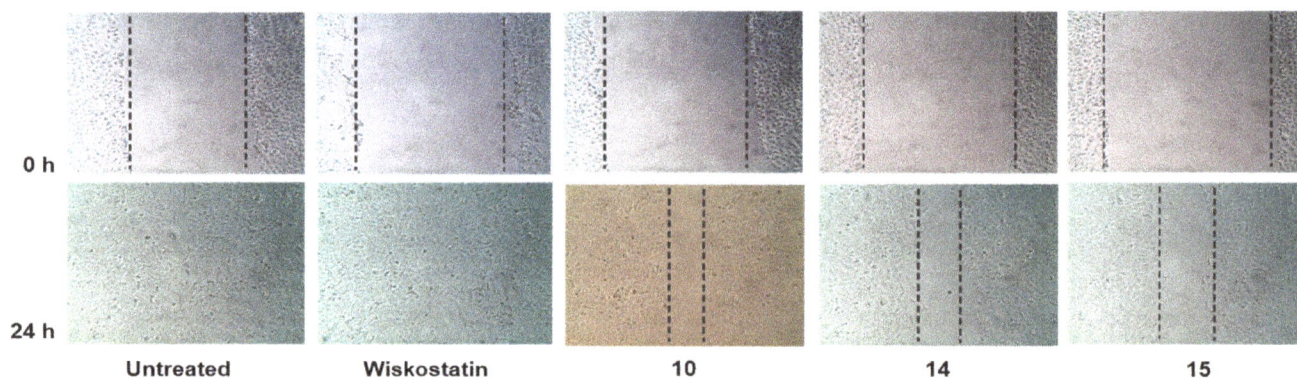

Figure 3. Inhibitory effect of compounds **10**, **14**, **15**, and Wiskostatin on MDA-MB-231 cells migration detected by wound-healing assay. MDA-MB-231 cells were treated with vehicle or with compounds **10**, **14**, **15**, and Wiskostatin. The photomicrographs were obtained at 0 and 24 h. Percent relative migration values are the average of three independent experiments. Dotted lines show the area occupied by the initial scraping for 0 h, and the wound edge for 24 h.

The Rho GTPases are believed to stimulate plasma membrane protrusion by inducing actin filament nucleation and polymerization on or close to membranes [43]. In particular, the Rho GTPase protein Cdc42, through activation of N-WASP/Arp2/3 pathway, is an important mediator of actin polymerization and filopodium extension [44,45]. Therefore, compounds that interfere with this process might be potentially useful molecular probes for the study of cell migration and invasion. To determine changes in actin cytoskeletal structures, we treated MDA-MB-231 breast cancer cells with vehicle or compounds **10**, **14**, **15**, and Wiskostatin at 10 μM for 24 h (Figure 4).

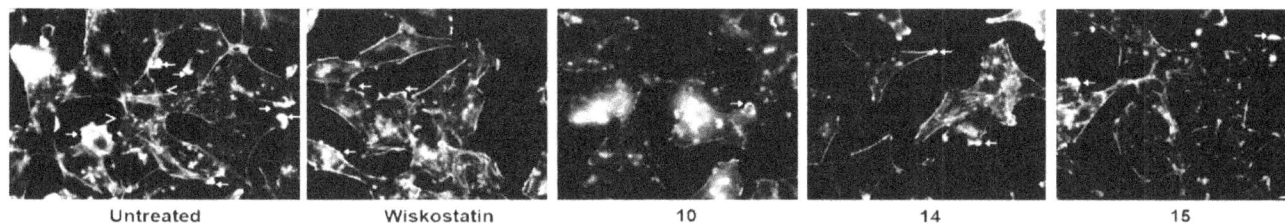

| Untreated | Wiskostatin | 10 | 14 | 15 |

Figure 4. Effect of Wiskostatin and compounds **10**, **14**, and **15** on actin cytoskeleton of metastatic cancer cell MDA-MB-231. MDA-MB-231 metastatic breast cancer cells were treated with vehicle or Wiskostatin (2 μM) and compounds **10**, **14**, or **15** at 10 μM for 24 h to determine changes in actin cytoskeletal structures. Cells were fixed, permeabilized, and stained with rhodamine phalloidin to visualize F-actin. Arrows, lamellipodia; arrowheads, filopodia.

To identify F-actin based cell surface extensions, cells were stained with rhodamine phalloidin to localize F-actin. The results showed that untreated cells (control) demonstrated a strong formation of lamellipodia extensions, membrane ruffles, and stress fibers, with few filopodia. Wiskostatin and compounds **14** and **15** moderately reduced lamellipodia extensions when compared with control cells at concentrations that do not affect cell viability. In addition, compound **10**, at concentrations that inhibit 13% cell migration (2 μM), exhibited a marked reduction in lamellipodia formation when compared to vehicle, and in particular with Wiskostatin, which inhibits cell migration in 5% at 2 μM (Table 1). Compound **15** demonstrates a marked reduction in polymerized actin indicating inhibition of Arp2/3 mediated actin nucleation. Specific inhibition of filopodia, as would be predicted by WASP inhibition, could not be determined since the vehicle control cells exhibited more invadopodia and lamellipodia than filopodia. In general, these results suggest that new N-alkyl-3,6-dibromocarbazoles and compounds derivatives of Wiskostatin can be explored as new probes to study actin dynamics in cancer cells, or to further develop new anti-cancer and anti-metastatic drugs.

2.2. N-alkyl-5-Bromoindole Derivatives

To further explore the N-alkyl-5-bromoindole butyramide derivative series, we synthesized several compounds in which the carbazole core was replaced by a 5-bromoindole ring (Scheme 2). The strategy is to analyze the effect of using a smaller ring system as a core connected to the C3 linker side chain and the amide group. The synthesis of N-alkyl-5-bromoindole derivatives is described in Scheme 2. The 5-bromoindole **28** was reacted with ethyl 4-bromobutyrate, followed by hydrolysis to yield the corresponding 5-bromoindole-4-butyric acid **29**. Since N-alkylation in indoles is more difficult than in carbazoles, the reaction rate to obtain **29** was improved by using Cs_2CO_3 as a base over K_2CO_3, where Cs_2CO_3 solubility is ten times higher in organic solvents than K_2CO_3. For the generation of 5-bromoindole-4-butyramide derivative **30**, carboxylic acid **29** was therefore used as starting material, which reacted with different amines via an amide coupling reaction using reaction conditions similar as described in Scheme 1 (see the Supplementary Materials for representative ^{1}H and ^{13}C NMR spectral data).

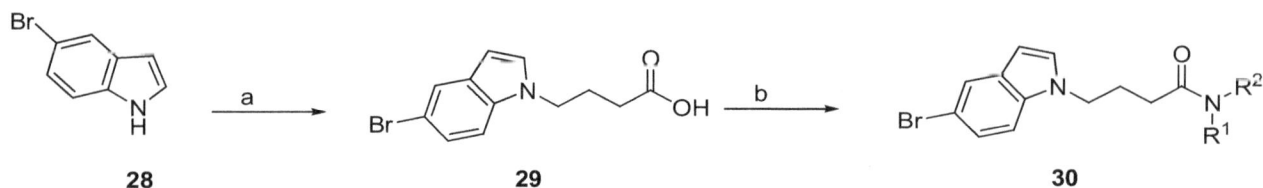

Scheme 2. General synthetic procedure of 5-bromoindole-4-butyramide derivative **30**. Reagents and conditions: (**a**) (i) Ethyl 4-bromobutyrate, Cs_2CO_3, DMF, 100 °C, 16 h; (ii) KOH, DMF/water, 80 °C, 2–6 h, 80%; (**b**) HOBt, EDAC, CH_2Cl_2, Et_3N, rt, amine: $R-NH_2$ or HNR^1R^2, 2-8 h.

The in vitro anti-proliferative and anti-migratory activities of compounds **31–34** are represented in Table 2. In this assay, the replacement of the rigid carbazole ring core by an indole resulted in loss of cytotoxic activity on both MCF-7 and MDA-MB-231 cell lines. For example, from the four representative 5-bromoindole derivatives synthesized, it can be observed that only compound **34** showed moderate cytotoxic effect on MCF-7 cells with GI_{50} of 18.4 μM, while GI_{50} value on MDA-MB-231 breast cancer cells was above 50 μM. Furthermore, the remaining compounds in that series had GI_{50}s above 50 μM in both breast cancer cell lines. Additionally, after 24 h treatment at 10 μM using the wound-healing assay in the MDA-MB-231 cell line, no migration inhibition could be observed. Hence, the absence of any activity of 5-bromoindole derivative series, together with the fact that several carbazole derivatives show promising activity, a structure-activity relationship (SAR) can be established. For example, it appears that the presence of a carbazole ring core, the C3 linker region, and amide group improve both anti-proliferative and anti-migratory activity.

Table 2. Cell growth inhibition and anti-migration activity of 5-bromoindole derivatives.

Comp.	R =	GI_{50} (μM)[a]		Migration (%)[b,c]
		MCF-7	MDA-MB-231	
31	(morpholine amide)	>50	>50	99 ± 0.05
32	(cyanopiperidine)	>50	>50	99 ± 7.78
33	(imidazole propylamide)	>50	>50	99 ± 0.02
34	(piperidine ethylamide)	18.4	>50	99 ± 6.60

[a] GI_{50} = compound concentration required to inhibit MDA-MB-231 proliferation by 50% after 48 h treatment. Values are expressed as the mean of triplicate experiments, and standard deviation (SD) is <10%. [b] After 24 h, MDA-MB-231 cellular migration was determined by measuring the distance traveled from the edge of the scratch toward the center of the scratch, relative to control. [c] Percent relative migration values at 10 μM. Results are presented as means ± SD of three independent experiments.

3. Materials and Methods

3.1. General Methods

All experiments were carried out in pre-dried glassware (≥1 h, 80–90 °C) under a nitrogen atmosphere. Nuclear magnetic resonance (NMR) spectra were obtained using a 400 MHz Bruker Avance UltraShield™ spectrometer. ^1H (400 MHz) and ^{13}C (100 MHz) NMR were recorded in CDCl$_3$ or DMSO-d_6, unless otherwise used, and the chemical shift was expressed in parts per million (ppm) relative to CDCl3 (δ 7.26 for ^1H and δ 77.0 for ^{13}C) or DMSO-d_6 (δ 2.50 for ^1H and δ 39.5 for ^{13}C) as the internal standard. ^1H NMR data is reported as position (δ), relative integral, multiplicity (s, singlet; d, doublet; t, triplet; q, quartet; dt, doublet of triplets; dd, doublet of doublets; dq, doublet of quartets; m, multiplet; br, broad peak), coupling constant (J) in hertz (Hz), and the assignment of the atom. The shift in ppm for multiplets correspond to the centermost value of the entire splitting pattern. ^{13}C NMR data are reported as position (δ) and assignment of the atom. Microwave reactions were conducted in a CEM Discovery Microwave for Drug Discovery, SP- 1445. High resolution electrospray ionization mass spectrometry (ESI-HRMS) data were obtained on a Thermo Scientific™ Q Exactive™ Hybrid Quadrupole-Orbitrap Mass Spectrometer with high performance liquid chromatography (HPLC) Agilent 1200 utilizing a Zorbax SB-C18 column (2.1 mm × 50 mm, 1.8μm) at 40 °C, and a mobile phase of acetonitrile containing 5% Milli Q water at a flow rate of 0.35 mL/min (run time: 6.5 min), and 1 μL injection volume.

3.2. Synthesis Methods

Progress of the reaction was monitored via TLC analysis using general purpose silica gel on glass 5 × 20 cm with UV indicator, 250 μm, 60 Å medium pore diameter, UV indicator, and visualized by UV fluorescent Spectroline E Series Ultraviolet lamps, in most cases followed by staining with I2. The compounds were purified via column chromatography over silica gel (70–230 mesh, 60 Å) with the appropriate size column (24/40, 12 in. × 0.5 in.) or (24/40, 12 in. × 0.72 in.). Wiskostatin compound was obtained from MilliporeSigma.

3.2.1. General Procedure for the Synthesis of 4-(3,6-Dibromo-Carbazol-9-yl)-Butyric Acid (2)

A 50 mL three-neck round-bottom flask, equipped with a reflux condenser, was charged with 3,6-dibromocarbazole 1 (0.325 g, 1.0 mmol), K_2CO_3 (0.1382 g, 1 mmol), and ethyl 4-bromobutyrate 2 (0.4436 mL, 3.1 mmol), dissolved in DMF (5 mL). After 15 min of stirring at room temperature, the reaction mixture was refluxed at 80 °C for 2 h. After completion of the reaction (analyzed by TLC), water (1 mL) and KOH (1.0 mmol) was added and the reaction mixture, refluxed at 80 °C for 2 h. After the reaction was completed (analyzed by TLC), the mixture was allowed to reach room temperature. The mixture was washed with water (20 mL) and the product was extracted using dichloromethane (3 × 10 mL). The organic layer was washed with brine and dried with Na2SO4, and filtered and concentrated under reduced pressure. The crude oil was purified via column chromatography over silica gel and 50% ethyl acetate in hexane, and the product obtained as a white solid for the precursor 4-(3,6-Dibromo-carbazol-9-yl)-butyric acid 2 (0.3535 g, 0.86 mmol, 86%). TLC analysis in ethyl acetate-hexane (1:1), R_f = 0.19. ^{1}H NMR (400 MHz, CDCl$_3$) δ 1.98 (2H, m), 2.27 (2H, t, J = 7.2 Hz), 4.41 (2H, t, J = 7.2 Hz), 7.30 (2H, d, J = 8.9 Hz), 7.56 (2H, dd, J = 2.0, 8.8 Hz), 8.14 (1H, d, J = 2.0 Hz); ^{13}C NMR (100 MHz, CDCl$_3$) 24.2, 31.1, 42.2, 111.8, 112.0, 123.4, 123.9, 139.5, 174.3. HR-FTMS (ESI) m/z calcd. for $C_{16}H_{13}Br_2NO_2$, [M + H]$^+$ 411.9365, found 411.9365.

3.2.2. Synthesis of 3,6-Dibromocarbazole-4-butyramide Derivatives (4–27)

3.2.3. General Procedure for the Synthesis of 4-(3,6-Dibromocarbazol-9-yl)-N-(2-Morpholin-4-Ylethyl)Butyramide (4), and for Compounds 5–27

A 50 mL three-neck round-bottom flask was charged with 4-(3,6-Dibromo-carbazol-9-yl)-butyric acid 2 (0.4111 g, 1.0 mmol), HOBT (0.2027 g, 1.5 mmol), and EDAC (0.2876 g, 1.5 mmol). The mixture was dissolved in CH$_2$Cl$_2$ (10 mL), stirred for 30 min, and 2-(4-morpholinyl)ethanamine 2 (0.133 g, 1.0 mmol) was added. After 15 min, Et$_3$N (0.43 mL, 3.0 mmol) was added and the mixture was stirred at room temperature for 16 h. After completion of the reaction (analyzed by TLC), water was added (30 mL) and the product was extracted using dichloromethane (3 × 10 mL). The organic layer was washed with brine and dried with Na$_2$SO$_4$, and filtered and concentrated under reduced pressure. The crude oil was purified via column chromatography over silica gel and 10% methanol in dichloromethane, and the product obtained as a white solid (0.382 g, 0.73 mmol, 73%). TLC analysis in CH$_2$Cl$_2$-MeOH (9:1), R_f = 0.26. ^{1}H NMR (400 MHz, CDCl$_3$) δ 2.0 (2H, m), 2.22 (2H, t, J = 6.8 Hz), 2.35 (2H, t, J = 4 Hz), 2.50 (4H, t, J = 1.6 Hz), 3.19 (2H, m), 3.56 (4H, t, J = 4.4 Hz), 4.39 (2H, t, J = 6.8 Hz),

7.60 (2H, d, J = 1.6 Hz), 8.0 (2H, bs), 8.46 (2H, bs); ^{13}C NMR (100 MHz, CDCl$_3$) 24.0, 31.2, 34.3, 41.8, 53.15, 53.2, 54.9, 57.2, 66.1, 111.3, 111.5, 122.9, 123.4, 128.8, 139.0, 161.0. HR-FTMS (ESI) m/z calcd. for C$_{22}$H$_{25}$Br$_2$N$_3$O$_2$, [M + H]$^+$ 524.0366, found 524.0367.

Synthesis of 4-(3,6-Dibromocarbazol-9-yl)-N-(2-methoxyethyl)butyramide (5)

The crude oil was purified via column chromatography over silica gel and 10% methanol in dichloromethane, and the product obtained as a white solid (0.096 g, 0.21 mmol, 63%). TLC analysis in CH$_2$Cl$_2$-MeOH (9:1), R_f = 0.56. ^{1}H NMR (400 MHz, CDCl$_3$) δ 1.63 (2H, bs), 2.15 (2H, t, J = 6.0 Hz), 2.21 (2H, m), 3.63 (3H, s), 3.46 (2H, d, J = 2.0 Hz), 4.39 (2H, t, J = 6.4 Hz), 7.35 (2H, d, J = 8.8 Hz), 7.57 (2H, dd, J = 1.6, 8.8 Hz), 8.16 (2H, d, J = 1.6 Hz); ^{13}C NMR (100 MHz, CDCl$_3$) 24.1, 32.4, 39.2, 42.3, 58.7, 71.0, 110.5, 112.1, 123.2, 123.4, 129.1, 139.2, 171.6. HR-FTMS (ESI) m/z calcd. for C$_{19}$H$_{20}$Br$_2$N2O$_2$, [M + H]$^+$ 468.9944, found 468.9947.

Synthesis of 4-(3,6-Dibromocarbazol-9-yl)-N-(3-imidazol-1-yl-propyl)butyramide (6)

The crude oil was purified via column chromatography over silica gel and 10% methanol in dichloromethane, and the product obtained as a white solid (0.078 g, 0.15 mmol, 49%). TLC analysis in CH$_2$Cl$_2$-MeOH (9:1), R_f = 0.22. ^{1}H NMR (400 MHz, CDCl$_3$) δ 1.96 (2H, t, J = 6.8 Hz), 2.07 (2H, t, J = 6.4 Hz), 2.20 (2H, m), 3.23 (2H, q, J = 6.4 Hz), 3.98 (2H, t, J = 6.8 Hz), 4.38 (2H, t, J = 6.8 Hz), 6.93 (1H, bs), 7.05 (1H, Bs), 7.33 (2H, d, J = 8.4 Hz), 7.51 (1H, bs), 7.56 (2H, dd, J = 2.0, 8.8 Hz), 8.15 (2H, d, J = 1.6 Hz); ^{13}C NMR (100 MHz, CDCl$_3$) 24.0, 31.0, 32.3, 36.9, 42.2, 44.8, 110.5, 112.2, 112.3, 123.3, 123.4, 129.1, 129.3, 129.4, 139.3, 171.9. HR-FTMS (ESI) m/z calcd. for C$_{22}$H$_{22}$Br$_2$N$_4$O, [M + H]$^+$ 519.0213, found 519.0211.

Synthesis of 4-(3,6-Dibromocarbazol-9-yl)-N-(2-piperidin-1-ylethyl)butyramide (7)

The crude oil was purified via column chromatography over silica gel and 10% methanol in dichloromethane, and the product obtained as a white solid (0.1033 g, 0.2 mmol, 59%). TLC analysis in CH$_2$Cl$_2$-MeOH (9:1), R_f = 0.47. ^{1}H NMR (400 MHz, CDCl$_3$) δ 1.43 (2H, q, J = 4. 9 Hz), 1.52 (4H, m), 2.11 (4H, dt, J = 3.3, 11.7 Hz), 2.34 (3H, bs), 2.38 (3H, t, J = 6.0 Hz), 3.31 (2H, q, J = 5.5 Hz), 4.29 (2H, t, J = 6.4 Hz), 6.05 (1H, bs), 7.28 (2H, d, J = 8.7 Hz), 7.5 (2H, dd, J = 1.9, 8.7 Hz), 8.06 (2H, d, J = 1.9 Hz); ^{13}C NMR (100 MHz, CDCl$_3$) 24.0, 24.2, 32.2, 35.9, 42.2, 54.2, 57.0, 110.5, 112.0, 123.1, 123.2, 128.9, 139.2, 171.4. HR-FTMS (ESI) m/z calcd. for C$_{23}$H$_{27}$Br$_2$N$_3$O, [M + H]$^+$ 522.0573, found 522.0572.

Synthesis of 4-(3,6-Dibromocarbazol-9-yl)-N-(2-piperazin-1-ylethyl)butyramide (8)

The crude oil was purified via column chromatography over silica gel and 10% methanol in dichloromethane, and the product obtained as a white solid (0.1425 g, 0.27 mmol, 71%). TLC analysis in CH$_2$Cl$_2$-MeOH (9:1), R_f = 0.23. ^{1}H NMR (400 MHz, CDCl$_3$) δ 1.9 (1H, bs), 2.11 (2H, t, J = 6.4 Hz), 2.20 (2H, m), 2.38 (3H, bs), 2.42 (4H, t, J = 5.9 Hz), 2.84 (4H, t, J = 4.7 Hz), 3.32 (2H, q, J = 5.4 Hz), 4.38 (2H, t, J = 6.7 Hz), 7.33 (2H, d, J = 8.7 Hz), 7.54 (2H, dd, J = 1.9, 10.6 Hz), 8.14 (2H, s); ^{13}C NMR (100 MHz, CDCl$_3$) 24.0, 32.2, 35.6, 42.4, 45.9, 54.1, 57.0, 110.6, 112.1, 123.2, 123.5, 139.4, 171.4. HR-FTMS (ESI) m/z calcd. for C$_{23}$H$_{27}$Br$_2$N$_3$O, [M + H]$^+$ 523.0526, found 523.0526.

Synthesis of 4-(3,6-Dibromocarbazol-9-yl)-N-(3-morpholin-4-ylpropyl)butyramide (9)

The crude oil was purified via column chromatography over silica gel and 10% methanol in dichloromethane, and the product obtained as a white solid (0.1496 g, 0.28 mmol, 69%). TLC analysis in CH$_2$Cl$_2$-MeOH (9:1), R_f = 0.59. ^{1}H NMR (400 MHz, CDCl$_3$) δ 1.56 (2H, m, J = 6.0 Hz), 1.95 (2H, t, J = 6.8 Hz), 2.14 (4H, m), 2.23 (2H, bs), 2.36 (2H, t, J = 6.4 Hz), 3.25 (2H, q, J = 5.6 Hz), 3.42 (1H, bs), 4.31 (2H, t, J = 6.8 Hz), 7.31 (2H, d, J = 8.8 Hz), 7.54 (2H, dd, J = 2.0, 8.8 Hz), 8.12 (2H, d, J = 1.6 Hz); ^{13}C NMR (100 MHz, CDCl$_3$) 24.0, 24.4, 32.3, 39.6, 42.1, 53.5, 58.0, 66.8, 110.6, 112.1, 123.2, 123.4, 129.1, 139.3, 171.1. HR-FTMS (ESI) m/z calcd. for C$_{23}$H$_{27}$Br$_2$N$_3$O$_2$, [M + H]$^+$ 538.0522, found 538.0521.

Synthesis, Anti-Cancer and Anti-Migratory Evaluation of 3,6-Dibromocarbazole and 5-Bromoindole Derivatives

43

Synthesis of 4-(3,6-Dibromocarbazol-9-yl)-N-(4-diethylamino-1-methylbutyl)butyramide (**10**)

The crude oil was purified via column chromatography over silica gel and 10% methanol in dichloromethane, and the product obtained as a white solid (0.0063 g, 0.040 mmol, 9.1%). TLC analysis in CH$_2$Cl$_2$-MeOH (9:1), R_f = 0.21. ^{1}H NMR (400 MHz, CDCl$_3$) δ 0.89 (2H, m), 1.19 (6H, t, J = 7.6 Hz), 1.64 (2H, m), 2.20 (3H, bs), 2.25 (2H, t, J = 6.8 Hz), 2.62 (2H, t, J = 6.4 Hz), 3.29 (4H, m), 3.60 (2H, t, J = 7.20 Hz), 4.37 (2H, t, J = 7.20 Hz), 7.33 (2H, d, J = 8.8 Hz), 7.55 (2H, dd, J = 2.0, 8.8 Hz), 8.13 (2H, d, J = 2.0 Hz), 9.28 (1H, bs); ^{13}C NMR (100 MHz, CDCl$_3$) 8.5, 21.2, 21.3, 24.4, 29.7, 32.7, 33.6, 42.6, 44.6, 47.0, 52.3, 110.7, 112.0, 123.2, 123.5, 129.1, 139.4, 172.0. HR-FTMS (ESI) m/z calcd. for C$_{25}$H$_{33}$Br$_2$N$_3$O$_2$, [M + H]$^+$ 552.1043, found 552.1044.

Synthesis of 4-[4-(3,6-Dibromocarbazol-9-yl)-butyrylamino]piperidine-1-carboxylic acid ethyl ester (**11**)

The crude oil was purified via column chromatography over silica gel and 10% methanol in dichloromethane, and the product obtained as a white solid (0.1254 g, 0.22 mmol, 85.3%). TLC analysis in CH$_2$Cl$_2$-MeOH (9:1), R_f = 0.63. ^{1}H NMR (400 MHz, CDCl$_3$) δ 1.25 (3H, t, J = 7.2 Hz), 1.88 (2H, dd, J = 2.8, 12.4 Hz), 2.08 (2H, t, J = 6.4 Hz), 2.19 (2H, m, J = 6.8 Hz), 2.88 (2H, t, J = 12.0 Hz), 3.92 (1H, m, J = 3.6 Hz), 4.12 (4H, q, J = 6.8 Hz), 4.37 (2H, t, J = 6.8 Hz), 5.16 (1H, d, J = 7.6 Hz), 7.32 (2H, d, J = 8.8 Hz), 7.55 (2H, dd, J = 2.0, 8.8 Hz), 8.14 (2H, d, J = 1.6 Hz); ^{13}C NMR (100 MHz, CDCl$_3$) 14.7, 24.0, 32.0, 32.4, 42.2, 42.7, 46.8, 61.4, 110.5, 112.2, 123.3, 123.5, 129.2, 139.3, 155.4, 170.1. HR-FTMS (ESI) m/z calcd. for C$_{24}$H$_{27}$Br$_2$N$_3$O$_3$, [M + H]$^+$ 566.0471, found 566.0470.

Synthesis of 4-(3,6-Dibromocarbazol-9-yl)-1-morpholin-4-ylbutan-1-one (**12**)

The crude oil was purified via column chromatography over silica gel and 10% methanol in dichloromethane, and the product obtained as a white solid (0.0768 g, 0.16 mmol, 52%). TLC analysis in CH$_2$Cl$_2$-MeOH (9:1), R_f = 0.94. ^{1}H NMR (400 MHz, CDCl$_3$) δ 2.15 (4H, t, J = 6.0 Hz), 2.21 (2H, m, J = 6.8 Hz), 3.16 (2H, t, J = 4.8 Hz), 3.50 (2H, t, J = 4.4 Hz), 3.64 (4H, dt, J = 2.8, 6.4 Hz), 7.31 (2H, d, J = 8.8 Hz), 7.55 (2H, dd, J = 1.6, 8.4 Hz), 8.14 (2H, d, J = 1.6 Hz); ^{13}C NMR (100 MHz, CDCl$_3$) 23.6, 28.6, 41.5, 41.9, 45.1, 65.9, 66.0, 111.3, 111.5, 122.9, 123.41, 128.8, 139.0, 170.0. HR-FTMS (ESI) m/z calcd. for C$_{20}$H$_{20}$Br$_2$N$_2$O$_2$, [M + H]$^+$ 480.9944, found 480.9945.

Synthesis of 4-(3,6-Dibromocarbazol-9-yl)-1-thiomorpholin-4-ylbutan-1-one (**13**)

The crude oil was purified via column chromatography over silica gel and 10% methanol in dichloromethane, and the product obtained as a white solid (0.0712 g, 0.41 mmol, 35%). TLC analysis in CH$_2$Cl$_2$-MeOH (9:1), R_f = 0.60. ^{1}H NMR (400 MHz, CDCl$_3$) δ 2.11 (2H, t, J = 6.3 Hz), 2.21 (2H, m), 2.34 (2H, t, J = 5.0 Hz), 2.62 (2H, t, J = 5.2 Hz), 3.46 (2H, t, J = 5.0 Hz), 3.89 (2H, t, J = 5.0 Hz), 4.41 (2H, t, J = 6.7 Hz), 7.32 (2H, d, J = 8.6 Hz), 7.56 (2H, dd, J = 1.9, 8.7 Hz), 8.15 (2H, d, J = 1.7 Hz); ^{13}C NMR (100 MHz, CDCl$_3$) 23.5, 27.3, 27.4, 29.0, 42.1, 44.3, 47.8, 110.6, 112.2, 123.3, 123.5, 129.1, 139.4, 169.9. HR-FTMS (ESI) m/z calcd. for C$_{20}$H$_{20}$Br$_2$N$_3$OS, [M + H]$^+$ 496.9715, found 496.9713.

Synthesis of 1-[4-(3,6-Dibromocarbazol-9-yl)butyryl]piperidine-4-carbonitrile (**14**)

The crude oil was purified via column chromatography over silica gel and 10% methanol in dichloromethane, and the product obtained as a white solid (0.0775 g, 0.16 mmol, 44%). TLC analysis in CH$_2$Cl$_2$-MeOH (9:1), R_f = 0.97. ^{1}H NMR (400 MHz, CDCl$_3$) δ 1.63 (2H, t, J = 5.6 Hz), 1.85 (1H, m), 2.15 (2H, m), 2.84 (2H, m), 3.14 (2H, dt, J = 5.2, 13.6 Hz), 3.35 (2H, dt, J = 6.0, 14.4 Hz), 3.63 (2H, dq, J = 4.4, 13.6 Hz), 3.76 (2H, dq, J = 3.2, 13.6 Hz), 4.41 (2H, m), 7.31 (2H, d, J = 8.4 Hz), 7.54 (2H, dd, J = 1.6, 8.4 Hz), 8.14 (2H, d, J = 1.6 Hz); ^{13}C NMR (100 MHz, CDCl$_3$) 23.4, 26.2, 28.1, 28.6, 28.7, 39.5, 42.1, 43.0, 110.6, 112.2, 120.5, 123.3, 123.5, 129.1, 139.4, 169.8. HR-FTMS (ESI) m/z calcd. for C$_{22}$H$_{21}$Br$_2$N$_3$O, [M + H]$^+$ 504.0104, found 504.0104.

Synthesis of 4-(3,6-Dibromocarbazol-9-yl)-1-(4-phenylpiperazin-1-yl)butan-1-one (15)

The crude oil was purified via column chromatography over silica gel and 10% methanol in dichloromethane, and the product obtained as a white solid (0.2658 g, 0.27 mmol, 69%). TLC analysis in CH_2Cl_2-MeOH (9:1), R_f = 0.53. ^{1}H NMR (400 MHz, $CDCl_3$) δ 1.55 (2H, bs), 2.22 (2H, m), 2.97 (2H, t, J = 5.3 Hz), 3.15 (2H, t, J = 4.9 Hz), 3.34 (2H, t, J = 4.5 Hz), 3.30 (2H, t, J = 4.7 Hz), 4.43 (2H, t, J = 3.4 Hz), 6.92 (2H, t, J = 7.9 Hz), 7.29 (3H, t, J = 7.9 Hz), 7.34 (2H, d, J = 8.7 Hz), 7.54 (2H, dd, J = 1.8, 8.6 Hz), 8.15 (2H, d, J = 1.7 Hz); ^{13}C NMR (100 MHz, $CDCl_3$) 23.6, 28.9, 41.6, 42.2, 45.1, 49.4, 49.5, 110.6, 112.1, 116.8, 120.7, 123.3, 123.5, 129.2, 129.3, 139.4, 150.9, 170.0. HR-FTMS (ESI) m/z calcd. for $C_{26}H_{25}Br_2N_3O$, [M + H]$^+$ 556.0417, found 556.0417.

Synthesis of 1-(4-Acetylpiperazin-1-yl)-4-(3,6-dibromocarbazol-9-yl)butan-1-one (16)

The crude oil was purified via column chromatography over silica gel and 10% methanol in dichloromethane, and the product obtained as a white solid (0.0775 g, 0.15 mmol, 62%). TLC analysis in CH_2Cl_2-MeOH (9:1), R_f = 0.67. ^{1}H NMR (400 MHz, $CDCl_3$) δ 1.57 (3H, s), 2.08 (2H, bs), 2.12 (2H, bs), 2.21 (2H, bs), 3.19 (2H, t, J = 5.3 Hz), 3.45 (2H, t, J = 6.2), 3.64 (2H, t, J = 5.0 Hz), 4.42 (2H, t, J = 6.6 Hz), 7.32 (2H, dd, J = 4.2, 8.7 Hz), 7.54 (2H, dd, J = 1.9, 8.7 Hz), 8.14 (2H, d, J = 1.8 Hz); ^{13}C NMR (100 MHz, $CDCl_3$) 21.4, 28.8, 31.0, 41.5, 42.0, 42.2, 44.8, 45.9, 110.5, 112.2, 123.4, 129.1, 139.3, 169.3, 170.4. HR-FTMS (ESI) m/z calcd. for $C_{22}H_{23}Br_2N_3O_2$, [M + H]$^+$ 522.0209, found 522.0209.

Synthesis of 4-[4-(3,6-Dibromocarbazol-9-yl)butyryl]piperazine-1-carboxylic acid tert-butyl ester (17)

The crude oil was purified via column chromatography over silica gel and hexane-ethyl acetate (1:1) as the mobile phase, and the product obtained as a white solid (0.1977 g, 0.4 mmol, 80%). TLC analysis in hexane-ethyl acetate (1:1), R_f = 0.35. ^{1}H NMR (400 MHz, $CDCl_3$) δ 1.47 (9H, s), 2.20 (4H, m), 3.16 (2H, bs), 3.26 (2H, bs), 3.40 (2H, t, J = 5.2 Hz), 3.60 (2H, t, J = 4.4 Hz), 4.41 (2H, t, J = 6.4 Hz), 7.32 (2H, d, J = 8.4 Hz), 7.54 (2H, dd, J = 1.6, 8.4 Hz), 8.14 (2H, d, J = 2.0 Hz); ^{13}C NMR (100 MHz, $CDCl_3$) 23.5, 28.4, 29.0, 41.4, 42.2, 45.0, 80.4, 110.5, 112.2, 123.3, 123.5, 129.1, 139.4, 154.5, 170.2. HR-FTMS (ESI) m/z calcd. for $C_{25}H_{29}Br_2N_3O_3$, [M + Na]$^+$ 602.0447, found 602.0446.

Synthesis of 4-(3,6-Dibromocarbazol-9-yl)-1-piperazin-1-ylbutan-1-one (18)

The crude oil was purified via column chromatography over silica gel and 10% methanol in dichloromethane, and the product obtained as a white solid (0.0383 g, 0.080 mmol, 80%). TLC analysis in CH_2Cl_2-MeOH (9:1), R_f = 0.38. ^{1}H NMR (400 MHz, $CDCl_3$) δ 1.25 (1H, s), 2.18 (4H, m), 2.68 (2H, t, J = 4.8 Hz), 2.84 (2H, t, J = 5.2 Hz), 3.16 (2H, t, J = 4.8 Hz), 3.61 (2H, t, J = 5.2 Hz), 4.41 (2H, t, J = 6.4 Hz), 7.32 (2H, d, J = 8.4 Hz), 7.54 (2H, dd, J = 2.0, 8.8 Hz), 8.14 (2H, d, J = 1.6 Hz); ^{13}C NMR (100 MHz, $CDCl_3$) 22.6, 23.6, 42.2, 42.7, 45.8, 46.0, 46.3, 110.6, 112.1, 123.3, 123.5, 129.1, 139.4, 170.0. HR-FTMS (ESI) m/z calcd. for $C_{20}H_{21}Br_2N_3O$, [M + H]$^+$ 480.0104, found 480.0101.

Synthesis of 4-(3,6-Dibromocarbazol-9-yl)-1-[4-(2-morpholin-4-ylethyl)piperazin-1-yl]butan-1-one (19)

The crude oil was purified via column chromatography over silica gel and 10% methanol in dichloromethane, and the product obtained as a white solid (0.2036 g, 0.34 mmol, 76.4%). TLC analysis in CH_2Cl_2-MeOH (9:1), R_f = 0.52. ^{1}H NMR (400 MHz, $CDCl_3$) δ 2.12 (2H, t, J = 6.0 Hz), 2.18 (2H, t, J = 7.2 Hz), 2.24 (2H, m), 2.44 (2H, t, J = 5.2 Hz), 2.48 (4H, t, J = 4.4 Hz), 3.17 (2H, t, J = 4.8 Hz), 3.63 (2H, t, J = 5.2 Hz), 3.70 (4H, t, J = 4.8 Hz), 4.41 (2H, t, J = 6.4 Hz), 7.28 (2H, d, J = 6.0 Hz), 7.37 (2H, dd, J = 6.4 Hz, 8.8 Hz), 8.15 (2H, d, J = 2.1 Hz); ^{13}C NMR (100 MHz, $CDCl_3$) 23.5, 28.7, 41.6, 42.1, 45.0, 53.2, 53.3, 54.1, 55.4, 56.3, 66.9, 110.7, 112.1, 123.3, 123.4, 129.2, 139.4, 169.8. HR-FTMS (ESI) m/z calcd. for $C_{26}H_{32}Br_2N_4O_2$, [M + H]$^+$ 593.0944, found 593.0945.

Synthesis of 2-{4-[4-(3,6-Dibromocarbazol-9-yl)-butyryl]piperazin-1-yl}-N-isopropylacetamide (**20**)

The crude oil was purified via column chromatography over silica gel and 10% methanol in dichloromethane, and the product obtained as a white solid (0.2273 g, 0.39 mmol, 87.3%). TLC analysis in CH_2Cl_2-MeOH (9:1), R_f = 0.68. ^{1}H NMR (400 MHz, $CDCl_3$) δ 1.17 (6H, d, J = 6.6 Hz), 2.10 (2H, t, J = 6.3 Hz), 2.21 (2H, m), 2.26 (2H, t, J = 4.7 Hz), 2.47 (2H, t, J = 4.5 Hz), 3.15 (2H, t, J = 4.5 Hz), 3.64 (2H, t, J = 4.5 Hz), 4.10 (1H, m), 4.43 (2H, t, J = 6.6 Hz), 6.73 (1H, bs), 7.31 (2H, d, J = 8.7 Hz), 7.54 (2H, dd, J = 1.9, 8.7 Hz), 8.14 (2H, d, J = 1.9 Hz); ^{13}C NMR (100 MHz, $CDCl_3$) 22.8, 23.4, 28.7, 40.8, 41.6, 42.0, 45.0, 53.0, 53.1, 61.5, 110.64, 112.1, 123.3, 123.5, 129.2, 139.4, 168.4, 170.0. HR-FTMS (ESI) m/z calcd. for $C_{25}H_{30}Br_2N_4O_2$, $[M + H]^+$ 579.0788, found 579.0790.

Synthesis of 4-(3,6-Dibromocarbazol-9-yl)-1-[4-(2-dimethylaminoethyl)piperazin-1-yl]butan-1-one (**21**)

The crude oil was purified via column chromatography over silica gel and 10% methanol in dichloromethane, and the product obtained as a white solid (0.0228 g, 0.04 mmol, 7%). TLC analysis in CH_2Cl_2-MeOH (9:1), R_f = 0.50. ^{1}H NMR (400 MHz, $CDCl_3$) δ 1.25 (6H, s), 2.12 (2H, t, J = 6.0 Hz), 2.19 (2H, m), 2.24 (4H, t, J = 5.6 Hz), 2.43 (4H, t, J = 4.8 Hz), 3.19 (2H, t, J = 4.4 Hz), 3.64 (2H, t, J = 4.4 Hz), 4.40 (2H, t, J = 6.4 Hz), 7.31 (2H, d, J = 8.8 Hz), 7.53 (2H, dd, J = 1.6, 8.4 Hz,), 8.21 (2H, d, J = 2.0 Hz); ^{13}C NMR (100 MHz, $CDCl_3$) 23.5, 28.7, 41.5, 42.1, 45.0, 45.6, 53.1, 53.3, 56.1, 56.5, 110.6, 112.1, 123.2, 123.4, 129.2, 139.4, 170.0. HR-FTMS (ESI) m/z calcd. for $C_{24}H_{30}Br_2N_4O$, $[M + H]^+$ 551.0839, found 551.0842.

Synthesis of 4-(3,6-Dibromocarbazol-9-yl)-N-(4-morpholin-4-ylphenyl)butyramide (**22**)

The crude oil was purified via column chromatography over silica gel and 10% methanol in dichloromethane, and the product obtained as a white solid (0.0689 g, 0.12 mmol, 40%). TLC analysis in CH_2Cl_2-MeOH (9:1), R_f = 0.80. ^{1}H NMR (400 MHz, DMSO-d_6) δ 2.05 (2H, t, J = 6.8 Hz), 2.30 (2H, m), 3.02 (4H, t, J = 4.8 Hz), 3.71 (4H, t, J = 4.4 Hz), 4.44 (2H, t, J = 6.8 Hz), 6.86 (2H, d, J = 8.8 Hz), 7.41 (2H, d, J = 8.8 Hz), 7.61 (2H, dd, J = 0.8, 8.8 Hz), 7.64 (2H, d, J = 8.4 Hz), 8.48 (2H, s), 9.62 (1H, s); ^{13}C NMR (100 MHz, DMSO-d_6) 24.1, 32.7, 42.0, 48.9, 66.1, 111.3, 111.6, 115.4, 120.3, 122.9, 123.4,128.8, 131.5, 139.0, 147.0, 169.7. HR-FTMS (ESI) m/z calcd. for $C_{26}H_{25}Br_2N_3O_2$, $[M + H]^+$ 572.0366, found 572.0365.

Synthesis of 4-(3,6-Dibromocarbazol-9-yl)-N-(3,4,5-trimethoxyphenyl)butyramide (**23**)

The crude oil was purified via column chromatography over silica gel and 10% methanol in dichloromethane, and the product obtained as a white solid (0.051 g, 0.10 mmol, 30%). TLC analysis in CH_2Cl_2-MeOH (9:1), R_f = 0.17. ^{1}H NMR (400 MHz, DMSO-d_6) δ 2.08 (2H, m), 2.28 (2H, t, J = 7.2 Hz), 3.60 (3H, s), 3.71 (3H, s), 3.72 (3H, s), 4.46 (2H, t, J = 6.8 Hz), 6.90 (2H, s), 7.60 (2H, dd, J = 1.6, 8.4 Hz), 7.64 (2H, d, J = 8.8 Hz), 8.47 (2H, d, J = 1.6 Hz), 9.71 (1H, s); ^{13}C NMR (100 MHz, DMSO-d_6) 6.96, 24.0, 32.0, 42.0, 55.6, 60.0, 96.9, 111.3, 111.6, 122.9, 123.4, 128.8, 133.3, 135.2, 139.1, 152.6, 170.1. HR-FTMS (ESI) m/z calcd. for $C_{25}H_{24}Br_2N_2O_4$, $[M + H]^+$ 577.0155, found 577.0142.

Synthesis of 4-(3,6-Dibromocarbazol-9-yl)-N-quinolin-3-ylbutyramide (**24**)

The crude oil was purified via column chromatography over silica gel and 10% methanol in dichloromethane, and the product obtained as a white solid (0.0275 g, 0.052 mmol, 15%). TLC analysis in hexane-ethyl acetate (1:1), R_f = 0.20. ^{1}H NMR (400 MHz, DMSO-d_6) δ 2.13 (2H, m), 2.44 (2H, t, J = 6.8 Hz), 4.50 (2H, t, J = 6.5 Hz), 7.41 (1H, t, J = 7.4 Hz), 7.54 (1H, t, J = 8.0 Hz), 7.62 (1H, t, J = 7.9 Hz), 7.67 (1H, d, J = 8.6 Hz), 7.71 (1H, d, J = 8.3 Hz), 7.92 (2H, t, J = 8.4 Hz), 7.98 (2H, d, J = 8.4 Hz), 8.47 (2H, s), 8.64 (1H, s), 8.82 (1H, s), 10.3 (1H, s); ^{13}C NMR (100 MHz, DMSO-d_6) 23.9. 32.9, 42.0, 109.6, 111.4, 111.7, 119.2, 122.0, 123.0, 123.5, 124.5, 127.0, 127.4, 127.6, 127.7, 127.8, 128.5, 128.9, 132.8, 139.1, 144.1, 144.5, 171.3. HR-FTMS (ESI) m/z calcd. for $C_{25}H_{19}Br_2N_3O$, $[M + H]^+$ 537.9947, found 537.9946.

Synthesis of 4-(3,6-Dibromocarbazol-9-yl)-N-(1H-indol-6-yl)butyramide (25)

The crude oil was purified via column chromatography over silica gel and 10% methanol in dichloromethane, and the product obtained as a white solid (0.1152 g, 0.22 mmol, 38%). TLC analysis in hexane-ethyl acetate (1:1), $R_f = 0.50$. ^{1}H NMR (400 MHz, DMSO-d_6) δ 2.08 (2H, m), 2.35 (2H, t, $J = 7.1$ Hz), 4.47 (2H, t, $J = 7.0$ Hz), 6.33 (1H, s), 6.97, (1H, d, $J = 9.1$ Hz), 7.24 (1H, s), 7.40 (1H, d, $J = 8.4$ Hz), 7.61 (2H, d, $J = 7.2$ Hz), 7.66 (2H, d, $J = 8.7$ Hz), 7.95 (1H, s), 8.49 (2H, s), 9.75 (1H, s); ^{13}C NMR (100 MHz, DMSO-d_6) 24.2, 32.9, 42.1, 100.9, 102.2, 111.3, 111.6, 112.3, 119.7, 123.0, 123.5, 123.7, 124.8, 128.9, 133.3, 135.9, 139.1. HR-FTMS (ESI) m/z calcd. for $C_{24}H_{19}Br_2N_3O$, $[M + H]^+$ 525.9947, found 9946.

Synthesis of N-(3H-Benzoimidazol-5-yl)-4-(3,6-dibromocarbazol-9-yl)butyramide (26)

The crude oil was purified via column chromatography over silica gel and 10% methanol in dichloromethane, and the product obtained as a white solid (0.100 g, 0.20 mmol, 44%). TLC analysis in hexane-ethyl acetate (1:1), $R_f = 0.70$. ^{1}H NMR (400 MHz, DMSO-d_6) δ 2.16 (2H, m, $J = 7.2$ Hz), 3.18 (2H, t, $J = 7.6$ Hz), 4.52 (2H, t, $J = 7.2$ Hz), 6.66 (1H, dd, $J = 2.0, 8.8$ Hz), 7.60 (1H, dd, $J = 2.0, 8.8$ Hz), 7.68 (1H, d, $J = 8.8$ Hz), 8.05 (1H, s), 8.47 (1H, dd, $J = 1.6, 8.0$ Hz); ^{13}C NMR (100 MHz, DMSO-d_6) 23.6, 32.0, 42.3, 97.2, 111.8, 112.0, 114.3, 117.2, 122.3, 123.5, 124.0, 129.4, 139.5, 141.0, 141.2, 151.7, 173.0. HR-FTMS (ESI) m/z calcd. for $C_{23}H_{18}Br_2N_4O$, $[M + H]^+$ 526.9900, found 526.9904.

Synthesis of 4-(3,6-Dibromocarbazol-9-yl)-N-(4-methoxyphenyl)butyramide (27)

The crude oil was purified via column chromatography over silica gel and 10% methanol in dichloromethane, and the product obtained as a white solid (0.1830 g, 0.35 mmol, 94%). TLC analysis in hexane-ethyl acetate (1:1), $R_f = 0.64$. ^{1}H NMR (400 MHz, DMSO-d_6) δ 2.05 (2H, m), 2.30 (2H, t, $J = 7.2$ Hz), 3.70 (3H, s), 4.45 (2H, t, $J = 7.2$ Hz), 6.84 (2H, d, $J = 9.2$ Hz), 7.44 (2H, d, $J = 9.2$ Hz), 7.60 (2H, dd, $J = 2.0, 8.8$ Hz), 7.65 (2H, d, $J = 8.8$ Hz), 8.48 (2H, d, $J = 2.0$ Hz), 9.68 (1H, s); ^{13}C NMR (100 MHz, DMSO-d_6) 24.1, 32.7, 42.0, 55.1, 111.3, 111.6, 113.8, 120.7, 123.0, 123.5, 128.7, 132.3, 139.1, 155.1, 169.9. HR-FTMS (ESI) m/z calcd. for $C_{23}H_{20}Br_2N_2O_2$, $[M + H]^+$ 516.9944, found 516.9941.

3.2.4. Synthesis of N-Alkyl-5-Bromoindole Derivatives (31–34)

3.2.5. General Procedure for the Synthesis of 4-(5-Bromoindol-1-yl)Butyric Acid (29)

A 50 mL three-neck round-bottom flask, equipped with a reflux condenser, was charged with 5-bromoindole 28 (0.1960 g, 1.0 mmol), Cs$_2$CO$_3$ (0.9770 g, 3 mmol) and ethyl 4-bromobutyrate (0.43 mL, 3.0 mmol), dissolved in DMF (3 mL). After 15 min of stirring at room temperature, the reaction mixture was refluxed at 100 °C for 16 h. After completion of the reaction (analyzed by TLC), water (1 mL) and KOH (1.0 mmol) were added and the reaction mixture refluxed at 80 °C for 2 h. After the reaction was completed (analyzed by TLC), the mixture was allowed to reach room temperature and 1N HCl solution was added until reach neutral pH. The mixture was washed with water (20 mL) and the product was extracted using dichloromethane (3 × 10 mL). The organic layer was washed with brine and dried with Na$_2$SO$_4$, and filtered and concentrated under reduced pressure. The crude oil was purified via column chromatography over silica gel and 10% CH$_2$Cl$_2$ in MeOH, and the product obtained as a white solid for the precursor 4-(5-Bromoindol-1-yl)Butyric acid 29 (0.2260 g, 0.801 mmol, 80%). TLC analysis in CH$_2$Cl$_2$-MeOH (9:1), $R_f = 0.25$. ^{1}H NMR (400 MHz, CDCl$_3$) δ 2.16 (2H, m), 2.34 (2H, t, $J = 7.2$ Hz), 4.20 (2H, t, $J = 6.80$ Hz), 6.44 (1H, d, $J = 2.4$ Hz), 7.08 (1H, 2, $J = 3.2$ Hz), 7.22 (1H, d, $J = 6.4$ Hz), 7.29 (1H, dd, $J = 2.0, 8.8$ Hz), 7.74 (1H, d, $J = 1.6$ Hz); ^{13}C NMR (100 MHz, CDCl$_3$) 25.1, 30.5, 45.3, 101.1, 110.7, 112.8, 123.5, 124.5, 128.9, 130.3, 134.6, 177.4. HR-FTMS (ESI) m/z calcd. for $C_{12}H_{12}BrNO_2$, $[M + H]^+$ 284.0104, found 284.0102.

3.2.6. General Procedure for the Synthesis of 4-(5-Bromoindol-1-yl)-N-(3-Morpholin-4-ylpropyl)Butyramide (**31**), and for Compounds **32–34**

A 50 mL three-neck round-bottom flask was charged with 4-(5-Bromoindol-1-yl)Butyric acid **29** (0.098 g, 0.35 mmol), HOBT (0.2027 g, 1.5 mmol), and EDAC (0.2876 g, 1.5 mmol). The mixture was dissolved in DMF (5 mL), stirred for 30 min, and 3-morpholinopropylamine (0.0512 mL, 0.35 mmol) was added. After 15 min, Et_3N (0.43 mL, 3.0 mmol) was added and the mixture stirred at room temperature for 16 h. After the reaction was completed (analyzed by TLC), water was added (30 mL) and the product was extracted using dichloromethane (3×10 mL). The organic layer was washed with brine and dried with Na_2SO_4, and filtered and concentrated under reduced pressure. The crude oil was purified via column chromatography over silica gel and 10% methanol in dichloromethane, and the product obtained as a white solid (0.0748 g, 0.18 mmol, 53%). TLC analysis in hexane-ethyl acetate (1:1), $R_f = 0.36$. ^{1}H NMR (400 MHz, $CDCl_3$) δ 1.62 (2H, m), 2.01 (2H, t, $J = 6.8$ Hz), 2.21 (2H, m), 2.35 (4H, bs), 2.42 (2H, t, $J = 6.4$ Hz), 3.32 (2H, q, $J = 5.6$ Hz), 3.47 (4H, bs), 4.39 (2H, t, $J = 6.8$ Hz), 7.0 (1H, bs), 7.26 (1H, d, $J = 1.2$ Hz), 7.32 (1H, d, $J = 8.8$ Hz), 7.55 (1H, dd, $J = 2.0, 8.8$ Hz), 8.14 (1H, d, $J = 1.6$ Hz); ^{13}C NMR (100 MHz, $CDCl_3$) 24.5, 25.8, 32.6, 39.6, 45.2, 53.6, 58.0, 67.0, 101.1, 110.9, 112.6, 123.4, 124.3, 128.8, 130.2, 134.9, 171.2. HR-FTMS (ESI) m/z calcd. for $C_{19}H_{26}BrN_3O_2$, $[M + H]^+$ 410.1261, found 410.1257.

Synthesis of 1-[4-(5-Bromoindol-1-yl)butyryl]piperidine-4-carbonitrile (**32**)

The crude oil was purified via column chromatography over silica gel and 10% methanol in dichloromethane, and the product obtained as a white solid (0.0356 g, 0.10 mmol, 24.4%). TLC analysis in CH_2Cl_2-MeOH (9:1), $R_f = 0.76$. ^{1}H NMR (400 MHz, DMSO-d_6) δ 1.58 (4H, m), 1.81 (2H, bs), 1.94 (2H, t, $J = 7.2$ Hz), 2.26 (2H, t, $J = 7.2$ Hz), 3.07 (1H, m), 3.50 (2H, dt, $J = 4.8, 15.2$ Hz), 3.78 (2H, dt, $J = 4.8, 13.6$Hz), 4.18 (2H, t, $J = 6.8$Hz), 6.42 (1H, d, $J = 3.2$ Hz), 7.24 (1H, dd, $J = 2.0, 8.4$ Hz), 7.41 (1H, d, $J = 3.2$ Hz), 7.47 (1H, d, $J = 8.8$ Hz), 7.73 (1H, d, $J = 2.0$ Hz); ^{13}C NMR (100 MHz, DMSO-d_6) 22.7, 25.3, 28.2, 29.4, 29.7, 39.5, 43.1, 45.3, 101.0, 111.0, 112.7, 120.6, 123.5, 124.4, 128.9, 130.2, 134.9, 169.9. HR-FTMS (ESI) m/z calcd. for $C_{18}H_{20}BrN_3O$, $[M + H]^+$ 376.0842, found 376.0837.

Synthesis of 4-(5-Bromoindol-1-yl)-N-(3-imidazol-1-yl-propyl)butyramide (**33**)

The crude oil was purified via column chromatography over silica gel and 10% methanol in dichloromethane, and the product obtained as a white solid (0.1255 g, 0.32 mmol, 57%). TLC analysis in CH_2Cl_2-MeOH (9:1), $R_f = 0.44$. ^{1}H NMR (400 MHz, $CDCl_3$) δ 1.81 (2H, m, $J = 6.8$ Hz), 1.98 (2H, m, $J = 6.8$ Hz), 2.06 (2H, t, $J = 6.4$ Hz), 3.01 (2H, q, $J = 5.6$ Hz), 3.95 (2H, t, $J = 6.8$ Hz), 4.17 (2H, t, $J = 7.2$ Hz), 6.42 (1H, d, $J = 2.8$ Hz), 6.95 (1H, bs), 7.23 (2H, dd, $J = 1.6, 8.4$ Hz), 7.40 (1H, d, $J = 2.8$ Hz), 7.45 (1H, d, $J = 8.8$ Hz), 7.72 (1H, d, $J = 2.0$ Hz), 7.90 (1H, t, $J = 5.2$ Hz); ^{13}C NMR (100 MHz, $CDCl_3$) 25.7, 31.0, 32.2, 36.5, 44.2, 45.6, 101.0, 111.0, 112.5, 119.1, 123.3, 124.4, 128.7, 128.8, 130.2, 134.7, 136.9, 172.4. HR-FTMS (ESI) m/z calcd. for $C_{18}H_{21}BrN_4O$, $[M + H]^+$ 391.0951, found 391.0956.

Synthesis of 4-(5-Bromoindol-1-yl)-N-(2-piperidin-1-ylethyl)butyramide (**34**)

The crude oil was purified via column chromatography over silica gel and 10% methanol in dichloromethane, and the product obtained as a white solid (0.1967 g, 0.50 mmol, 50%). TLC analysis in CH_2Cl_2-MeOH (9:1), $R_f = 0.47$. ^{1}H NMR (400 MHz, DMSO-d_6) δ 1.35 (2H, m, $J = 5.2$ Hz), 1.47 (4H, m, $J = 5.6$ Hz), 1.96 (2H, m, $J = 6.4$ Hz), 2.01 (2H, t, $J = 6.0$ Hz), 2.30 (2H, t, $J = 6.8$ Hz), 2.35 (2H, bs), 3.13 (2H, q, $J = 6.4$ Hz), 4.18 (2H, t, $J = 6.4$ Hz) 7.35 (1H, dd, $J = 2.0, 8.8$ Hz), 7.54 (2H, d, $J = 2.4$ Hz), 7.56 (1H, s), 7.68 (1H, s), 7.71 (1H, t, $J = 5.6$ Hz); ^{13}C NMR (100 MHz, DMSO-d_6) 24.1, 25.5, 25.7, 32.4, 35.7, 45.8, 54.3, 57.2, 100.8, 109.4, 111.0, 118.5, 120.3, 128.9, 129.0, 134.7, 171.7. HR-FTMS (ESI) m/z calcd. for $C_{25}H_{30}Br_2N_4O_2$, $[M + H]^+$ 394.1312, found 394.1313.

3.3. Biological Evaluation

3.3.1. Cell Culture

MCF-7 and MDA-MB-231 cells were cultured in Minimum Essential Medium Eagle (MEME) 10% FBS supplemented with Earle's Balanced Salt Solution (EBSS), Non-essential Amino Acids (NEAA), Sodium Pyruvate, Pen/Strep, and L-glutamine 37 °C in 5% CO_2.

3.3.2. Sulforhodamine B (SRB) Assay

A stock solution of compounds was prepared at 50 mM in 100% DMSO. For cell preparation, a flask of 75 cm^2 or 25 cm^2 was used for 2.6×10^5 cells/mL or 1.44×10^5 cells/mL, respectively, with an 80–90% confluence. Cells were washed with PBS and trypsinized. The concentration of cells was determined using a 1:2 dilution with Trypan Blue and a hemocytometer. After cell count, the concentration was adjusted to have a $7.0–10.0 \times 10^4$ cells/mL. Approximately 100 μL of cells suspension, compounds, control positive and control negative were added in triplicates to a 96 well plate. The positive control used was doxorubicin, and the negative control was DMSO 0.1%. All compounds at 50, 25, 12.5, 6.3, and 1.6 μM were incubated with cells at 37 °C for 48 hrs. For fixation, cold TCA 50% was used and incubated at 4 °C for 1 hr. Wells were washed and dried prior to tincture with 100 μL of SRB 0.4%. To remove excess SRB, acetic acid was used. For analysis, TRIS-Base Solution (pH = 10.5) was used and shaken prior to reading using an ELISA reader at 540 nm and the software SoftMax Pro 4.8. For each compound, 50% growth inhibition (GI_{50}) was calculated from sigmoidal dose-response curves (variable-slope) that were generated with data obtained from experiments carried out in triplicates (GI_{50} values were generated with GraphPad Prism V. 6.02, GraphPad Software, Inc.).

3.3.3. Wound Healing Assay (Scratch Method) Using MDA-MB-231 Cancer Cells

Prior to assays, cells were grown until 80–90% confluence was observed. We used a 75 cm^2 flask for 2.6×10^5 cells/mL in 10 mL, and for a 25 cm^2 flask 1.44×10^5 cells/mL in 5 mL. The cells were washed with PBS to remove all traces of FBS. We added trypsin at 2 mL for a 25 cm^2 flask or 4 mL for a 75 cm^2 flask, and incubated 5–10 min at 37 °C. At the end of the incubation time, cells were re-suspended and counted with hemocytometer using 1:2 dilutions with Trypan Blue. Subsequently, cell viability was calculated. In a 12 multiwell plate. Cells were seeded at $1.5–2.2 \times 10^5$ cells/mL in 1 mL and incubated for 24 h. Cells were then rinsed with PBS and incubated in starving media (0.5% FBS) overnight. All controls and drugs were tested in triplicate. The vehicle control for each drug was prepared according to the drug's DMSO concentration. Drugs were diluted and the final concentration at each well was 10 μM (or $GI_{50}/5$ on MDA-MB-231 cells). The wound was made using a sterile pipette tip of 200 μL. Cells were then rinsed very gently with media without FBS and media with vehicle controls or drugs were added. After a 24 h incubation, the gap distance was evaluated using the software Lumera Infinity Analyze 6.4.0. Pictures were taken at 0, 8, 12, and 24 h using a 10X objective in an Inverted Laboratory Microscope Leica DM IL LED, and an Infinity1-3 3.1 Megapixel USB 2.0 camera CMOS. The percentage of migration was calculated using the following formula:

$100 - [(X_0/\ddot{X}_0)]*100$ for time 0 h measurements
$100 - [(X_{24}/\ddot{X}_0)]*100$ for time 24 h measurements

3.3.4. Actin Polymerization Assay

MDA-MB-231 cells were treated with vehicle or compound derivatives at 10 μM (or at concentrations that do not affect cell viability) for 24 h at 37 °C in 5% CO_2. Cells were fixed in 3.7% of formaldehyde, permeabilized using 0.2% Triton, and stained with Rhodamine Phalloidin to visualize F-actin. Fluorescence micrographs were acquired at 60x in an Eclipse E400 fluorescence microscope using a DS-Qi2 monochrome digital camera from Nikon for fluorescence imaging.

4. Conclusions

In this study, a new series of N-alkyl-3,6-dibromocarbazole and N-alkyl-5-bromoindole derivatives were designed, synthesized, and biologically evaluated for their anti-cancer and anti-migration effect on MCF-7 and MDA-MB-231 cancer cells. In addition, the effect of compounds on the actin cytoskeleton of MDA-MB-231 cancer cells was explored. From the results, we have established the Structure-Activity Relationships of novel derivatives of the lead compound Wiskostatin. We found that the carbazole moiety is needed for in vitro anti-cancer and anti-migratory potency. The replacement of the carbazole by an indole ring resulted in loss of activity. Moreover, the aliphatic or aromatic amide group was extended 3-carbon atoms away from the carbazole moiety. The most potent anti-proliferative compounds were those bearing a 3,6-dibromocarbazole group with GI_{50} values between 7–32 μM and 4.7–23 μM on MCF-7 and MDA-MB-231 cancer cells, respectively. The most promising results in terms of anti-migratory effect was exhibited by carbazole derivatives **10**, **23**, **14–16**, and **24** with migration inhibition in the range of 10–20% on the highly metastatic breast cancer cells MDA-MB-231. Future studies will improve these derivatives and also test their effects at higher concentrations and shorter times of migration to reduce potential cytotoxic effects, which may confound inhibition of cell migration. The carbazole derivatives **10**, **14**, and **15** were further examined as actin polymerization inhibitors and results demonstrated reduction in actin polymerization and extension of F-actin based structures. Further studies of mechanism of actions focused on the effect of these novel compounds in the Cdc42/N-WASP/Arp2/3 pathway is needed to fully characterize and analyze the potential of this new series of compounds as in vitro and in vivo anti-metastatic drugs.

Author Contributions: K.B., Z.R., and A.F. performed the experiments and data collection; J.B. performed data analysis of GCMS; S.D. developed a methodology for actin assay experiments; and E.H. supervised, administrated, and was in charge of funding acquisition of the project. All authors read and approved the final manuscript.

Acknowledgments: We thank Fernando González-Illán from the US FDA for assisting with the high-resolution electrospray ionization mass spectrometry data and analysis.

References

1. Gupta, G.P.; Massagué, J. Cancer Metastasis: Building a Framework. *Cell* **2006**, *127*, 679–695. [CrossRef] [PubMed]

2. Walker, C.; Mojares, E.; Hernández, A.D.R. Role of Extracellular Matrix in Development and Cancer Progression. *Int. J. Mol. Sci.* **2018**, *19*, 3028. [CrossRef] [PubMed]

3. Chen, W.T. Proteolytic activity of specialized surface protrusions formed at rosette contact sites of transformed cells. *J. Exp. Zool.* **1989**, *251*, 167–185. [CrossRef] [PubMed]

4. Pollard, T.D.; Borisy, G.G. Cellular Motility Driven by Assembly and Disassembly of Actin Filaments. *Cell* **2003**, *113*, 549. [CrossRef]

5. Wertheimer, E.; Gutierrez-Uzquiza, A.; Rosemblit, C.; Lopez-Haber, C.; Sosa, M.S.; Kazanietz, M.G. Rac signaling in breast cancer: A tale of GEFs and GAPs. *Cell. Signal.* **2012**, *24*, 353–362. [CrossRef] [PubMed]

6. Muise, A.M.; Walters, T.; Xu, W.; Shen-Tu, G.; Guo, C.H.; Fattouh, R.; Lam, G.Y.; Wolters, V.M.; Bennitz, J.; Van Limbergen, J.; et al. Single nucleotide polymorphisms that increase expression of the guanosine triphosphatase RAC1 are associated with ulcerative colitis. *Gastroenterology* **2011**, *141*, 633–641.

7. (a) Worthylake, R.A.; Lemoine, S.; Watson, J.M.; Burridge, K. RhoA is required for monocyte tail retraction during transendothelial migration. *J. Cell Biol.* **2001**, *154*, 147–160, (b) Takenawa, T.; Miki, H. WASP and WAVE family proteins: key molecules for rapid rearrangement of cortical actin filaments and cell movement. *J. Cell Sci.* **2001**, *114*, 1801–1809. [CrossRef]

8. Rohatgi, R.; Ma, L.; Miki, H.; Lopez, M.; Kirchhausen, T.; Takenawa, T.; Kirschner, M.W. The Interaction between N-WASP and the Arp2/3 Complex Links Cdc42-Dependent Signals to Actin Assembly. *Cell* **1999**, *97*, 221–231. [CrossRef]

9.   Vlaar, C.P.; Castillo-Pichardo, L.; Medina, J.I.; Marrero-Serra, C.M.; Velez, E.; Ramos, Z.; Hernández, E. Design, synthesis and biological evaluation of new carbazole derivatives as anti-cancer and anti-migratory agents. *Biorganic. Med. Chem.* **2018**, *26*, 884–890. [CrossRef]

10. Montalvo-Ortiz, B.L.; Castillo-Pichardo, L.; Hernández, E.; Humphries-Bickley, T.; De La Mota-Peynado, A.; Cubano, L.A.; Vlaar, C.P.; Dharmawardhane, S. Characterization of EHop-016, novel small molecule inhibitor of Rac GTPase. *J. Biol. Chem.* **2012**, *287*, 13228–13238. [CrossRef]

11. Castillo-Pichardo, L.; Humphries-Bickley, T.; De La Parra, C.; Forestier-Roman, I.; Martinez-Ferrer, M.; Hernandez, E.; Vlaar, C.; Ferrer-Acosta, Y.; Washington, A.V.; Cubano, L.A.; et al. The Rac inhibitor EHop-016 inhibits mammary tumor growth and metastasis in a nude mouse model. *Transl. Oncol.* **2014**, *7*, 546–555. [CrossRef] [PubMed]

12. Dharmawardhane, S.; Hernandez, E.; Vlaar, C. Development of EHop-016: a small molecule inhibitor of Rac. *Enzymes* **2013**, *33*, 117–146. [PubMed]

13. Humphries-Bickley, T.; Castillo-Pichardo, L.; Corujo-Carro, F.; Duconge, J.; Hernandez-O'Farrill, E.; Vlaar, C.; Rodriguez-Orengo, J.F.; Cubano, L.; Dharmawardhane, S. Pharmacokinetics of Rac inhibitor EHop-016 in mice by ultra-performance liquid chromatography tandem mass spectrometry. *J. Chromatogr. B* **2015**, *981*, 19–26. [CrossRef] [PubMed]

14. Głuszyńska, A. Biological potential of carbazole derivatives. *Eur. J. Med. Chem.* **2015**, *94*, 405–426. [CrossRef] [PubMed]

15. Guillonneau, C.; Pierré, A.; Charton, Y.; Guilbaud, N.; Kraus-Berthier, L.; Léonce, S.; Michel, A.; Bisagni, E.; Atassi, G. Synthesis of 9-*O*-substituted derivatives of 9-hydroxy-5,6-dimethyl-6*H*-pyrido[4,3-*b*]carbazole-1-carboxylic acid (2-(Dimethylamino)-ethyl) amide and their 10-and 11-methyl analogues with improved antitumor activity. *J. Med. Chem.* **1999**, *42*, 2191–2203. [CrossRef] [PubMed]

16. Saturnino, C.; Iacopetta, D.; Sinicropi, M.; Rosano, C.; Caruso, A.; Caporale, A.; Marra, N.; Marengo, B.; Pronzato, M.; Parisi, O.; et al. N-alkyl carbazole derivatives as new tools for Alzheimer's disease: preliminary studies. *Molecules* **2014**, *19*, 9307–9317. [CrossRef] [PubMed]

17. Bandgar, B.P.; Adsul, L.K.; Chavan, H.V.; Jalde, S.S.; Shringare, S.N.; Shaikh, R.; Meshram, R.J.; Gacche, R.N.; Masand, V. Synthesis, biological evaluation, and docking studies of 3-(substituted)-aryl-5-(9-methyl-3-carbazole)-1H-2-pyrazolines as potent anti-inflammatory and antioxidant agents. *Bioorganic Med. Chem. Lett.* **2012**, *22*, 5839–5844. [CrossRef] [PubMed]

18. Biamonte, M.A.; Wanner, J.; Le Roch, K.G. Recent advances in malaria drug discovery. *Bioorganic Med. Chem. Lett.* **2013**, *23*, 2829–2843. [CrossRef]

19. Caruso, A.; Voisin-Chiret, A.S.; Lancelot, J.-C.; Sinicropi, M.S.; Garofalo, A.; Rault, S. Efficient and Simple Synthesis of 6-Aryl-1,4-dimethyl-9H-carbazoles. *Molecules* **2008**, *13*, 1312–1320. [CrossRef] [PubMed]

20. Chakrabarty, M.; Ghosh, N.; Harigaya, Y. A clay-mediated, regioselective synthesis of 2-(aryl/alkyl) amino-thiazolo [4, 5-c] carbazoles. *Tetrahedron Lett.* **2004**, *45*, 4955–4957. [CrossRef]

21. Caruso, A.; Sinicropi, M.S.; Lancelot, J.C.; El-Kashef, H.; Saturnino, C.; Aubert, G.; Ballandonne, C.; Lesnard, A.; Cresteil, T.; Dallemagne, P.; et al. Synthesis and evaluation of cytotoxic activities of new guanidines derived from carbazoles. *Bioorganic Med. Chem. Lett.* **2014**, *24*, 467–472. [CrossRef] [PubMed]

22. Iacopetta, D.; Rosano, C.; Puoci, F.; Parisi, O.I.; Saturnino, C.; Caruso, A.; Longo, P.; Ceramella, J.; Malzert-Fréon, A.; Dallemagne, P.; et al. Multifaceted properties of 1, 4-dimethylcarbazoles: Focus on trimethoxybenzamide and trimethoxyphenylurea derivatives as novel human topoisomerase II inhibitors. *Eur. J. Pharm. Sci.* **2017**, *96*, 263–272. [CrossRef] [PubMed]

23. Saturnino, C.; Palladino, C.; Napoli, M.; Sinicropi, M.S.; Botta, A.; Sala, M.; Carcereri de Prati, A.; Novellino, E.; Suzuki, H. Synthesis and biological evaluation of new N-alkylcarbazole derivatives as STAT3 inhibitors: Preliminary study. *Eur. J. Pharm. Sci.* **2013**, *60*, 112–119. [CrossRef] [PubMed]

24. Rizza, P.; Pellegrino, M.; Caruso, A.; Iacopetta, D.; Sinicropi, M.S.; Rault, S.; Lancelot, J.C.; El-Kashef, H.; Lesnard, A.; Rochais, C.; et al. 3-(Dipropylamino)-5-hydroxybenzofuro [2, 3-f] quinazolin-1 (2H)-one (DPA-HBFQ-1) plays an inhibitory role on breast cancer cell growth and progression. *Eur. J. Pharm. Sci.* **2016**, *107*, 275–287. [CrossRef] [PubMed]

25. Issa, S.; Walchshofer, N.; Kassab, I.; Termoss, H.; Chamat, S.; Geahchan, A.; Bouaziz, Z. Synthesis and antiproliferative activity of oxazinocarbazole and N,N-bis(carbazolylmethyl)amine derivatives. *Eur. J. Med. Chem.* **2010**, *45*, 2567–2577. [CrossRef] [PubMed]

26. Danish, I.A.; Prasad, K.J.R. A one-pot synthesis of 1, 2, 4, 5-tetraazaspiro [5.5]-6, 7, 8, 9-tetrahydrocarbazol-3-thiones and their antibacterial activities. *Indian J. Heterocycl. Chemstry* **2004**, *14*, 19–22.

27. Indumathi, T.; Fronczek, F.R.; Prasad, K.R. Synthesis of 2-amino-8-chloro-4-phenyl-5, 11-dihydro-6H-pyrido[2,3-a]carbazole-3-carbonitrile: Structural and biological evaluation. *J. Mol. Struct.* **2012**, *1016*, 134–139. [CrossRef]

28. Kantevari, S.; Yempala, T.; Surineni, G.; Sridhar, B.; Yogeeswari, P.; Sriram, D. Synthesis and antitubercular evaluation of novel dibenzo[b,d]furan and 9-methyl-9H-carbazole derived hexahydro-2H-pyrano[3,2-c]quinolines via Povarov reaction. *Eur. J. Med. Chem.* **2011**, *46*, 4827–4833. [CrossRef] [PubMed]

29. Woon, K.L.; Ariffin, A.; Ho, K.W.; Chen, S.-A. Effect of conjugation and aromaticity of 3,6 di-substituted carbazoles on triplet energy and the implication of triplet energy in multiple-cyclic aromatic compounds. *RSC Adv.* **2018**, *8*, 9850–9857. [CrossRef]

30. Bashir, M.; Bano, A.; Ijaz, A.S.; Chaudhary, B.A. Recent Developments and Biological Activities of N-Substituted Carbazole Derivatives: A Review. *Molecules* **2015**, *20*, 13496–13517. [CrossRef]

31. Mac Millan, K.S.; Naidoo, J.; Liang, J.; Melito, L.; Williams, L.S.; Morlock, L.; Huntington, P.J.; Estill, S.J.; Longood, J.; Becker, G.; et al. Development of Proneurogenic, Neuroprotective Small Molecules. *J. Am. Chem. Soc.* **2011**, *133*, 1428–1437. [CrossRef] [PubMed]

32. Molette, J.; Routier, J.; Abla, N.; Besson, D.; Bombrun, A.; Brun, R.; Burt, H.; Georgi, K.; Kaiser, M.; Nwaka, S.; et al. Identification and Optimization of an Aminoalcohol-Carbazole Series with Antimalarial Properties. *ACS Med. Chem. Lett.* **2013**, *4*, 1037–1041.

33. Saturnino, C.; Caruso, A.; Iacopetta, D.; Rosano, C.; Caramella, J.; Muia, N.; Mariconda, A.; Grazia Bonomo, M.; Ponassi, M.; Rosace, G.; et al. Inhibition of Human Topoisomerase II by N,N,N-Trimethylethanammonium Iodide Alkylcarbazole Derivatives. *Chem. Med. Chem.* **2018**, *13*, 2635–2643. [CrossRef] [PubMed]

34. Caruso, A.; Iacopetta, D.; Pouci, F.; Cappello, A.R.; Saturnino, C.; Sinicropi, M.S. Carbazole derivatives: A promising scenario for breast cancer treatment. *Mini Rev. Med. Chem.* **2016**, *16*, 630. [CrossRef] [PubMed]

35. Bombrun, A.; Gerber, P.; Casi, G.; Terradillos, O.; Antonsson, B.; Halazy, S. 3,6-dibromocarbazole piperazine derivatives of 2-propanol as first inhibitors of cytochrome c release via Bax channel modulation. *J. Med. Chem.* **2003**, *46*, 4365–4368. [CrossRef] [PubMed]

36. Zhang, Y.; Tangadanchu, V.K.R.; Cheng, Y.; Yang, R.G.; Lin, J.M.; Zhou, C.H. Potential Antimicrobial Isopropanol-Conjugated Carbazole Azoles as Dual Targeting Inhibitors of Enterococcus faecalis. *ACS Med. Chem. Lett.* **2018**, *9*, 244–249. [CrossRef]

37. Pieper, A.A.; Xie, S.; Capota, E.; Estill, S.J.; Zhong, J.; Long, J.M.; Becker, G.L.; Huntington, P.; Goldman, S.E.; Shen, C.-H.; et al. Discovery of a proneurogenic, neuroprotective chemical. *Cell* **2010**, *142*, 39. [CrossRef]

38. Peterson, J.R.; Bickford, L.C.; Morgan, D.; Kim, A.S.; Ouerfelli, O.; Kirschner, M.W.; Rosen, M.K. Chemical inhibition of N-WASP by stabilization of a native autoinhibited conformation. *Nat. Struct. Mol. Boil.* **2004**, *11*, 747–755. [CrossRef]

39. Guerriero, C.J.; Weisz, O.A. N-WASP inhibitor wiskostatin non-selectively perturbs membrane transport by decreasing cellular ATP levels. *Am. J. Physiol. Cell Physiol.* **2007**, *292*, C1562–C1566. [CrossRef]

40. Orellana, E.A.; Kasinski, A.L. Sulforhodamine B (SRB) Assay in Cell Culture to Investigate Cell Proliferation. *Bio-protocol* **2016**, *6*, e1984. [CrossRef]

41. Liang, C.C.; Park, A.Y.; Guan, J.L. In vitro scratch assay: A convenient and inexpensive method for analysis of cell migration in vitro. *Nat. Protoc.* **2007**, *2*, 329–333. [CrossRef] [PubMed]

42. Olson, M.F.; Sahai, E. The actin cytoskeleton in cancer cell motility. *Clin. Exp. Metastasis* **2009**, *26*, 273. [CrossRef] [PubMed]

43. Ridley, A.J. Rho GTPases and actin dynamics in membrane protrusions and vesicle trafficking. *Trends Cell Boil.* **2006**, *16*, 522–529. [CrossRef] [PubMed]

44. Takenawa, T.; Suetsugu, S. The WASP–WAVE protein network: Connecting the membrane to the cytoskeleton. *Nat. Rev. Mol. Cell Boil.* **2007**, *8*, 37–48. [CrossRef]

45. Frugtniet, B.; Jiang, W.G.; Martin, T.A.; Martin, T. Role of the WASP and WAVE family proteins in breast cancer invasion and metastasis. *Breast Cancer: Targets Ther.* **2015**, *7*, 99–109.

Macrocybin, a Natural Mushroom Triglyceride, Reduces Tumor Growth In Vitro and In Vivo through Caveolin-Mediated Interference with the Actin Cytoskeleton

Marcos Vilariño [1], Josune García-Sanmartín [1], Laura Ochoa-Callejero [1], Alberto López-Rodríguez [2], Jaime Blanco-Urgoiti [2] and Alfredo Martínez [1,*]

[1] Oncology Area, Center for Biomedical Research of La Rioja (CIBIR), 26006 Logroño, Spain; mvilarino@riojasalud.es (M.V.); jgarcias@riojasalud.es (J.G.-S.); locallejero@riojasalud.es (L.O.-C.)

[2] CsFlowchem, Campus Universidad San Pablo CEU, Boadilla del Monte, 28668 Madrid, Spain; alberto.lopez@csflowchem.com (A.L.-R.); jaime.blanco@csflowchem.com (J.B.-U.)

* Correspondence: amartinezr@riojasalud.es;

Academic Editor: Thomas J. Schmidt

Abstract: Mushrooms have been used for millennia as cancer remedies. Our goal was to screen several mushroom species from the rainforests of Costa Rica, looking for new antitumor molecules. Mushroom extracts were screened using two human cell lines: A549 (lung adenocarcinoma) and NL20 (immortalized normal lung epithelium). Extracts able to kill tumor cells while preserving non-tumor cells were considered "anticancer". The mushroom with better properties was *Macrocybe titans*. Positive extracts were fractionated further and tested for biological activity on the cell lines. The chemical structure of the active compound was partially elucidated through nuclear magnetic resonance, mass spectrometry, and other ancillary techniques. Chemical analysis showed that the active molecule was a triglyceride containing oleic acid, palmitic acid, and a more complex fatty acid with two double bonds. The synthesis of all possible triglycerides and biological testing identified the natural compound, which was named Macrocybin. A xenograft study showed that Macrocybin significantly reduces A549 tumor growth. In addition, Macrocybin treatment resulted in the upregulation of Caveolin-1 expression and the disassembly of the actin cytoskeleton in tumor cells (but not in normal cells). In conclusion, we have shown that Macrocybin constitutes a new biologically active compound that may be taken into consideration for cancer treatment.

Keywords: natural product; therapeutic triglyceride; xenograft study; Caveolin-1; actin cytoskeleton

1. Introduction

The discovery of new anticancer drugs can be accomplished through different approaches, including the screening of natural products, and the testing of synthetic compound libraries, computer-assisted design, and machine learning, among others [1]. Living organisms constitute an almost unlimited source of compounds with potential biological activity and, so far, have provided the majority of currently approved therapies for the treatment of cancer [2,3]. A few examples include taxol, which was obtained from the bark of the Pacific Yew tree [4,5], vinblastine and related alkaloids from *Vinca* [6], camptothecin from the bark of a Chinese tree [7], or trabectedin and other drugs which were purified from marine organisms [8]. In addition, many natural products are the basis for further chemical development and the rational design of synthetic drugs [9].

The mechanisms of action by which natural products reduce cancer cell growth are diverse. In the case of taxanes, direct interaction with tubulin results in cytoskeleton hyperpolymerization and mitosis arrest [10]; vinblastine has the reverse effect, depolymerizing the cytoskeleton, but achieves the same final outcome, stopping cell division [10]; others, such as some mushroom extracts, induce immunomodulation [11,12], or affect other cancer hallmarks [13].

Mushrooms have been used for millennia in Eastern traditional medicine as cancer remedies [13,14] and recent scientific publications have corroborated the presence of anticancer molecules in mushroom extracts. For instance, some polysaccharides from *Ganoderma* possess anticancer activity through immunomodulatory, anti-proliferative, pro-apoptotic, anti-metastatic, and anti-angiogenic effects [15]; lentinan, a β-glucan from *Lentinus* is licensed as a drug for treating gastric cancer where it activates the complement system [16]; other β-glucans from *Ganoderma* and *Grifola* [17] also show great potential as modulators of the immune system; lectins from *Clitocybe* provide distinct carbohydrate-binding specificities, showing immunostimulatory and adhesion-/phagocytosis-promoting properties [18]; furthermore, triterpenoids from *Inonotus* have been shown to induce apoptosis in lung cancer cell lines [19]. In addition, the immense number of mushroom species around the world [20], and their sessile nature, suggests that many fungal natural products may still be waiting for discovery.

Our goal in this study was to screen a number of scarcely known mushroom species collected in the rain forest of Costa Rica looking for new antitumor molecules. The most potent extract was found in specimens of *Macrocybe titans*, a local mushroom of very large proportions which usually grows in the anthills of leaf cutter ants [21]. The molecule responsible for the anticancer activity was isolated, characterized, and synthesized, and its "anticancer" properties were demonstrated both in vitro and in vivo.

2. Results

Several mushroom species were collected in the rainforests of Costa Rica, classified by expert botanists, and brought to the laboratory for extract preparation. Each specimen was subjected to several extraction procedures, including water- and ethanol-based techniques. All extracts were freeze-dried and sent to the Center for Biomedical Research of La Rioja (CIBIR) for anticancer activity testing in cell lines. Several extracts from different species showed some "anticancer" properties, defined as the ability to destroy cancer cells while being innocuous to nontumoral cells (Figure 1).

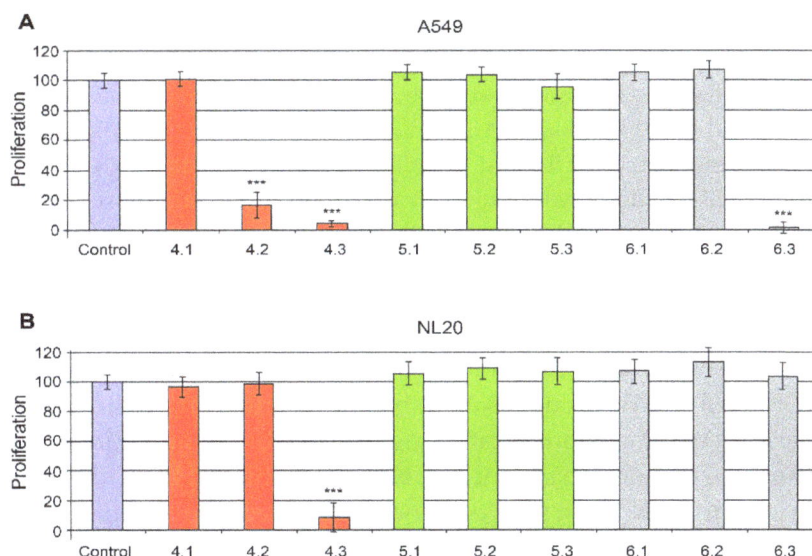

Figure 1. Toxicity of different mushroom extracts on cell lines A549 (**A**) and NL20 (**B**). All extracts were added at 0.3 mg/mL in a growth medium containing 1% FBS and incubated for 5 days. Comparing extract effects in both cell lines, three behaviors can be identified: (i) no effect on either cell line (extract 4.1, for example), (ii) toxic for both cell lines (extract 4.3), and (iii) "antitumoral" effect (toxic for A549 and nontoxic for NL20, extracts 4.2 and 6.3). Bars represent the mean ± SD of 8 independent measures. ***: $p < 0.001$ vs. control.

The most promising sample was the precipitated phase of a 95% ethanol extract from the mushroom *Macrocybe titans*. Specifically, we began with 3.5 Kg of fresh mushroom specimens. These were dried to obtain 367.2 g of dry mushroom powder, which was extracted with two washes, 30 min each, in 500 mL 95% ethanol at room temperature, with ultrasounds. The ethanol extracts were kept at −20 °C for 24 h and, then, the soluble phase was separated from the precipitate. This species was chosen for further analysis.

The initial extract was fractionated following different techniques and the resulting fractions were tested again in the cell lines to follow the anticancer activity. The finally successful strategy consisted of an initial alkaloidal separation, followed by column chromatography with polymeric resin (HP20-SS) using different mobile phases. The best ratio of selectivity was obtained with an IPA:CH2Cl2 8:2 mobile phase at pH 12.0 (Figure 2).

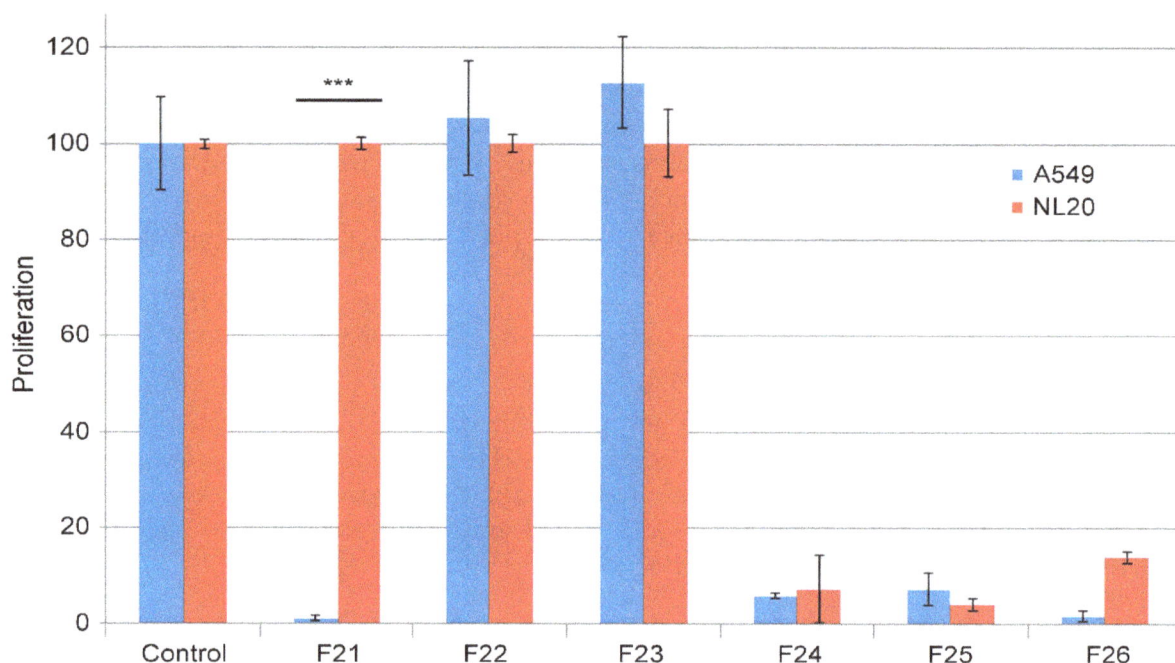

Figure 2. Toxicity of several fractions obtained by chromatography of the initial *M. titans* extract on cell lines A549 (blue bars) and NL20 (red bars). All extracts were added at 0.3 mg/mL in a growth medium containing 1% FBS and incubated for 5 days. Fraction 21 (F21) presents the desired characteristics of destroying the cancer cells while preserving the nontumoral cells. Bars represent the mean ± SD of 8 independent measures. ***: $p < 0.001$ between cell lines.

Once the molecule responsible for the differential growth inhibitory activity was pure enough, the final fraction was subjected to nuclear magnetic resonance (NMR), mass spectrometry, and 2D-COSY (Supplementary Materials, Natural extract characterization) to determine its chemical structure.

Data analysis identified our molecule as a triglyceride containing palmitic acid, oleic acid, and a more complex fatty acid of 18–20 carbons containing two double bonds. Since the final structure was impossible to determine, we decided to synthesize all compatible triglycerides (Table 1) and test them for biological activity with the cell lines. The presence of the two double bonds provides the molecule with optical activity. Some molecules were synthesized as racemic mixtures. For other molecules, both enantiomers were synthesized and tested. From the 10 triglycerides that were synthesized (Table 1) only one exerted differential growth inhibitory activity, specifically the R enantiomer of TG (C18:2, 9z,12z; C16:0; C18:1, 9z) (Supplementary Materials, Growth modulatory activity of synthetic triglycerides). A search of the Chemical Abstract database came out negative, indicating that this is a new structure. This triglyceride was named Macrocybin because of its origin from the *Macrocybe titans* mushroom.

Table 1. Triglycerides synthesized for this study and the chemical structure of Macrocybin. The structure of the other triglycerides is shown in Supplementary Materials (Triglyceride synthesis).

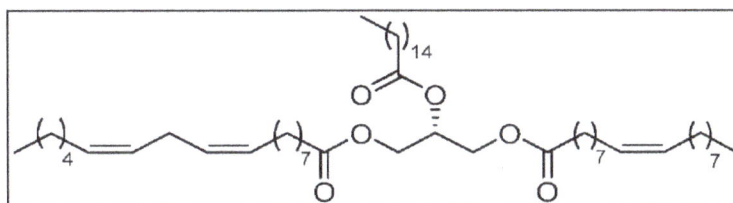

Internal Code	Chemical Formula
TG1	TG (C16:0; C18:1, 9z; C20:2, 11z,14z)
TG2	TG (C16:0; C20:2, 11z,14z; C18:1, 9z)
TG3	TG (C16:0; C18:1, 9z; C18:1, 9z)
TG4	TG (C18:0; C18:1, 9z; C18:2, 9z,12z)
TG5	2S-TG (C20:2, 11z,14z; C18:1, 9z; C16:0)
TG6	2R-TG (C20:2, 11z,14z; C18:1, 9z; C16:0)
TG7	2S-TG (C20:2, 11z,14z; C16:0; C18:1, 9z)
TG8	2R-TG (C20:2, 11z,14z; C16:0; C18:1, 9z)
TG9	2S-TG (C18:2, 9z,12z; C16:0; C18:1, 9z)
TG10 (Macrocybin)	2R-TG (C18:2, 9z,12z; C16:0; C18:1, 9z)

To determine the similarities between the synthetic molecule and the mushroom fraction, their NMR spectra were compared (Figure 3) and they were very similar.

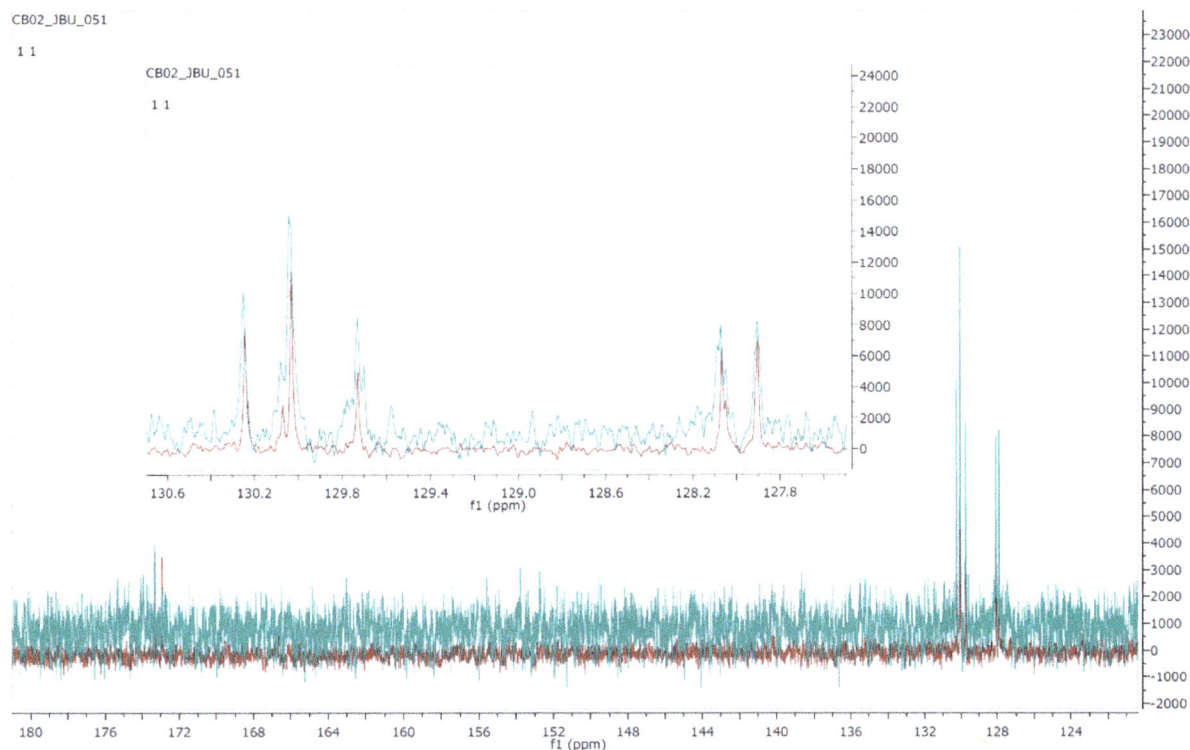

Figure 3. Comparison of ^{13}C-NMR spectra of olefinic carbons of the synthetic triglyceride TG10 (red) and the natural extract (green). Spectra comparing the aliphatic carbons are shown in Supplementary Materials.

Toxicity assays for TG10 demonstrated a wide ratio of selectivity between A549 and NL20, with IC_{50} values of 13.4 and 50.1 μg/mL, respectively (Figure 4), thus confirming the in vitro anticancer activity of the synthetic triglyceride, Macrocybin.

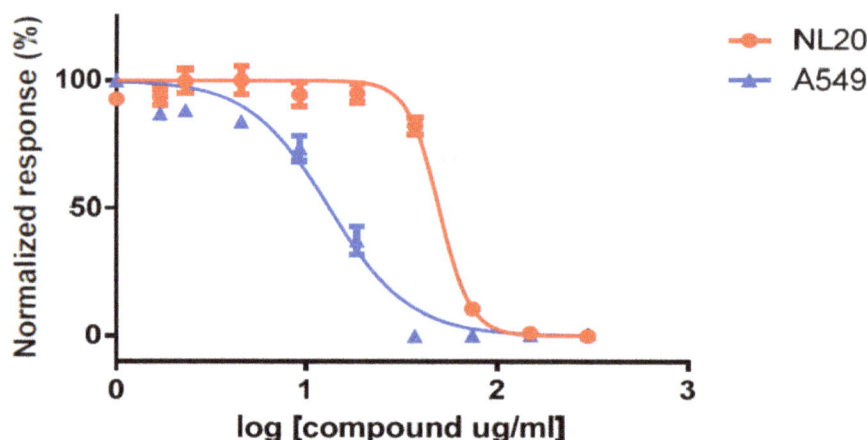

Figure 4. Concentration-dependent toxicity of synthetic Macrocybin on cell lines A549 (blue triangles) and NL20 (red circles). The synthetic triglyceride is more toxic for tumor cells than for nontumoral cells. Error bars represent the SD of 8 independent measures.

To determine whether this new molecule had antitumor properties in vivo, a xenograft study was performed, using A549 as the tumor-initiating cell. Tumors of mice receiving vehicle injections grew progressively until they reached the maximum volume allowed for humane reasons and the mice had to be sacrificed. On the other hand, tumors injected with Macrocybin grew somewhat more slowly ($p < 0.05$ after 40 days of treatment), indicating a therapeutic function for the triglyceride (Figure 5).

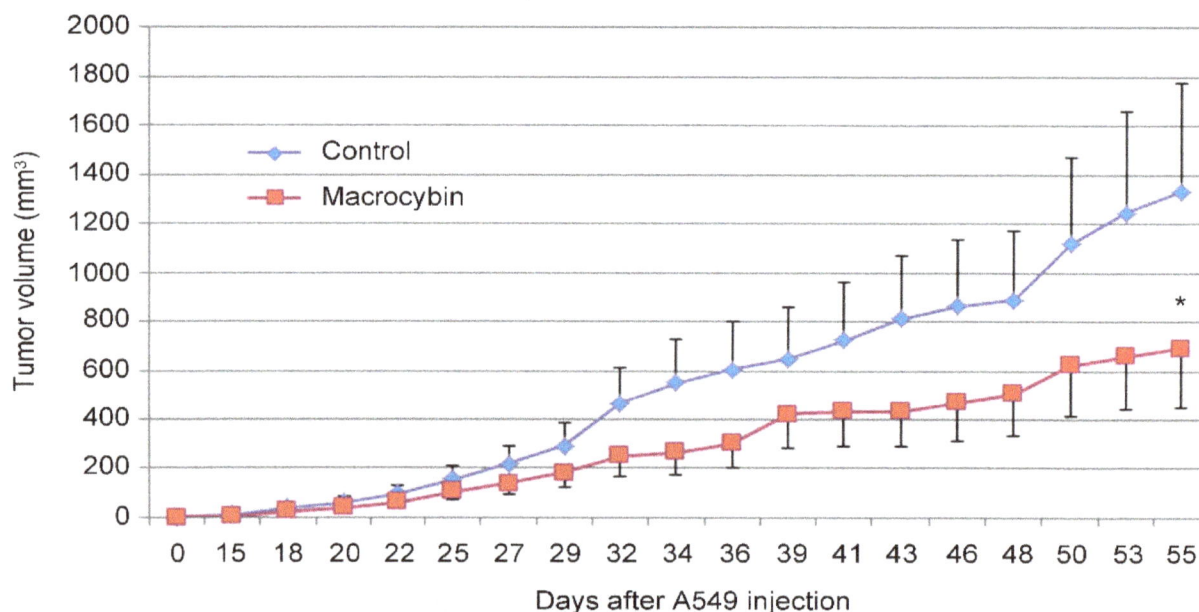

Figure 5. Xenograft experiment. Evolution of tumor volume in control (blue diamonds) and Macrocybin treated (red squares) A549 tumors grown in the flank of experimental mice. Cell injection was performed on day 0, and intratumoral injection began on day 15. There was a significant difference between treatments (ANOVA, $p < 0.05$). Each point represents the mean ± SD for 10 mice. *: $p < 0.05$ between treatments. Raw data values are shown in the Supplementary Materials.

To investigate the potential mechanism of action driving this antitumor activity, A549 and NL20 cells were stained with cytoskeleton-labeling moieties after exposure to Macrocybin. No differences were found in the tubulin cytoskeleton (results not shown) but the actin cytoskeleton, as stained with phallacidin, was dismantled in A549 tumor cells by the triglyceride, whereas it was unaffected in NL20 cells. The actin molecules of A549 translocated to the cell membrane forming filopodia (Figure 6).

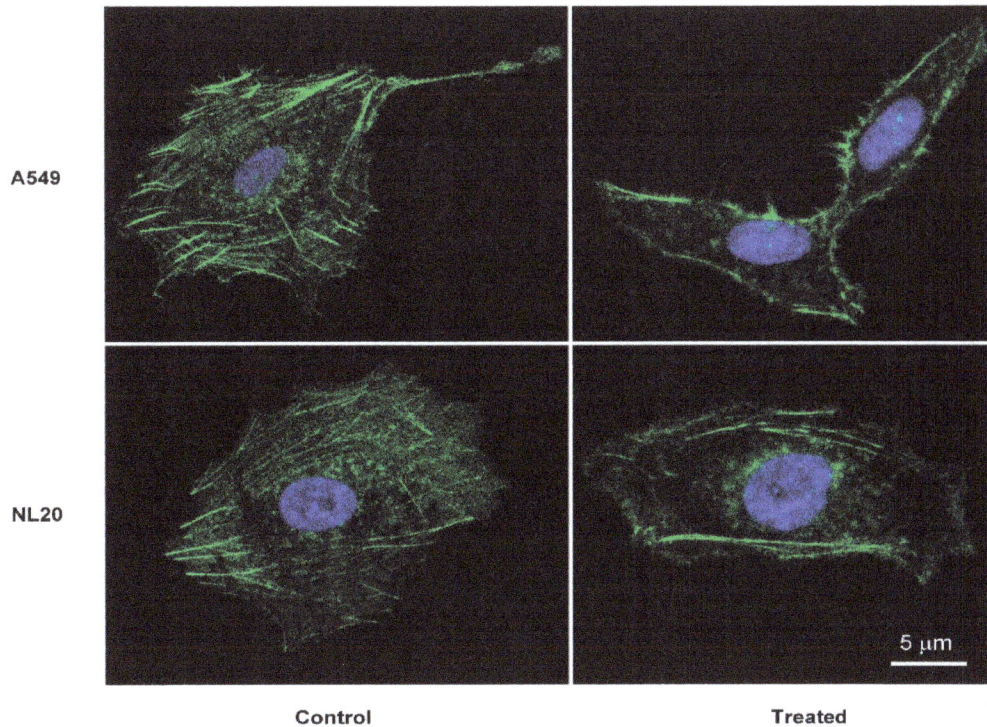

Figure 6. Representative confocal microscopy images of A549 and NL20 cells treated, or not (control), with 37 μg/mL Macrocybin for 24 h. The actin cytoskeleton was stained with Bodipy-phallacidin (green) and the nuclei with DAPI (blue). Following treatment, A549 cells lose their stress fibers and actin migrates to the cell membrane to produce small filopodia. Scale bar = 5 μm.

Macrocybin is a complex lipid and, as such, could be internalized into the cell through a number of lipid transport mechanisms [22]. To investigate whether a preferential transport into tumoral cells takes place, we analyzed Macrocybin-induced changes in lipid transport molecules (Table 2) through qRT-PCR. A549 and NL20 cells were seeded in 6-well plates and Macrocybin (or PBS as the vehicle) was added at 37 μg/mL for 6 h. The only significant differences were found for Caveolin-1 whose expression increased significantly ($p < 0.05$) in Macrocybin-treated A549 cells over the untreated controls. In contrast, Macrocybin did not affect Caveolin-1 expression in NL20 cells (Figure 7).

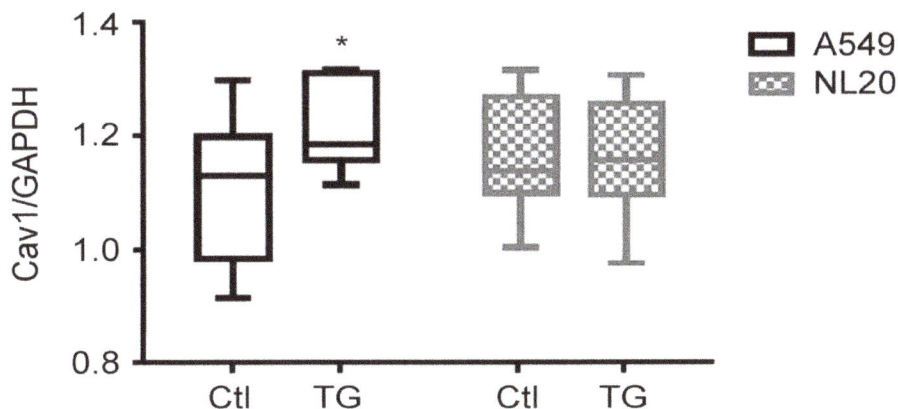

Figure 7. Gene expression for A549 and NL20 cells that were treated with 37 μg/mL Macrocybin (or control) for 6 h. Several lipid membrane transport proteins were analyzed by qRT-PCR. The only changes were observed in the expression of Caveolin-1 (Cav1) on treated A549 cells. Caveolin expression values were relativized to the housekeeping gene GAPDH. *: $p < 0.05$ vs. control (CTL). This is a representative example of 3 independent experiments. Raw data values are provided in the Supplementary Materials.

3. Discussion

We have shown that the Costa Rican mushroom *Macrocybe titans* has "anticancer" properties. The molecule responsible for this activity was isolated to purity and identified as a complex triglyceride with formula 2R-TG (C18:2, 9z,12z; C16:0; C18:1, 9z). This molecule was named Macrocybin and was synthesized in the laboratory. The synthetic molecule retained the "anticancer" properties both in vitro and in a xenograft model in vivo. The mechanism of action of the new molecule involves Caveolin-1 overexpression and actin cytoskeleton disorganization in the cancer cells.

The mushroom *M. titans* is a species that inhabits the tropical and subtropical regions of America and has been found between Florida and Argentina [23]. Other species of the same genus are found in tropical regions around the world, and include *M. gigantea* (India), *M. crassa* (Sri Lanka), *M. lobayensis* (Ghana), and *M. spectabilis* (Mauritius), among others [21]. *Macrocybe titans* arguably produces the largest carpophores in the world of fungi, with some specimens reaching 100 cm in diameter and weighing up to 20 Kg [21]. Interestingly, the specimens found in Costa Rica appear predominantly in the vicinity of the nests of gardening ants (*Atta cephalotes*) suggesting a potential symbiotic relationship between these two species [21]. All members of the *Macrocybe* genus are considered edible [24]. Although these mushrooms have not been reported as medicinal remedies in traditional pharmacopeia, recent studies have found that some polysaccharides of *M. titans* inhibit melanoma cell migration [25] and that the fruiting body of *M. gigantea* contains antimicrobial compounds [26]. These discoveries underscore the need for preserving biodiversity as a source for novel drugs and drug precursors [27].

The idea of a triglyceride acting as a therapy against cancer may seem rather counterintuitive. High levels of triglycerides in the blood constitute a clear risk for cancer initiation and progression since they provide a rich source of energy for developing tumors [28] and may increase metastatic potential [29]. Nevertheless, there are some specific types of cancer, such as breast [30] or prostate [28], where high levels of circulating triglycerides correlate with a better prognosis. In addition, a few studies have identified specific lipids with therapeutic functions. For instance, conjugated linoleic acid has been described as a natural anticarcinogenic compound [31].

Our studies testing the anticancer efficacy of different synthetic candidates indicate a high level of specificity in the anticancer actions of Macrocybin. Even the S enantiomer of Macrocybin was devoid of physiological activity. This indicates that the anticancer activity is dependent on a very specific interaction of Macrocybin with biological components (receptors and/or membrane transporters) of the tumor cells, rather than a bulk role, such as energy provider (a role that generic blood triglycerides may play).

Macrocybin was able to reduce tumor growth in a xenograft model of human lung cancer. As a triglyceride, Macrocybin has a modest solubility in water-based vehicles. Perhaps future formulations using micelles [32] or nanoparticles [33] may increase Macrocybin biodisponibility and antitumor efficacy. Furthermore, combinations of Macrocybin with other chemotherapeutic or immunotherapeutic drugs may represent promising avenues to reduce tumor burden [34].

Our results show that Macrocybin differentially affects the actin cytoskeleton of tumor vs. nontumor cells and that this mechanism is mediated by changes in the expression of Caveolin-1. Caveolin-1 has been shown as a lipid transporter in a variety of cell types [35–37]. Changes in the expression of this protein have been related to lung cancer prognosis [38], although some studies suggest that this relationship may be context-dependent [39]. This protein may constitute the entry point for Macrocybin into the cell and the fact that its expression is affected in tumor cells but not in nontumor cells may partially explain the preferential toxicity of the triglyceride for cancer cells.

Disruption of the actin cytoskeleton is a common mechanism of action for many natural products with antitumor properties. For instance, proteoglucans extracted from *Grifola* mushrooms affect actin cytoskeleton rearrangements, thus decreasing breast cancer cell motility [40]. Cucurbitacin I disrupts actin filaments in A549 cells, resulting in a reduction in lung cancer cell growth [41]. Enterolactone, a flaxseed-derived lignan, alters Focal Adhesion Kinase-Sarcoma Protein (FAK-Src) signaling and disorganizes the actin cytoskeleton, suppressing the migration and invasion of lung cancer cells [42]. Another example is narciclasine, an isocarbostyril alkaloid isolated from *Amaryllidaceae* plants, which impairs actin cytoskeleton organization and induces apoptosis in brain cancers [43]. All these studies suggest that interfering with the actin cytoskeleton of tumor cells provides a useful approach to induce tumor cell death and to prevent metastasis by reducing tumor cell motility.

Given the ubiquity among cancer cells of Caveolin-1 and the actin cytoskeleton, Macrocybin may constitute a common therapeutic agent for a variety of cancers. Many further investigations will be necessary to evaluate, in more detail, the usefulness of Macrocybin as an antitumoral drug or lead structure. These studies must include, among others, studies on the systemic applicability of Macrocybin. Future studies would also have to investigate whether other tumors are also susceptible to this new antitumor compound.

4. Materials and Methods

4.1. Mushroom Collection and Extract Preparation

Several mushroom specimens belonging to different species were collected in the rainforests of Costa Rica by expert personnel of the Instituto Nacional de Biodiversidad de Costa Rica (INBio, Santo Domingo, Costa Rica), under a specific permit issued by the Costa Rican Government (Oficina Técnica de la Comisión Nacional de la Gestión de la Biodiversidad, CONAGEBIO, San José, Costa Rica). Mushroom fragments were subjected to different extraction procedures, including crude extracts, extraction in hot water (80 °C) for several 30 min incubations, or in 95% ethanol at 50 °C for several 30 min incubations, with different exposures to ultrasound treatments. Final fractions, including the pellet and supernatant of each extraction, were freeze-dried and sent to CIBIR for screening. Voucher samples (FRS 01) of the fungal collection are kept at INBio (Santo Domingo, Costa Rica).

4.2. Anticancer Screening Strategy (Toxicity Assays)

Two human cell lines were used to screen the "anticancer" properties of the mushroom extracts: lung adenocarcinoma A549, and non-tumoral immortalized bronchiolar epithelial cell line NL20 (ATCC). Both cell lines were exposed in parallel to different concentrations of particular extracts for 5 days, and cytotoxicity was measured by the MTS method (Cell Titer, Promega, Madison, WI, USA), as reported in [44]. To identify a sample as having "anticancer" properties, it had to destroy cancer cells while preserving non-tumoral cells (or at least showing a wide therapeutic window between both lines). This strategy was used iteratively to guide extract purification until the final molecule could be identified.

Following ATCC's protocols, A549 cells were maintained in Ham's F12 medium containing 10% fetal bovine serum (FBS) and NL20 cells in complete medium (Ham's F12 with 2 mM L-glutamine, 1.5 g/L sodium bicarbonate, 2.7 g/L D-glucose, 0.1 mM NEAA, 0.005 mg/mL insulin, 10 ng/mL EGF, 0.001 mg/mL transferrin, 500 ng/mL hydrocortisone, and 4% FBS).

Before starting the project, optimization of the toxicity assay was performed, testing different numbers of cells per well, days of incubation with the extracts, and FBS contents. We wanted all cells to receive the same number of extracts in the same medium. We, therefore, chose the NL20 medium, which is the most complex and restrictive. FBS concentration was reduced to 1% to allow for a 5-day incubation period. Specifically, A549 and NL20 were seeded in 96-well plates at different densities (2000 and 10,000 cells/well, respectively) in a complete NL20 medium containing 1% FBS, in a final volume of 50 μL/well, and incubated at 37 °C in a humidified atmosphere, containing 5% CO_2. The next day, extracts were added at the indicated concentrations, in another 50 μL/well, in the same medium, and incubated for 5 days. At the end of this period, 15 μL of Cell Titer were added per well and, after an additional incubation of 4 h, color intensity was assessed in a plate reader (POLARstar Omega, BMG Labtech, Ortenberg, Germany) at 490 nm.

To determine IC_{50} values, treatments were diluted at 0.6 mg/mL in test medium and 8 serial double dilutions were prepared. These solutions were added to cells and incubated as above. For each concentration point, 8 independent repeats were performed. Graphs and IC_{50} values were obtained with GraphPad Prism 8.3.0 software.

Cell lines were authenticated by STR profiling (IDEXX BioAnalytics, Westbroock, ME, USA).

4.3. Fractionation Strategies

The mushroom with the highest anticancer activity was chosen for further analysis. The initial extract was subjected to different fractionation protocols, which included different chromatographic techniques. Each time new fractions were separated, they were analyzed for their "anticancer" properties through cell line screening (as above) and the positive fractions were subjected to further fractionation until a pure enough compound, that could be identified through analytical chemistry methods, was obtained.

Many combinations were tested, but the one that resulted in final successful purification included alkaloidal separation, followed by column chromatography with polymeric resin HP20-SS, using different mobile phases.

4.4. Elucidation of the Compound's Chemical Structure

The final extract was subjected to analytical techniques, including ^{1}H-nuclear magnetic resonance (NMR), ^{13}C-NMR, DEPT-135-NMR, mass spectroscopy (Q-TOF), and bidimensional experiments heteronuclear multiplke-quantum correlation (HMQC) and correlation spectroscopy (COSY). Interpretation of the data indicated that the new compound was a triglyceride and the component fatty acids were identified to a certain degree of confidence, but the exact location of the fatty acids in the triglyceride, and the position of the two double bonds in the more complex fatty acid, could not be completely determined. Therefore, we synthesized the most probable molecules (Table 1) and tested them with our cell line screening strategy. Given the presence of two double bonds in one of the fatty acids, the triglyceride demonstrated optical activity. Therefore, both enantiomers were synthesized (Table 1) and tested.

4.5. Triglyceride Synthesis

The molecules in Table 1 were synthesized following standard techniques. The details are shown in the Supplementary Materials (Triglyceride synthesis).

4.6. Anticancer Activity in a Xenograft Model

Once the active synthetic molecule (Macrocybin) was available, it was tested in vivo following standard protocols [45]. Briefly, 10×10^6 A549 cells were injected in the flank of twenty 8-week-old non-obese diabetic (NOD) *scid* gamma mice (NSG, Stock No. 005557, The Jackson Laboratory). Animals were randomly divided into 2 experimental groups and when tumors became palpable, they were injected intratumorally with 100 µL of the vehicle (PBS) in the control group ($n = 10$), or with 0.1 mg/mL Macrocybin in 100 µL of PBS in the treatment group ($n = 10$), three times a week. Just before injection, tumor volume was estimated with a caliper by measuring the maximum length and width of the tumor and by applying the following formula: Volume = $(width)^2 \times length/2$ [46]. When tumor volume reached 2000 mm^3, mice were sacrificed for ethical consideration.

All procedures involving animals were carried out in accordance with the European Communities Council Directive (2010/63/UE), and Spanish legislation (RD53/2013) on animal experiments, and with approval from CIBIR's committee on the ethical use of animals (Órgano Encargado del Bienestar Animal del Centro de Investigación Biomédica de La Rioja, OEBA-CIBIR).

4.7. Cytoskeleton Staining and Confocal Microscopy

To test whether Macrocybin, like other natural products, acts through cytoskeleton interactions, A549 and NL20 cells were seeded in 8-well chamber slides (Lab-Tek II), treated with different concentrations of Macrocybin (or the vehicle) for 24 h, washed, fixed with 10% formalin, and permeabilized for 10 min with 0.1% Triton X-100. For cytoskeleton imaging, cells were exposed to 1:1000 mouse anti-tubulin antibody (T6074, Sigma-Aldrich, Sant Louis, MI, USA) overnight at 4 °C, washed with PBS, incubated with a mixture of 1:200 Bodipy-phallacidin (Molecular Probes) and 1:400 goat-anti mouse IgG labeled with Alexa Fluor 633 (A-21052, Invitrogen, Waltham, MA, USA), and washed again. Nuclear staining was achieved with DAPI (ProLong Gold Antifade Mountant, Invitrogen). Slides were observed with a confocal microscope (TCS SP5, Leica, Badalona, Spain).

4.8. Gene Expression

To identify the cellular pathways potentially involved in Macrocybin action, mRNA was extracted from treated and untreated A549 and NL20 cells using the RNeasy MiniKit (Qiagen, Hilden, Germany). Total RNA (1 µg) was reverse transcribed using the SuperScriptR III Reverse Transcriptase Kit (Thermo Fisher Scientific, Waltham, MA, USA), and quantitative real-time PCR was performed as described [47]. Specific primers are shown in Table 2. GAPDH was used as a housekeeping gene.

Table 2. Primers used for qRT-PCR in this study. Annealing temperature was 60 °C for all primers. GAPDH was used as a housekeeping gene.

Target Gene	Forward Primer	Reverse Primer	Amplicon Size
CAV1	GCGACCCTAAACACCTCAAC	CAGCAAGCGGTAAAACCAGT	149
hGOT2_F (=FABPpm)	TGGTGCCTACCGGGATGATA	GGCAGAAAGACATCTCGGCT	153
hSLC27A1_F (=FATP1)	GCCAAATCGGGGAGTTCTAC	TTGAAACCACAGGAGCCGA	85
hSLC27A4_F (=FATP4)	CAAGACCATCAGGCGCGATA	CCGAACGGTAGAGGCAAACA	118
GAPDH	AAATCCCATCACCATCTTCC	GACTCCACGACGTACTCAGC	81

4.9. Statistical Analysis

All datasets were tested for normalcy and homoscedasticity. Normally distributed data were evaluated by Student's t test or by ANOVA followed by the Dunnet's post hoc test while data not following a normal distribution were analyzed with the Kruskal–Wallis test followed by the Mann–Whitney U test. All data were analyzed with GraphPad Prism 8.3.0 software and were considered statistically significant when $p < 0.05$.

5. Conclusions

In conclusion, we have shown that the natural mushroom product, Macrocybin, is a new, biologically active compound that reduces tumor growth by disassembling the actin cytoskeleton, providing a potential new strategy to fight cancer.

Author Contributions: Conceptualization, M.V., and A.M.; methodology, J.G.-S., L.O.-C., A.L.-R., and J.B.-U.; formal analysis, J.G.-S., L.O.-C., A.L.-R., and J.B.-U.; investigation, M.V., J.G.-S., L.O.-C., A.L.-R., and J.B.-U.; data curation, J.G.-S., L.O.-C., J.B.-U., and A.M.; writing—original draft preparation, A.M.; writing—review and editing, A.M.; supervision, A.M. All authors have read and agreed to the published version of the manuscript.

Acknowledgments: The authors gratefully acknowledge the work of Kattia Rosales and her colleagues collecting specimens at the Instituto Nacional de Biodiversidad de Costa Rica (INBio).

References

1.   Hu, Y.; Zhao, T.; Zhang, N.; Zhang, Y.; Cheng, L. A Review of Recent Advances and Research on Drug Target Identification Methods. *Curr. Drug Metab.* **2019**, *20*, 209–216. [CrossRef] [PubMed]

2.   Rates, S. Plants as source of drugs. *Toxicon* **2001**, *39*, 603–613. [CrossRef]

3.   Newman, D.J.; Cragg, G.M. Natural Products as Sources of New Drugs over the Last 25 Years. *J. Nat. Prod.* **2007**, *70*, 461–477. [CrossRef] [PubMed]

4.   Guéritte-Voegelein, F.; Guenard, D.; Potier, P. Taxol and Derivatives: A Biogenetic Hypothesis. *J. Nat. Prod.* **1987**, *50*, 9–18. [CrossRef]

5.   Barbuti, A.M.; Chen, Z.-S. Paclitaxel Through the Ages of Anticancer Therapy: Exploring Its Role in Chemoresistance and Radiation Therapy. *Cancers* **2015**, *7*, 2360–2371. [CrossRef]

6.   Martino, E.; Casamassima, G.; Castiglione, S.; Cellupica, E.; Pantalone, S.; Papagni, F.; Rui, M.; Siciliano, A.M.; Collina, S. Vinca alkaloids and analogues as anti-cancer agents: Looking back, peering ahead. *Bioorg. Med. Chem. Lett.* **2018**, *28*, 2816–2826. [CrossRef]

7.   Wall, M.E.; Wani, M.C.; Cook, C.E.; Palmer, K.H.; McPhail, A.T.; Sim, G.A. Plant Antitumor Agents. I. The Isolation and Structure of Camptothecin, a Novel Alkaloidal Leukemia and Tumor Inhibitor from Camptotheca acuminata1,2. *J. Am. Chem. Soc.* **2005**, *88*, 3888–3890. [CrossRef]

8.   Jimenez, P.; Wilke, D.V.; Branco, P.C.; Bauermeister, A.; Rezende-Teixeira, P.; Susana, G.; Costa-Lotufo, L.V. Enriching cancer pharmacology with drugs of marine origin. *Br. J. Pharmacol.* **2020**, *177*, 3–27. [CrossRef]

9.   Hamburger, M.; Hostettmann, K. 7. Bioactivity in plants: The link between phytochemistry and medicine. *Phytochemistry* **1991**, *30*, 3864–3874. [CrossRef]

10. Matson, D.R.; Stukenberg, P.T. Spindle Poisons and Cell Fate: A Tale of Two Pathways. *Mol. Interv.* **2011**, *11*, 141–150. [CrossRef]

11. Guggenheim, A.G.; Wright, K.M.; Zwickey, H.L. Immune Modulation From Five Major Mushrooms: Application to Integrative Oncology. *Integr. Med.* **2014**, *13*, 32–44.

12. Benson, K.F.; Stamets, P.; Davis, R.; Nally, R.; Taylor, A.; Slater, S.; Jensen, G.S. The mycelium of the Trametes versicolor (Turkey tail) mushroom and its fermented substrate each show potent and complementary immune activating properties in vitro. *BMC Complement. Altern. Med.* **2019**, *19*, 1–14. [CrossRef] [PubMed]

13. Blagodatski, A.; Yatsunskaya, M.; Mikhailova, V.; Tiasto, V.; Kagansky, A.; Katanaev, V.L. Medicinal mushrooms as an attractive new source of natural compounds for future cancer therapy. *Oncotarget* **2018**, *9*, 29259–29274. [CrossRef] [PubMed]

14. Sullivan, R.; Smith, J.E.; Rowan, N.J. Medicinal Mushrooms and Cancer Therapy: Translating a traditional practice into Western medicine. *Perspect. Biol. Med.* **2006**, *49*, 159–170. [CrossRef] [PubMed]

15. Sohretoglu, D. Ganoderma lucidum Polysaccharides as An Anti-cancer Agent. *Anti-Cancer Agents Med. Chem.* **2018**, *18*, 667–674. [CrossRef] [PubMed]

16. Ina, K.; Kataoka, T.; Ando, T. The Use of Lentinan for Treating Gastric Cancer. *Anti-Cancer Agents Med. Chem.* **2013**, *13*, 681–688. [CrossRef]

17. Rossi, P.; Difrancia, R.; Quagliariello, V.; Savino, E.; Tralongo, P.; Randazzo, C.L.; Berretta, M. B-glucans from Grifola frondosa and Ganoderma lucidum in breast cancer: An example of complementary and integrative medicine. *Oncotarget* **2018**, *9*, 24837–24856. [CrossRef]

18. Pohleven, J.; Kos, J.; Sabotic, J. Medicinal Properties of the Genus Clitocybe and of Lectins from the Clouded Funnel Cap Mushroom, C. nebularis (Agaricomycetes): A Review. *Int. J. Med. Mushrooms* **2016**, *18*, 965–975. [CrossRef]

19. Baek, J.; Roh, H.-S.; Baek, K.; Lee, S.; Lee, S.; Song, S.-S.; Kim, K.H. Bioactivity-based analysis and chemical characterization of cytotoxic constituents from Chaga mushroom (Inonotus obliquus) that induce apoptosis in human lung adenocarcinoma cells. *J. Ethnopharmacol.* **2018**, *224*, 63–75. [CrossRef]

20. Mueller, G.M.; Schmit, J.P. Fungal biodiversity: What do we know? What can we predict? *Biodivers. Conserv.* **2007**, *16*, 1–5. [CrossRef]

21. Pegler, D.N.; Lodge, D.J.; Nakasone, K.K. The Pantropical Genus Macrocybe Gen. nov. *Mycologia* **1998**, *90*, 494. [CrossRef]

22. Lev, S. Non-vesicular lipid transport by lipid-transfer proteins and beyond. *Nat. Rev. Mol. Cell Biol.* **2010**, *11*, 739–750. [CrossRef] [PubMed]

23. Ramirez, N.A.; Niveiro, N.; Michlig, A.; Popoff, O. First record of Macrocybe titans (Tricholomataceae, Basidiomycota) in Argentina. *Check List.* **2017**, *13*, 153–158. [CrossRef]

24. Razaq, A.; Nawaz, R.; Khalid, A.N. An Asian edible mushroom, Macrocybe gigantea: Its distribution and ITS-rDNA based phylogeny. *Mycosphere* **2016**, *7*, 525–530. [CrossRef]

25. Milhorini, S.D.S.; Smiderle, F.R.; Biscaia, S.M.P.; Rosado, F.R.; Trindade, E.S.; Iacomini, M. Fucogalactan from the giant mushroom Macrocybe titans inhibits melanoma cells migration. *Carbohydr. Polym.* **2018**, *190*, 50–56. [CrossRef]

26. Gaur, T.; Rao, P.B. Analysis of Antibacterial Activity and Bioactive Compounds of the Giant Mushroom, Macrocybe gigantea (Agaricomycetes), from India. *Int. J. Med. Mushrooms* **2017**, *19*, 1083–1092. [CrossRef]

27. Sen, T.; Samanta, S.K. Medicinal plants, human health and biodiversity: A broad review. *Adv. Biochem. Eng. Biotechnol.* **2015**, *147*, 59–110.

28. Ulmer, H.; Borena, W.; Rapp, K.; Klenk, J.; Strasak, A.; Diem, G.; Concin, H.; Nagel, G. Serum triglyceride concentrations and cancer risk in a large cohort study in Austria. *Br. J. Cancer* **2009**, *101*, 1202–1206. [CrossRef]

29. Shen, Y.; Wang, C.; Ren, Y.; Ye, J. A comprehensive look at the role of hyperlipidemia in promoting colorectal cancer liver metastasis. *J. Cancer* **2018**, *9*, 2981–2986. [CrossRef]

30. Ni, H.; Liu, H.; Gao, R. Serum Lipids and Breast Cancer Risk: A Meta-Analysis of Prospective Cohort Studies. *PLoS ONE* **2015**, *10*, e0142669. [CrossRef]

31. Cannella, C.; Giusti, A. Conjugated linoleic acid: A natural anticarcinogenic substance from animal food. *Ital. J. Food Sci.* **2000**, *12*, 123–127.

32. Hanafy, N.A.N.; El-Kemary, M.; Leporatti, S. Micelles structure development as a strategy to improve smart cancer therapy. *Cancers* **2018**, *10*, 238. [CrossRef] [PubMed]

33. Nicolas, J.; Couvreur, P. Polymer nanoparticles for the delivery of anticancer drug. *Med. Sci.* **2017**, *33*, 11–17.

34. Joshi, S.; Durden, D.L. Combinatorial Approach to Improve Cancer Immunotherapy: Rational Drug Design Strategy to Simultaneously Hit Multiple Targets to Kill Tumor Cells and to Activate the Immune System. *J. Oncol.* **2019**, *2019*, 1–18. [CrossRef] [PubMed]

35. Meshulam, T.; Simard, J.R.; Wharton, J.; Hamilton, J.A.; Pilch, P.F. Role of Caveolin-1 and Cholesterol in Transmembrane Fatty Acid Movement. *Biochemistry* **2006**, *45*, 2882–2893. [CrossRef] [PubMed]

36. Siddiqi, S.; Sheth, A.; Patel, F.; Barnes, M.; Mansbach, C.M. Intestinal caveolin-1 is important for dietary fatty acid absorption. *Biochim. Biophys. Acta* **2013**, *1831*, 1311–1321. [CrossRef] [PubMed]

37. Gerbod-Giannone, M.-C.; Dallet, L.; Naudin, G.; Sahin, A.; Decossas, M.; Poussard, S.; Lambert, O. Involvement of caveolin-1 and CD36 in native LDL endocytosis by endothelial cells. *Biochim. Biophys. Acta* **2019**, *1863*, 830–838. [CrossRef]

38. Chen, D.; Shen, C.; Du, H.; Zhou, Y.; Che, G.-W. Duplex value of caveolin-1 in non-small cell lung cancer: A meta analysis. *Fam. Cancer* **2014**, *13*, 449–457. [CrossRef]

39. Shi, Y.-B.; Li, J.; Lai, X.-N.; Jiang, R.; Zhao, R.-C.; Xiong, L.-X. Multifaceted Roles of Caveolin-1 in Lung Cancer: A New Investigation Focused on Tumor Occurrence, Development and Therapy. *Cancers* **2020**, *12*, 291. [CrossRef]

40. Alonso, E.N.; Ferronato, M.J.; Fermento, M.E.; Gandini, N.A.; Romero, A.L.; Guevara, J.A.; Facchinetti, M.M.; Curino, A.C. Antitumoral and antimetastatic activity of Maitake D-Fraction in triple-negative breast cancer cells. *Oncotarget* **2018**, *9*, 23396–23412. [CrossRef]

41. Guo, H.; Kuang, S.; Song, Q.-L.; Liu, M.; Sun, X.-X.; Yu, Q. Cucurbitacin I inhibits STAT3, but enhances STAT1 signaling in human cancer cells in vitro through disrupting actin filaments. *Acta Pharmacol. Sin.* **2018**, *39*, 425–437. [CrossRef] [PubMed]

42. Chikara, S.; Lindsey, K.; Borowicz, P.; Christofidou-Solomidou, M.; Reindl, K. Enterolactone alters FAK-Src signaling and suppresses migration and invasion of lung cancer cell lines. *BMC Complement. Altern. Med.* **2017**, *17*, 1–12. [CrossRef] [PubMed]

43. Van Goietsenoven, G.; Mathieu, V.; Lefranc, F.; Kornienko, A.; Evidente, A.; Kiss, R. Narciclasine as well as other Amaryllidaceae Isocarbostyrils are Promising GTP-ase Targeting Agents against Brain Cancers. *Med. Res. Rev.* **2013**, *33*, 439–455. [CrossRef] [PubMed]

44. Iwai, N.; Martinez, A.; Miller, M.-J.; Vos, M.; Mulshine, J.L.; Treston, A.M. Autocrine growth loops dependent on peptidyl α-amidating enzyme as targets for novel tumor cell growth inhibitors. *Lung Cancer* **1999**, *23*, 209–222. [CrossRef]

45. Zitvogel, L.; Pitt, J.M.; Daillère, L.Z.J.M.P.R.; Smyth, M.J.; Kroemer, G. Mouse models in oncoimmunology. *Nat. Rev. Cancer* **2016**, *16*, 759–773. [CrossRef]

46. Monga, S.P.S.; Wadleigh, R.; Sharma, A.; Adib, H.; Strader, D.; Singh, G.; Harmon, J.W.; Berlin, M.; Monga, D.K.; Mishra, L. Intratumoral Therapy of Cisplatin/Epinephrine Injectable Gel for Palliation in Patients With Obstructive Esophageal Cancer. *Am. J. Clin. Oncol.* **2000**, *23*, 386–392. [CrossRef]

47. Ochoa-Callejero, L.; Garcia-Sanmartin, J.; Martínez-Herrero, S.; Rubio-Mediavilla, S.; Narro-Íñiguez, J.; Martinez, A. Small molecules related to adrenomedullin reduce tumor burden in a mouse model of colitis-associated colon cancer. *Sci. Rep.* **2017**, *7*, 17488. [CrossRef]

3-Vinylazetidin-2-Ones: Synthesis, Antiproliferative and Tubulin Destabilizing Activity in MCF-7 and MDA-MB-231 Breast Cancer Cells

Shu Wang [1], Azizah M. Malebari [2,†], Thomas F. Greene [1,†], Niamh M. O'Boyle [1], Darren Fayne [3], Seema M. Nathwani [3], Brendan Twamley [4], Thomas McCabe [4], Niall O. Keely [1], Daniela M. Zisterer [3] and Mary J. Meegan [1,*]

[1]   School of Pharmacy and Pharmaceutical Sciences, Trinity College Dublin, Trinity Biomedical Sciences Institute, 152-160 Pearse Street, Dublin 2 DO2R590, Ireland; wangsh@tcd.ie (S.W.); tgreene@tcd.ie (T.F.G.); Niamh.OBoyle@tcd.ie (N.M.O.); nkeely@tcd.ie (N.O.K.)

[2]   Department of Pharmaceutical Chemistry, College of Pharmacy, King Abdulaziz University, Jeddah 21589, Saudi Arabia; amelibary@kau.edu.sa

[3]   School of Biochemistry and Immunology, Trinity College Dublin, Trinity Biomedical Sciences Institute, 152-160 Pearse Street, Dublin 2 DO2R590, Ireland; FAYNED@tcd.ie (D.F.); seema.nathwani@outlook.com (S.M.N.); dzistrer@tcd.ie (D.M.Z.)

[4]   School of Chemistry, Trinity College Dublin, Dublin 2 DO2R590, Ireland; TWAMLEYB@tcd.ie (B.T.); TMCCABE@tcd.ie (T.M.)

*   Correspondence: mmeegan@tcd.ie;

†   These authors contributed equally to this work.

Abstract: Microtubule-targeted drugs are essential chemotherapeutic agents for various types of cancer. A series of 3-vinyl-β-lactams (2-azetidinones) were designed, synthesized and evaluated as potential tubulin polymerization inhibitors, and for their antiproliferative effects in breast cancer cells. These compounds showed potent activity in MCF-7 breast cancer cells with an IC_{50} value of 8 nM for compound **7s** 4-[3-Hydroxy-4-methoxyphenyl]-1-(3,4,5-trimethoxyphenyl)-3-vinylazetidin-2-one) which was comparable to the activity of Combretastatin A-4. Compound **7s** had minimal cytotoxicity against both non-tumorigenic HEK-293T cells and murine mammary epithelial cells. The compounds inhibited the polymerisation of tubulin in vitro with an 8.7-fold reduction in tubulin polymerization at 10 µM for compound **7s** and were shown to interact at the colchicine-binding site on tubulin, resulting in significant G2/M phase cell cycle arrest. Immunofluorescence staining of MCF-7 cells confirmed that β-lactam **7s** is targeting tubulin and resulted in mitotic catastrophe. A docking simulation indicated potential binding conformations for the 3-vinyl-β-lactam **7s** in the colchicine domain of tubulin. These compounds are promising candidates for development as antiproiferative microtubule-disrupting agents.

Keywords: Combretastatin A-4; β-lactam; 3-vinylazetidin-2-ones; antiproliferative activity; tubulin; antimitotic

1. Introduction

Antimitotic agents such as taxol and the vinca alkaloids vinblastine and vincristine are a major class of drugs used clinically in the treatment of many cancers [1–3]. Microtubule-destabilizing agents (e.g., vinblastine) typically bind with tubulin at the vinca alkaloid site [4], while colchicine **1** exerts its biological effects at the intrasubunit interface within a tubulin dimer [5]. Stilbene-based compounds have attracted the attention of chemists and pharmacologists due to their many biological properties such as anticancer, antioxidant and anti-inflammatory activities, and are often used in traditional medicine for a variety of therapeutic effects [6]. The combretastatins are a group of stilbenes isolated from the South African bush willow tree *Combretum caffrum* [7], and are shown to have outstanding potency in binding to the colchicine-binding site of tubulin and thus inhibiting the formation of the mitotic spindle [8]. Combretastatin A-4 **2a** and Combretastatin A-1 **2c** demonstrate exceptionally potent antiproliferative activity against a range of human cancer cell lines (Figure 1) [7]. Additionally, antivascular effects are produced by these compounds in vivo [9,10]. Although some combretastatin compounds have progressed to clinical trials[11,12], there are major problems associated with combretastatins including poor water solubility and *cis/trans* isomerization during administration or storage, which results in an extensive loss of potency. Water soluble prodrugs such as the combretastatin phosphate CA-4P, (fosbretabulin) **2b** [13,14] are currently in clinical trials for advanced anaplastic thyroid carcinoma [15], ovarian cancer [16], and in combination with Bevacizumab for patients with advanced cancer [17]. Recently, the potential combination therapy of CA-4P and vincristine in the treatment of hepatocellular carcinoma was reported to show a beneficial effect in reducing doses of drugs with narrow therapeutic windows [18]. Ombrabulin is a serine prodrug whose derivatives display the same activity as CA-4 and has completed a phase III clinical trial for the treatment of advanced stage soft tissue sarcoma [19,20]. There is ongoing interest in the clinical development of combretastatin A1 diphosphate (OXi 4503) **2d** [21]. The structurally related benzophenones phenstatin **3a**, phenstatin phosphate **3b** [22] and the lignin podophyllotoxin **4** also destabilize microtubules [23].

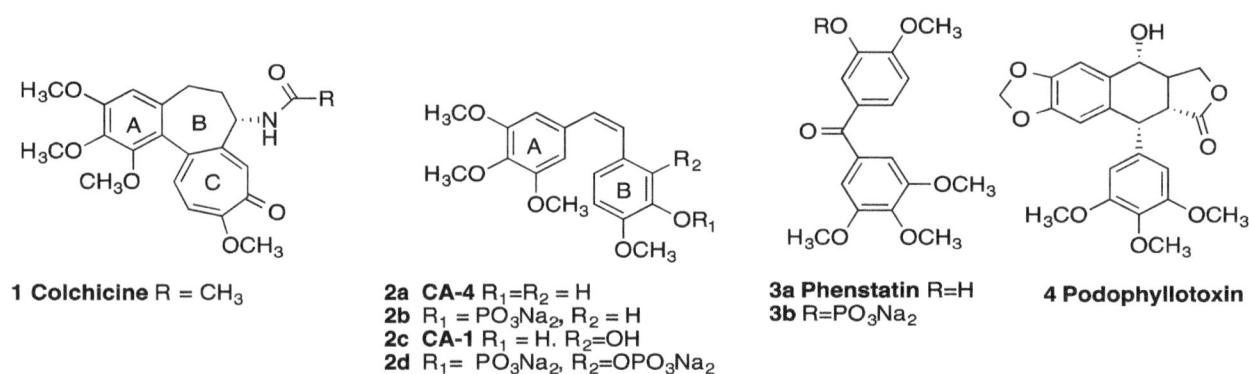

1 Colchicine R = CH₃

2a CA-4 R₁=R₂ = H
2b R₁ = PO₃Na₂, R₂ = H
2c CA-1 R₁ = H. R₂=OH
2d R₁= PO₃Na₂, R₂=OPO₃Na₂

3a Phenstatin R=H
3b R=PO₃Na₂

4 Podophyllotoxin

Figure 1. Colchicine (**1**), Combretastatins (**2a–2d**), phenstatins (**3a**, **3b**) and podophyllotoxin (**4**).

Many heterocyclic scaffold structures have been introduced to replace the alkene of the stilbene structure of CA-4 and to provide conformational restriction by locking the stilbene in the *cis* configuration (Rings A and B) required for biological activity [24]. Small molecule tubulin polymerization inhibitors have been reported in which the *cis* double bond of CA-4 has been replaced by various heterocycles such as furan [25], indole[26,27], imidazole [28], isoxazole [29], triazole [30], tetrazole [31], benzoxepine [32], pyrazole [33], pyridine [34], benzimidazole [35] and related heterocycles [36]. While β-lactam antibiotics have occupied a central role in the treatment of pathogenic bacteria, the antiproliferative activity of compounds containing the β-lactam (azetidin-2-one) ring has also been investigated [37–42]. The synthesis and antitumour activity of a number of chiral β-lactam bridged CA-4 analogues have been reported [37,38]. Additional impetus for research efforts on β-lactam chemistry has been provided by the use of β-lactams as synthetic intermediates in organic synthesis [43].

We have previously investigated the antiproliferative and SERM (selective estrogen receptor modulator) activity of the azetidin-2-one(β-lactam) scaffold [44] and also demonstrated the effectiveness of 1,4-diarylazetidin-2-ones in breast cancer cell lines as tubulin targeting agents. [45,46]. These compounds also demonstrated both anti-angiogenic effects in MDA-MB-231 breast adenocarcinoma cells. In addition, we established that these compounds inhibited the migration of MDA-MB-231 cells indicating a potential anti-metastatic function for these compounds [47]. To further our understanding of the antiproliferative activity of these compounds, we wished to investigate the design, synthesis and evaluation of a series of azetidin-2-ones containing a vinyl substituent at C3 of the azetidin-2-one ring, and to explore the effect of this hydrophobic substituent on the biological activity of these compounds in which the *cis* configuration (Rings A and B) is locked into the azetidin-2-one ring structure. The introduction of this vinyl substituent at C-3 also allowed us to examine further chemical transformations of the alkene, and to determine structure-activity relationships for the series. On this basis, we now aimed to investigate a new series of novel 3-vinylazetidinones compounds with an improved biochemical profile particularly in triple negative breast cancer for potential development in preclinical study of breast cancer as tubulin destabilising agents. Therefore, we focused our efforts on the preparation of a library of 1,4-diarylazetidin-2-ones which contain a vinyl substituent at C-3. The synthesis of phosphate esters and amino acid amide type prodrugs of the most potent 1,4-diarylazetidin-2-ones were examined, together with the antiproliferative and tubulin targeting effects.

2. Results and Discussion

2.1. Chemistry: Synthesis of β-lactams

There are many synthetic routes available for the construction of the β-lactam ring [43,48]. The choice of route depends on the structural features required in the final product. In the present work, the Staudinger reaction between an imine and a ketene was chosen for the formation of the β-lactam ring because of its ease of use, adaptability for use with structurally diverse imines and acid chlorides, and readily available starting materials. A series of analogues with a variety of substituents at C4 of the β-lactam ring B was synthesized from the appropriate imines. The preparation of the Schiff bases 5a–5r was achieved by the condensation of the appropriately substituted benzaldehyde with the 3,4,5-trimethoxyaniline in ethanol in the presence of a catalytic amount of sulphuric acid, (Scheme 1). The 3,4,5-trimethoxy substituted A-Ring of CA-4 plays an important role in inhibiting tubulin polymerisation, and is confirmed in the docking of CA-4 in tubulin [49]. The substituents located at the para-position of C-4 aryl Ring B included halogens (compounds 5a–5c), nitro (5d), dimethylamino (5e), methyl (5g), alkoxyl (5h–5j), phenoxy (5k), benzyloxy (5l), nitrile (5q) and thiomethyl (5r) together with naphthyl (compounds 5m and 5n). 5s was similarly obtained by reaction of 4-methoxybenzaldehyde with 3,5-dimethoxyaniline. For the synthesis of β-lactam derivatives with a phenolic hydroxy group to mimic Ring B of CA-4, it was necessary to use the benzyl ether 5l and *tert*-butyldimethylsilyl ether 5o. A further series of Schiff bases (6a–6k) was obtained from 3,4,5-trimethoxybenzaldehyde with appropriate anilines using the same procedure as above, (Scheme 1). An example of the crystal structure of the imine 6k is displayed in Figure 2, showing the *E* configuration of the imine N1-C2 bond (bond length 1.278(2) Å) (Table 1).

5a: R_1=F; R_2=R_3=H
5b: R_1=Cl; R_2=R_3=H
5c: R_1=Br; R_2=R_3=H
5d: R_1=NO_2; R_2=R_3=H
5e: R_1=$N(CH_3)_2$; R_2=R_3=H
5f: R_1= R_2=R_3=H
5g: R_1=CH_3; R_2=R_3=H
5h: R_1=OCH_3; R_2=R_3=H
5i: R_1=OCH_2CH_3; R_2=R_3=H
5j: R_1=$O(CH_2)_3CH_3$; R_2=R_3=H
5k: R_1=OPh; R_2=R_3=H
5l: R_1=OCH_2Ph; R_2 =R_3=H
5m: R_1=H, R_2R_3=CH=CH-CH=CH
5n: R_1R_2=CH=CH-CH=CH; R_3=H
5o: R_1=OCH_3; R_2=OTBDMS,, R_3=H
5p: R_1=OCH_3; R_2=NO_2, R_3=H
5q: R_1=CN, R_2=R_3=H
5r: R_1=SCH_3, R_2=R_3=H

5s

6a: R_1=F
6b: R_1=Cl
6c: R_1=Br
6d: R_1=NO_2
6e: R_1=$C(CH_3)_3$
6f: R_1=H
6g: R_1=CH_3
6h: R_1=CH_2CH_3
6i: R_1=OCH_3
6j: R_1=$NHCOCH_3$
6k: R_1=SCH_3

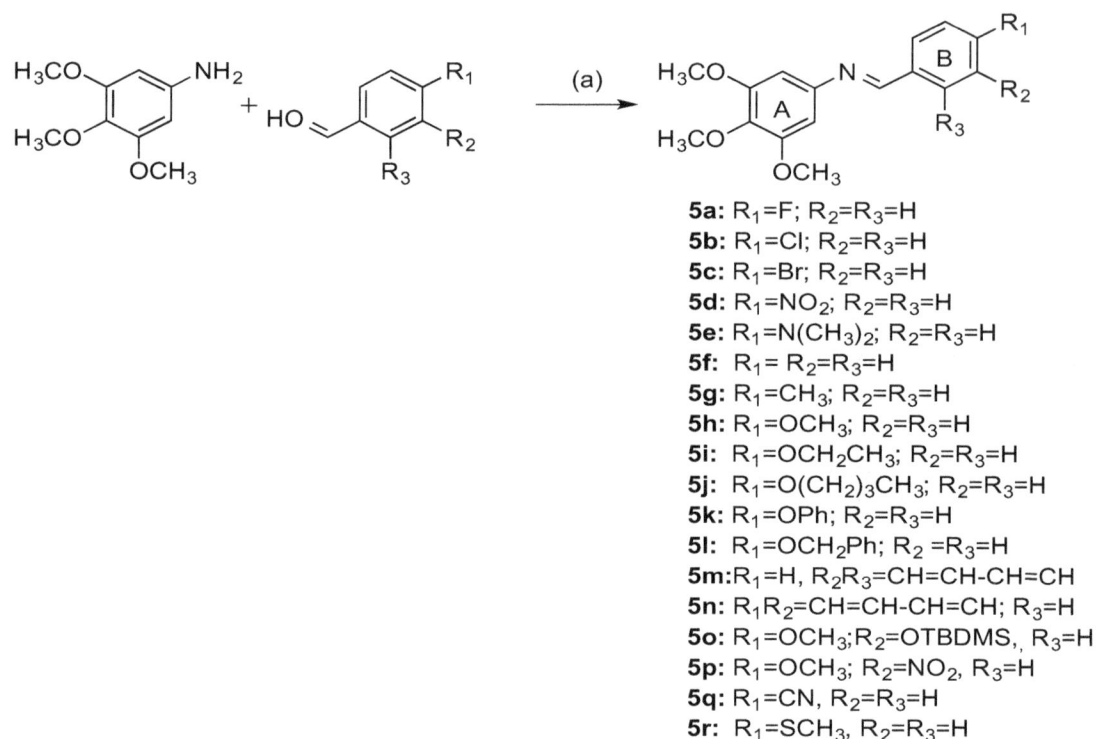

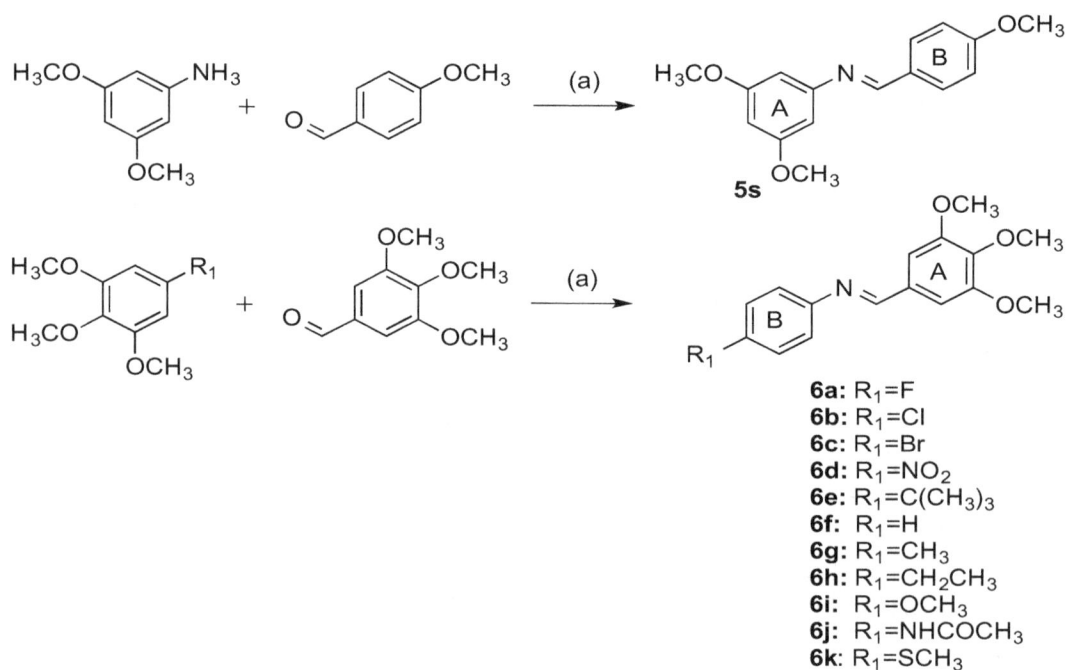

Scheme 1. Synthesis of imines **5a–5s**, **6a–6k**. Reagents and conditions: (a) EtOH, conc H_2SO_4, reflux, 4 h, (67–100%).

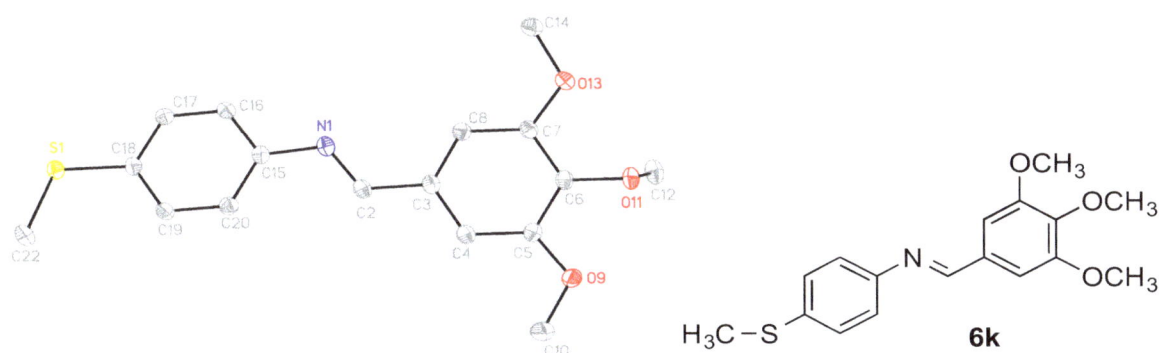

Figure 2. ORTEP representation of the X-ray crystal structure of compound **6k** with the thermal ellipsoids set at 50% probability.

Table 1. Crystal data, details of data collections and refinement **6k, 7h, 8h, 8i, 8k.**

Compound	6k	7h	8h	8i	8k
Empirical formula	$C_{17}H_{19}NO_3S$	$C_{21}H_{23}NO_5$	$C_{22}H_{25}NO_4$	$C_{21}H_{23}NO_5$	$C_{21}H_{23}NO_4S$
M (g/mol)	317.39	369.40	367.43	369.40	385.46
Crystal System	monoclinic	monoclinic	monoclinic	triclinic	triclinic
SG	$P2_1$ (No. 4)	$P2_1$ (No. 4)	$P2_1/n$ (No. 14)	$P\bar{1}$ (No. 2)	$P\bar{1}$ (No. 2)
a (Å)	7.8282(3)	20.1106(7)	7.2135(14)	10.9022(5)	8.2131(4)
b (Å)	7.7880(3)	9.1481(3)	26.440(5)	13.0315(6)	10.5047(5)
c (Å)	13.2937(6)	22.6378(8)	10.389(2)	14.9787(8)	12.5704(6)
α (°)	-	-	-	94.994(2)	107.9218(16)°
β (°)	106.4320(10)	110.6238(14)	101.41(3)	105.024(2)°	96.7759(18)°
γ (°)	-	-	-	108.284(2)°	103.3909(18)°
V (Å3)	777.36(6)	3897.9(2)	1942.3(7)	1918.37(16)	982.64(8)
T (K)	100(2)	100(2)	150(2)	100(2)	100(2)
Z	2	8	4	4	2
$Dcalc$ (g/cm^3)	1.356	1.259	1.256	1.279	1.303
μ (mm^{-1})	0.220 (Mo Kα)	0.738 (Cu Kα)	0.086 (Mo Kα)	0.091 (Mo Kα)	0.191 (Mo Kα)
Total reflns	27644	59468	14461	29738	14916
Indep. reflns	4394	14180	3492	9673	4903
R(int)	0.0258	0.0602	0.0565	0.0532	0.0304
S	1.058	1.047	1.188	1.006	1.038
R_1 * [I > 2σ(I)]	0.0251	0.0364	0.0666	0.0509	0.0388
wR_2 * [all data]	0.0676	0.0945	0.1509	0.1191	0.0918
Flack	0.027(12)				
CCDC number	1820354	1820355	1820358	1820356	1820357

$^* R_1 = \sum||F_o| - |F_c||/\sum|F_o|, wR_2 = [\sum w(F_o^2 - F_c^2)^2/\sum w(F_o^2)^2]^{1/2}.$

A series of novel β-lactams (**7a–7r**) was obtained by reaction of imines **5a–5r** with crotonyl chloride using Staudinger reaction conditions requiring the slow addition of a solution of the appropriate acid chloride to a refluxing solution of imine and TEA, (Scheme 2) [50,51]. One enantiomer is illustrated in each case and products are obtained as a racemic mixture. β-Lactam (**7s**) containing the required Ring B phenolic group of CA-4 was successfully synthesised from the silyl ether imine **5o** and crotonyl chloride to afford the silyl ether β-lactam **7o** which was deprotected in situ by treatment with tBAF to yield the phenol **7s** (Scheme 2). This series of compounds **7a–7r** differ only in the substituent pattern of aryl ring at C-4 of the β-lactam ring B.

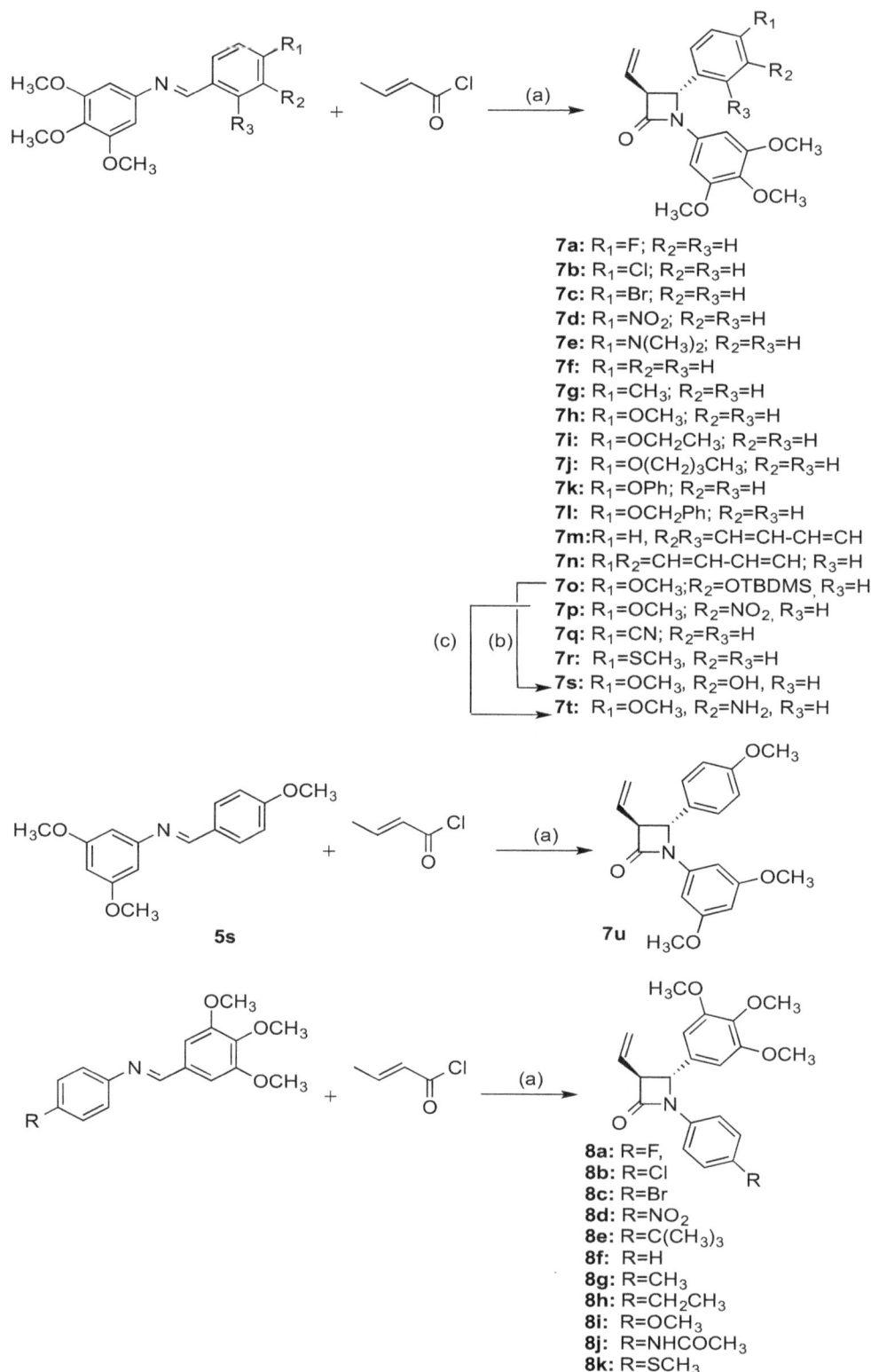

7a: R₁=F; R₂=R₃=H
7b: R₁=Cl; R₂=R₃=H
7c: R₁=Br; R₂=R₃=H
7d: R₁=NO₂; R₂=R₃=H
7e: R₁=N(CH₃)₂; R₂=R₃=H
7f: R₁=R₂=R₃=H
7g: R₁=CH₃; R₂=R₃=H
7h: R₁=OCH₃; R₂=R₃=H
7i: R₁=OCH₂CH₃; R₂=R₃=H
7j: R₁=O(CH₂)₃CH₃; R₂=R₃=H
7k: R₁=OPh; R₂=R₃=H
7l: R₁=OCH₂Ph; R₂=R₃=H
7m: R₁=H, R₂R₃=CH=CH-CH=CH
7n: R₁R₂=CH=CH-CH=CH; R₃=H
7o: R₁=OCH₃;R₂=OTBDMS, R₃=H
7p: R₁=OCH₃; R₂=NO₂, R₃=H
7q: R₁=CN; R₂=R₃=H
7r: R₁=SCH₃, R₂=R₃=H
7s: R₁=OCH₃, R₂=OH, R₃=H
7t: R₁=OCH₃, R₂=NH₂, R₃=H

5s   **7u**

8a: R=F,
8b: R=Cl
8c: R=Br
8d: R=NO₂
8e: R=C(CH₃)₃
8f: R=H
8g: R=CH₃
8h: R=CH₂CH₃
8i: R=OCH₃
8j: R=NHCOCH₃
8k: R=SCH₃

Scheme 2. Synthesis of β-lactams **7a–7u, 8a–8k**; Reagents and conditions: (a) triethylamine, CH₂Cl₂, reflux, 5 h, (17–61%); (b) TBAF, dry THF, 0 °C, 30 min, (20%); (c) Zn dust, acetic acid, 20 °C, 7 days, (43%).

Many potentially useful CA-4 derivatives contain the amino substituent replacing the phenol on ring B and have shown interesting biochemical activity[52]. We were interested in the preparation of β-lactam CA-4 type compounds containing an amino substituent in Ring B, and the subsequent conversion to a water-soluble prodrug by conjugation with an amino acid. The nitro containing C-3-vinyl-β-lactam **7p** was successfully reduced to the amino product **7t** using zinc dust in the presence of acetic acid (Scheme 2). To investigate the effect of replacement of the 3,4,5-trimethoxy ring A of CA-4 with 3,5-dimethoxy substituted ring A, the β-lactam **7u** was prepared in a similar route from the imine **5s**. Tripodi et al. reported that 3,5-dimethoxy substituted ring A compounds demonstrated comparable activity to the β-lactam compounds containing the 3,4,5-trimethoxy ring A of CA-4 [53]. A further series of β-lactam compounds (**8a–8k**), was also prepared containing the 3,4,5-trimethoxyphenyl substituent (Ring A of the Combretastatin A-4) at C-4 position, (Scheme 2).

The products of the Staudinger reaction with imines and crotonyl chloride show IR absorptions at approximately ν 1750 cm^{-1} characteristic of the carbonyl group of the β-lactam ring. All of the β-lactams were obtained with exclusively *trans* stereochemistry, with coupling constants of 1–3 Hz for the β-lactam ring protons (e.g., for compound **7s**, H-4 is identified as a doublet δ 4.69, $J_{3,4}$ = 2.52 Hz). Coupling constants of 5–6 Hz are usually observed for β-lactams with *cis* stereochemistry [46].

Subsequent to our initial biochemical evaluation of the 3-vinyl-β-lactam CA-4 analogues, a further series of 3-substituted β-lactams was prepared from 3-unsubstituted β-lactams by aldol type reaction with a suitable electrophile [54,55]. We were particularly interested in the introduction of modified alkene substituents at C-3, due to the exceptional biochemical activity displayed by the 3-vinyl β-lactam **7s**. Lithium enolates of 3-unsubstituted β-lactams **9a** and **9b** were reacted with selected aldehydes and ketones to provide alcohol products **10a–10i**, (Scheme 3). The β-lactams **9a** and **9b** were obtained via the Reformatsky reaction of ethyl bromoacetate with imines **5h** and **5o** using microwave conditions. Treatment of **9b** with tBAF afforded the phenol **9c**. Similarly, for the preparation of compounds **10a**, **10c**, **10d**, **10f**, **10g**, **10h** the initially obtained tBDMS ether intermediate was subsequently deprotected in situ using tBAF to yield the desired phenolic product. The enolate chemistry is stereoselective, favouring *trans* stereochemistry for the products. The presence of a diastereomeric mixture for products is confirmed from the ^{1}H NMR spectra (e.g., for **10h** where H-3 and H-4 appear as two sets of doublets, δ 3.20 and δ 4.83 respectively, with J = 2.4 Hz, ratio H$_3$/H$_4$ 1.14:1.00). To investigate the role of the alcohol group at C-5 in the biochemical activity of the products **10a–10h**, the alcohol **10i** was oxidised to the corresponding ketone **11** using pyridinium chlorochromate. An alternative route to **11** was identified where treatment of the 3-unsubstituted β-lactam **9b** with LDA followed by addition of acetyl chloride to gave the desired product **11** but only in low yields (11%) with the alcohol **10a** also isolated (22%), (Scheme 3).

To further investigate the role of the 3-vinyl substitution pattern in the biochemical activity of. β-lactams, a 3-ethylidene product **12** was investigated. The initial route attempted involved the chlorination of the alcohol **10i** using thionyl chloride followed by dehydrohalogentation with a suitable base such as DBU. However, a more successful method to give the 3-ethylidene β-lactams was the dehydration of the alcohol **10i** under Mitsunobu conditions and subsequent deprotection by treatment with tBAF to yield **12** in 63% yield overall, (Scheme 3). The Peterson olefination of 3-unsubstituted β-lactams has also been reported by Kano et al. as an alternative route to 3-ethylidene β-lactams [56], while the Mitsunobu reaction for the dehydration of alcohols has been described by Plantan et al. in the synthesis of a trinem β-lactamase inhibitor [57]. The product **12** was obtained as a mixture of Z/E isomers in a 1:1 ratio. The configuration of the separated isomers was determined by examining the chemical shifts associated with the C-6 methyl protons. The further downfield doublet signal (δ 2.05, J = 4.16 Hz) is more deshielded, and so is assigned to the Z isomer while the signal at δ 1.62, (J = 4.40 Hz) is assigned to the E isomer [51].

The introduction of a diol functionality at C-3 was now explored. The diol **13** was synthesised in 39% yield by the oxidation of the alkene **7s** with osmium tetroxide (Scheme 3). The ^{1}H NMR spectrum for **13** clearly illustrates the formation of a diastereomeric product. H-3 appears as a pair of double doublets at δ 3.16 (0.7H) and δ 3.19 (0.3H) with coupling constants of 2.42 Hz and 5.55 Hz, while H-4 appears as two separate doublets at δ 4.90 (0.3H) and δ 5.00 (0.7H), J = 2.37 Hz.

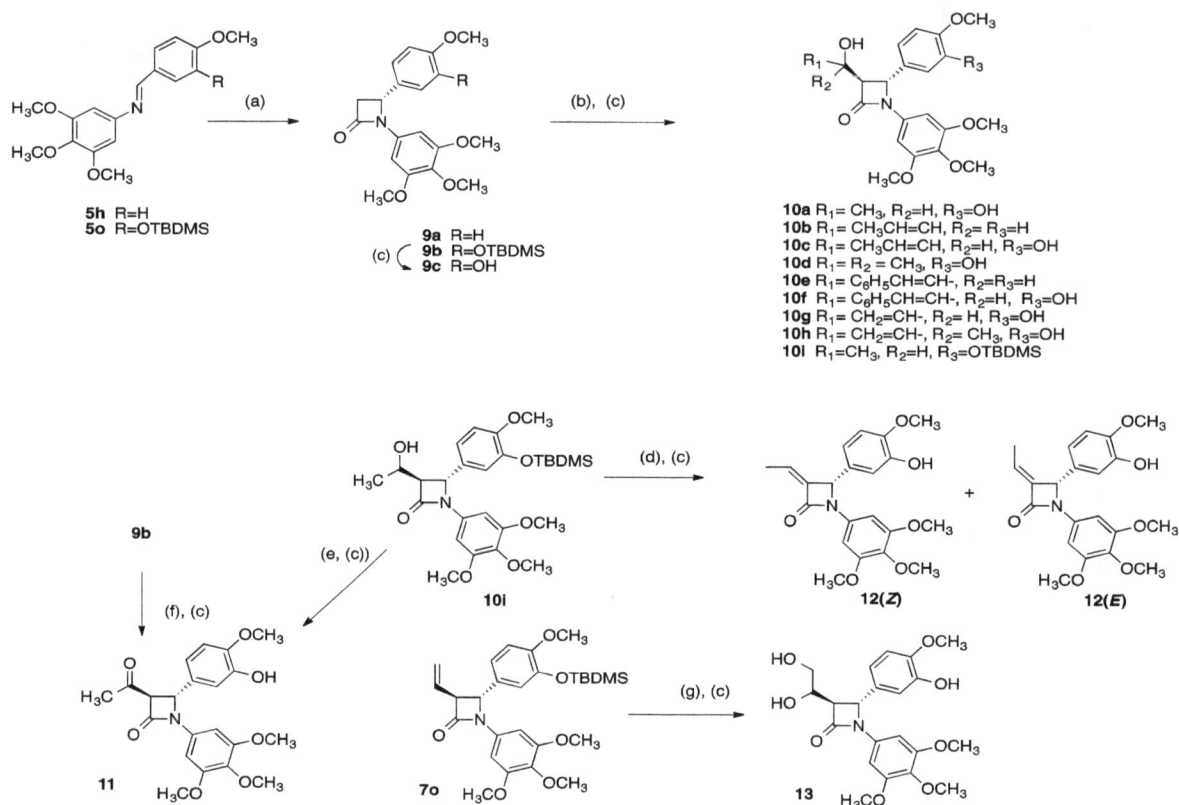

Scheme 3. Synthesis of azetidinones **10a–10i**, **11–13**. Scheme reagents and conditions: (a) Zn, BrCH$_2$CO$_2$Et, microwave, 100 °C, 30 min, (37–39%) (b) LDA, THF, R$_1$COR$_2$, −78 °C, 30 min, (17–38%); (c) TBAF, THF, 0 °C, 1.5 h (for compounds **10a, 10c, 10d, 10f, 10g, 10h, 11, 12, 13**), (17–52%); (d) Ph$_3$P, DEAD, CH$_2$Cl$_2$, 0 °C, 3 min, (52%); (e) PCC, CH$_2$Cl$_2$, 20 °C, 18 h, (7%) (f) LDA, THF, CH$_3$COCl, −78 °C, 30 min, (11%); (g) OsO$_4$, pyridine, 0 °C 1 min, then 20 °C, 22 h, (39%).

The amino acid alanine was chosen for prodrug formation of the β-lactam **7t** [58]. The protected amino acid prodrug **14** was obtained from **7t** using the coupling agent DCC with HOBt in dry DMF (Scheme 4). The FMOC protecting group was easily removed from **14** by treatment with 2N sodium hydroxide over 24 h to afford the amino acid prodrug conjugate **15** (57%). Controlled esterification of the phenolic β-lactams **7s** and **9c** with dibenzyl phosphite using diisopropylethylamine and dimethylaminopyridine afforded dibenzyl phosphate β-lactams **16a** and **16b** respectively, (Scheme 4). The dimethyl and diethylethyl phosphate esters of compound **9c**, **16c** and **16d** respectively, were also prepared (Scheme 4). The phosphate **17a** was obtained by treatment of dibenzylphosphate ester **16a** with bromotrimethylsilane. Hydrogenation of the dibenzylphosphate ester **16b** with palladium/carbon catalyst removed the dibenzyl protecting groups and also reduced the double bond at C-3 position of the β-lactam ring to afford phosphate **17c**. For the preparation of compound **17b**, where removal of the benzyl protecting groups and retention of the double bond was required, reaction of the dibenzyl phosphate ester **16b** with bromotrimethylsilane was effective.

Preliminary stability studies of the representative β-lactam **7s** were carried out at acidic, neutral and basic conditions (pH 4, 7.4 and 9) and in plasma using HPLC. The half-life ($t_{\frac{1}{2}}$) was determined to be greater than 24 h at pH 4, 7.4 and 9 and in plasma for compound **7s**. The phosphate esters **17b** and **17c** were also found to be stable over the range of pH and in plasma, with half-life ($t_{\frac{1}{2}}$) determined to be greater than 24 h. The cleavage of phosphate prodrugs **17b** and **17c** was also investigated in whole blood. They were cleaved much more rapidly in whole blood (62% and 34% remaining after 6 h respectively) than in human plasma (94% and 92% remaining after 6 h respectively). Based on this stability study the β-lactam **7s** would be suitable for further development.

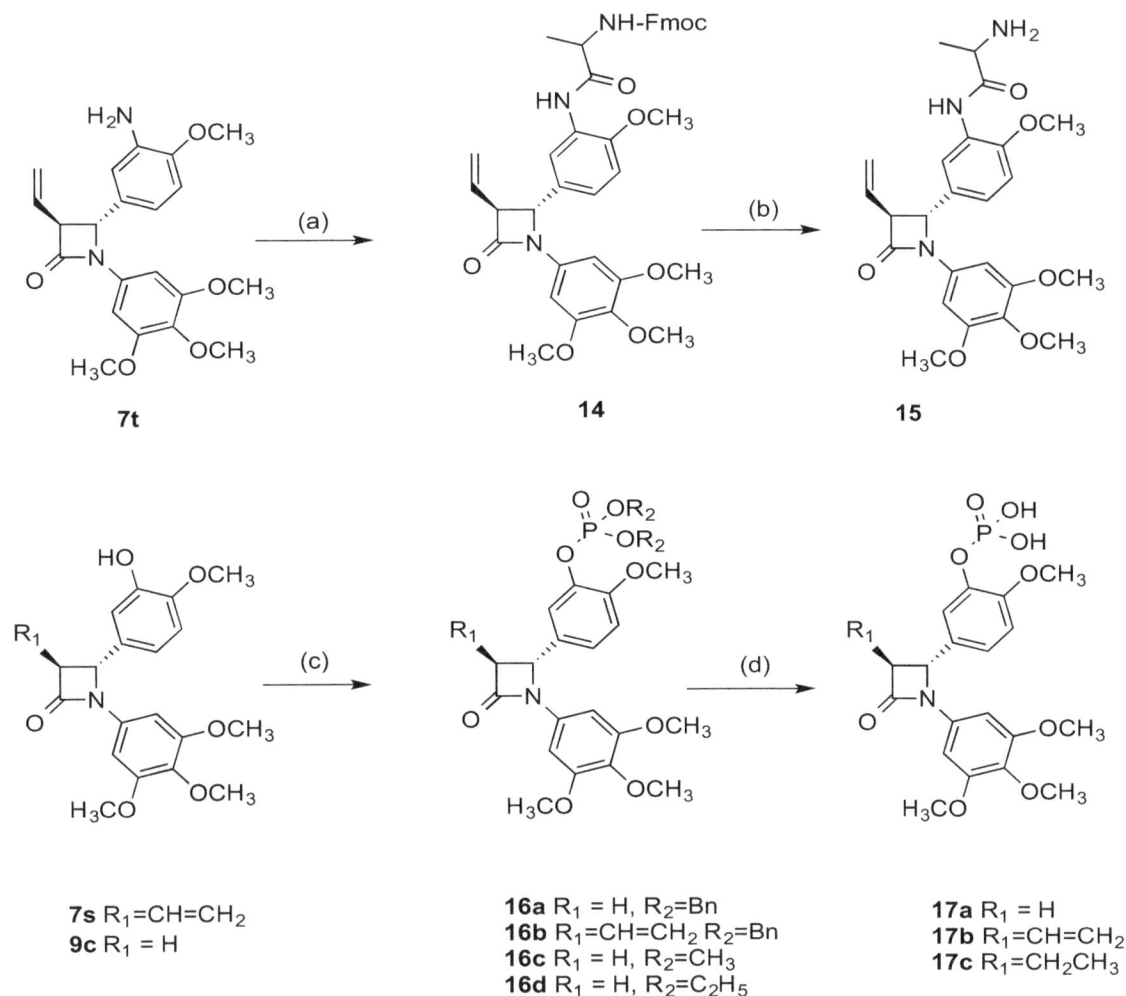

Scheme 4. Synthesis of amino acid prodrugs **15**, **17a–c**. Reagents and conditions: (a) Fmoc-L-alanine, anhydrous DMF, DCC, HOBt.H$_2$O, 20 °C, 24 h (58%); (b) 2N NaOH aq, CH$_3$OH, CH$_2$Cl$_2$, 20 °C, 24 h (57%); (c) for compounds **16a–16b**, dibenzyl phosphate, DIPEA, DMAP, CCl$_4$, CH$_3$CN, −10 °C–20 °C, 3h (60–61%); for compound **16c**, dimethyl phosphate, DIPEA, DMAP, CCl$_4$, CH$_3$CN, −10 °C–20 °C, 3h (52%); for compound **16d** diethyl phosphate, DIPEA, DMAP, CCl$_4$, CH$_3$CN, −10 °C–20 °C, 3h (79%); (d) for compounds **17a**, **17b**: bromotrimethylsilane, dry DCM, 45 min, 0 °C, (91–63%); for compound **17c**: H$_2$/Pd/C, ethanol-ethyl acetate, 1:1, 3 h, 20 °C, (98%).

2.2. X-Ray Structural Study

The X-ray crystal structures of compounds **7h, 8i, 8k** and **8h** are displayed in Figure 3 and confirm the structural assignment. The crystal data for the compounds are shown in Tables 1 and 2. For each compound the two aryl rings at N-1 and C-4 position are in a pseudo *cis* arrangement while the phenyl ring at C4 and the alkene group are on opposite sides of the β-lactam (*trans* configuration). The structure of the compounds **7h, 8h, 8i** and **8k** clearly demonstrated a non-coplanar configuration for rings A and B of the β-lactams, with the β-lactam ring providing a rigid scaffold. For compound **7h** even though both enantiomers are present, the compound crystallizes out in a chiral space group. The *trans* configuration of the aryl rings A and B at C-3 and C-4 is also evident. The dihedral angle H3/H4 is observed for compounds **7h, 8h, 8i** and **8k** respectively, which is consistent with the small *trans* coupling constant observed in the ^{1}H NMR spectrum of 2.00 Hz, 2.52 Hz, 2.48 Hz and 2.44 Hz respectively for these compounds. The β-lactam C=O bond lengths are 1.209(3) Å, 1.214(3) Å, 1.2077(17) Å and 1.2077(17) Å for compounds **7h, 8h, 8i** and **8k** respectively, which is consistent with data previously reported for the carbonyl bond length of monocyclic β-lactams of 1.217(3) Å [59] and 1.207(2) Å [60].

The ring A/B torsional angles for compounds **7h**, **8h**, **8i** and **8k** were observed as −59.5°, 59.7°, −73.5° and −77.0° respectively; these values are significantly greater than those observed for the corresponding rings A/B in the DAMA-colchicine **1b** [5], Combretastatin A-4 **2a** [61] and related 4-arylcoumarin [62] as 53°, 55° and 48.3° respectively (Table 2). The azetidinone N1-C4 bond length was observed at 1.372(3) Å, 1.376(3) Å, 1.367(2) Å and 1.3767(18) Å for compounds **7h**, **8h**, **8i** and **8k** respectively, which compares with 1.334(4)Å reported for the alkene C=C of combretastatin A-4 [61]. The C26-C27 alkene bond length for **7h**, **8h**, **8i** and **8k** were observed at 1.303(3) Å, 1.3174 Å, 1.308(3) Å and 1.316(2) Å respectively, while the alkene C=C bond length for *iso*-combretastatin CA-4 has been reported as 1.329(3) Å [63]. The C-N bonds lengths in the β-lactam ring are unequal with N1-C4 bond lengths of 1.487(3) Å, 1.483(3) Å, 1.4774(19) Å and 1.4801(17) Å for compounds **7h**, **8h**, **8i** and **8k** respectively, compared to 1.372(3) Å, 1.376(3) Å, 1.367(2) Å and 1.3767(18) Å for the N1/C2 bond in compounds **7h**, **8h**, **8i** and **8k** respectively, indicating some degree of amide resonance [59].

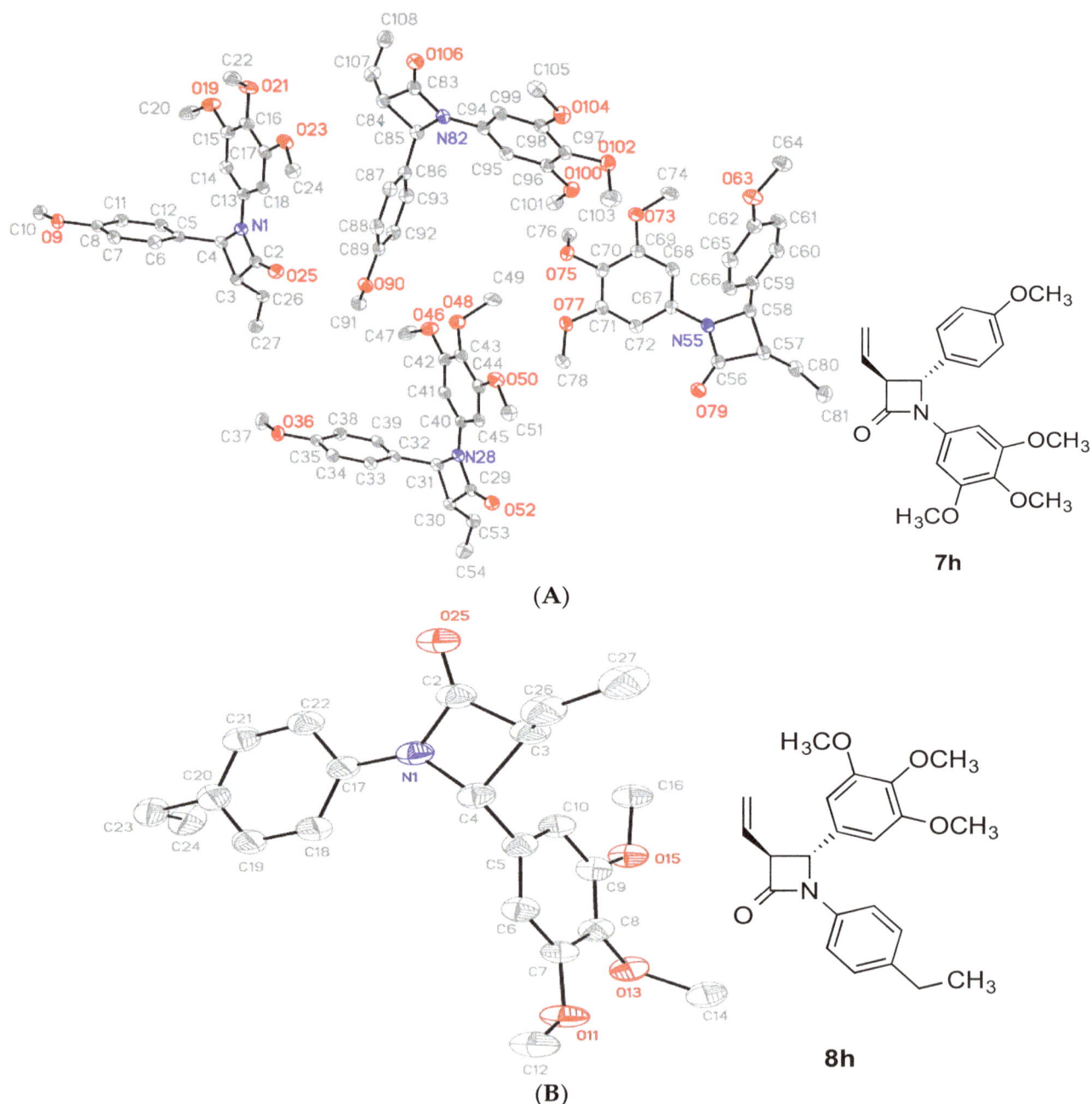

(A)

(B)

Figure 3. *Cont.*

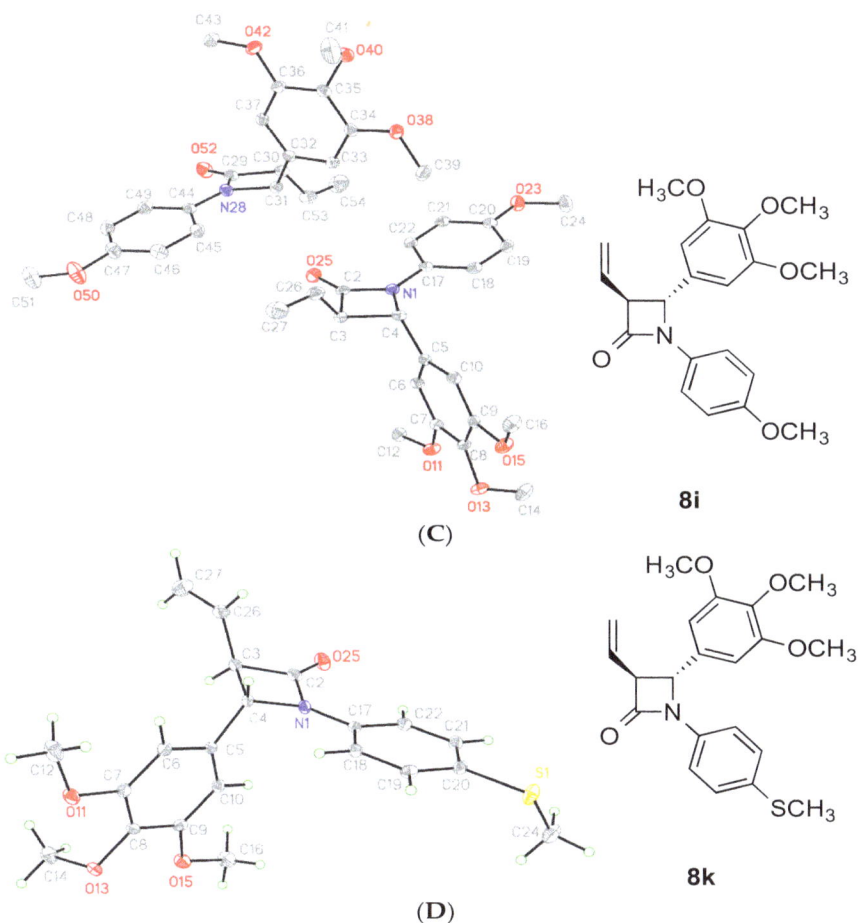

Figure 3. ORTEP representation of the X-ray crystal structure of (**A**) compound **7h**, (**B**) compound **8i**, (**C**) compound **8j** and (**D**) compound 8kwith the thermal ellipsoids set at 50% probability.

Table 2. X-Ray data and torsional angles for compounds **7h, 8h, 8i, 8k**.

Compound	Ring Plane Normal AB Angle(°)	Ring A to Central Torsion (°) [a]	Ring B to Central Torsion (°) [b]	RingAB Torsion (°) [c]	Ring B Vinyl Torsion (°) [d]
7h *	82.79(8)	177.0(2)	137.7(2)	−59.5(3)	124.8(2)
	75.19(8)	179.4(2)	137.1(2)	−53.8(5)	123.8(2)
	100.51(8)	177.6(2)	−136.1(2)	58.1(3)	−126.1(2)
	85.35(8)	−167.5(2)	−138.9(2)	59.7(3)	−120.9(2)
8h	93.14(7)	−171.6(3)	−130.1(2)	59.7(3)	−124.4(2)
8i §	86.28(5)	170.67(17)	150.21(14)	−73.5(2)	127.75(18)
	85.68(6)	165.62(18)	155.26(16)	−73.2(2)	127.49(16)
8k	85.60(5)	162.50(17)	156.94(13)	−77.0(2)	122.95(15)

a	b	c	d
C14-C13-N1-C2	C12-C5-C4-N1	C13-N1-C4-C5	C5-C4-C3-C26
C18-C17-N1-C2	C10-C5-C4-N1	C17-N1-C4-C5	C5-C4-C3-C26
C18-C17-N1-C2	C6-C5-C4-N1	C17-N1-C4-C5	C5-C4-C3-C26
C18-C17-N1-C2	C6-C5-C4-N1	C17-N1-C4-C5	C5-C4-C3-C26
C14-C13-N1-C2	C10-C5-C4-N1	C13-N1-C4-C5	C5-C4-C3-C26

* Four independent molecules in the asymmetric unit. § = 2 independent molecules in the asymmetric unit. Each angle given but only the first atom numbering scheme is outlined above.

2.3. Biological Results and Discussion

2.3.1. In vitro Antiproliferative Activities

The synthesized compounds were first evaluated for their antiproliferative activity against the human breast cancer cell line MCF-7 and compared with CA-4 as a reference compound (IC$_{50}$ = 3.9 nM) [64,65]. The results are shown in Table 3 (**7a–7n, 7p–7t, 8a–8k**), and Table 4 (**10a–h, 11–13, 15** and **17a–c**). All β-lactams were evaluated as the *trans* isomer. The most potent compounds were identified as **7s** and **7t**, with IC$_{50}$ values of 8 νM and 17 nM respectively. Compound **7s** is a direct analogue of CA-4, while **7t** is the corresponding amino compound and this type of substitution has been demonstrated to confer potency in many CA-4 analogues [52]. Compounds having the methoxy, ethoxy and thiomethyl substituents at C-4 of Ring B displayed potent antiproliferative effects, with IC$_{50}$ values of 20 nM, 37 nM and 51 nM respectively for compounds **7h, 7i** and **7r** respectively. The halo substituted compounds, **7b** and **7c** and 4-methyl compound **7g** were less effective with IC$_{50}$ values of 690 nM, 445 nM and 355 nM respectively. Selectivity in antiproliferative effect was demonstrated by the 1 and 2-naphthyl compounds **7m** (IC$_{50}$ = 1.738 µM) and **7n** (IC$_{50}$ = 68 nM). This result compares favourably with the naphthyl CA-4 analogues reported by Medarde et al. in which the 2-naphthalene ring directly replaces the Ring B of CA-4 [66].

The IC$_{50}$ of compound **7u** containing the 3,5-dimethoxyphenyl Ring A was determined as 170 nM in MCF-7 cells, demonstrating retention of antiproliferative potency with slightly reduced activity compared to the 3,4,5-trimethoxy ring A substituted compound **7h**. This observation could infer that the *para*-methoxy aryl group is less important for activity and the 3,5-dimethoxyaryl substituted Ring A is favourable for interaction of the molecule with the colchicine binding site of tubulin [53]. Compounds **8a–8k** containing the 3,4,5-trimethoxyphenyl substituent (Ring A of CA-4) at the C-4 position were generally observed to have poorer antiproliferative activity than the corresponding compounds **7a–7t**, containing the 3,4,5-trimethoxyphenyl substituent (Ring A of the Combretastatin A-4) at the N-1 position, (Table 3). The exceptions were compounds **8a** (4-fluoro) and **8j** (4-NHCOCH$_3$) with IC$_{50}$ values of 1.066 µM and 4.024 µM respectively. The relative positions of the 3,4,5-trimethoxyphenyl Ring A and Ring B on the β-lactam ring at positions N-1 and C-4 have a significant effect on the antiproliferative activity of the compounds as we previously reported [45].

The effects of various structural modifications on the activity of the more potent 3-vinylazetidinones were next explored, (Table 4). The most potent compound in this series is the 3-styryl containing compound **10f**, with IC$_{50}$ = 46 nM. The alcohol **10a** showed interesting activity (65 nM) while the introduction of an additional methyl group at C-5 to afford the alcohol **10d** resulted in reduced efficacy with IC$_{50}$ = 544 nM. The diol **13** also proved noteworthy with IC$_{50}$ = 69 nM. The 3-acetyl compound **11** and 3-ethylidene compound **12** resulted in similar antiproliferative effects (IC$_{50}$ = 414 nM and 502 nM respectively). Additional compounds containing the hydroxyalkene substituent at C-3 (e.g., compounds **10b, 10c, 10e, 10g, 10h**) were found to be moderately active (IC$_{50}$ values 288–570 nM).

The amino acid prodrug amide **15** was evaluated in MCF-7 breast cancer cells to determine if it retained any antiproliferative activity when compared with the parent compound **7t** which was extremely potent with IC$_{50}$ = 17 nM. The IC$_{50}$ for **15** (3.251 µM) was lower than expected; however metabolic activation in vivo may be required for the hydrolysis of the amide [67]. The phosphate esters **17a–17c** displayed impressive antiproliferative activity, with IC$_{50}$ values of 22 nM, 27 nM and 21 nM respectively (Table 4). The IC$_{50}$ values for the corresponding phenols **7s** and **9c** in MCF-7 cells are 8 nM and 17 nM respectively. Comparison of the 3-vinyl **17b** (IC$_{50}$ = 27 nM) with the 3-ethyl **17c** (IC$_{50}$ = 21 nM) indicated that introduction of the 3-vinyl or 3-ethyl substituent, together with the 3-unsubstituted **17a** (22 nM) retains potency and optimum activity. The potent activity displayed for the phosphate esters **17a–17c**, together with the predicted improvement in water solubility, indicate that these compounds are useful prodrugs for future development. Rapid in vivo dephosphorylation would be expected to occur for the β-lactam phosphates **17a–c** as observed for CA-4P [11].

Table 3. Antiproliferative activities of β-lactams **7a–7n**, **7p–7u**, **8a–8k** in human MCF-7 breast cancer cells.

Compound Number	Antiproliferative Activity IC_{50} (µM) [a]
7a	8.314 ± 1.40
7b	0.690 ± 0.11
7c	0.445 ± 0.07
7d	3.827 ± 0.53
7e	4.047 ± 0.45
7f	4.034 ± 0.42
7g	0.355 ± 0.03
7h	0.020 ± 0.0025
7i	0.037 ± 0.0033
7j	13.990 ± 1.81
7k	57.041 ± 3.72
7l	8.015 ± 0.63
7m	1.738 ± 0.17
7n	0.068 ± 0.01
7p	0.618 ± 0.10
7q	6.251 ± 5.05
7r	0.051 ± 0.001
7s	0.008 ± 0.00071
7t	0.017 ± 0.0018
7u	0.170 ± 0.07.
8a	1.066 ± 0.14
8b	29.150 ± 1.14
8c	10.400 ± 0.87
8d	59.150 ± 4.16
8e	68.840 ± 3.63
8f	50.460 ± 4.25
8g	43.130 ± 2.16
8h	36.400 ± 2.13
8i	65.120 ± 5.55
8j	4.024 ± 0.64
8k	>50
CA-4 [b]	0.0039 ± 0.00032

[a] IC_{50} values are half maximal inhibitory concentrations required to block the growth stimulation of MCF-7 cells. Values represent the mean ± SEM (error values × 10^{-6}) for at least three experiments performed in triplicate. [b] The IC_{50} value obtained for CA-4 (0.0039 µM for MCF-7) is in good agreement with the reported values [64,65].

Table 4. Antiproliferative activities of β-lactams **10a–h**, **11–13**, **15a** and **17a–c** in human MCF-7 breast cancer cells [a].

Compound Number	Antiproliferative Activity IC_{50} (nM) [a]
10a	65 ± 15
10b	292 ± 50
10c	5701 ± 246
10d	544 ± 310
10e	537 ± 80
10f	46 ± 41
10g	288 ± 76
10h	467 ± 0.253
11	414 ± 132
12	502 ± 212
13	69 ± 29
15	3251 ± 270
17a	22 ± 1.5
17b	27 ± 2
17c	21 ± 1.5
CA-4 [b]	39 ± 3.2

[a] IC_{50} values are half maximal inhibitory concentrations required to block the growth stimulation of MCF-7 cells. Values represent the mean ± SEM (error values × 10^{-6}) for at least three experiments performed in triplicate. [b] The IC_{50} value obtained for CA-4 (39 nM for MCF-7) is in good agreement with the reported values [64,65].

Triple-negative breast cancers (TNBC) are characterised by the absence of estrogen receptors (ER-), progesterone receptors (PR-) and human epidermal growth factor receptor 2 (HER2-). TNBC does not respond to hormonal therapy (such as tamoxifen or aromatase inhibitors) or therapies that target HER2 receptors, such as Herceptin. Treatment options are limited leading to poor prognosis, as indicated by low 5-year survival rates. A number of the more potent compounds were evaluated in the triple negative MDA-MB-231 cell line (Table 5). Compound **7s** was the most effective of the series with an IC_{50} value of 10 nM. Compounds **7h**, **7t**, **17a**, **17b** and **17c** were also seen to be effective with IC_{50} values of 31 nM, 30 nM, 30 nM, 49 nM and 44 nM respectively, and compared favourably with the positive CA-4 (control IC_{50} = 43 nM) [34,63,68].

Table 5. Antiproliferative activities of selected β-lactams in human MDA-MB-231 breast cancer cells [a].

Compound Number	Antiproliferative Activity IC_{50} (nM) [a]
7b	191 ± 16
7h [b]	31.7
7i	61 ± 7
7n	77 ± 9
7s [b]	10
7t	30 ± 2
17a	30 ± 4
17b [b]	48.6
17c	44 ± 7
CA-4 [c]	43

[a] IC_{50} values are half maximal inhibitory concentrations required to block the growth stimulation of MDA-MB-231 cells. Values represent the mean ± SEM (error values × 10^{-6}) for at least three experiments performed in triplicate. [b] Antiproliferative activity against MDA-MB-231 from NCI (see Supplementary Information). [c] The IC_{50} value obtained for CA-4 in this assay is 43 nM for MDA-MB-231 in good agreement with reported values for CA-4 in MTT assay on human MDA-MB-231 breast cancer cell line [34,63,68].

Compound **7h** was also evaluated in the triple-negative Hs578T breast cancer cell line and its isogenic subclone Hs578Ts(i)8 cells to examine the activity of β-lactams as CA-4 analogues and as anti-tubulin agents for metastasis. Hs578Ts(i)8 cells are 3-fold more invasive and 2.5-fold more migratory than the parental cell line (Hs578T). In addition, Hs578Ts(i)8 cells had 30% more CD44+/CD24-/low cells that could enhance the invasive properties but with a significantly increased capacity to proliferate, migrate and produce tumours in vivo in nude mice [69]. Compound **7h** exhibited an excellent anti-proliferative activity in Hs578T cells (IC_{50} 31 nM) and interestingly retained potency in invasive Hs578Ts(i)8 cells (IC_{50} 76 nM). The values for CA4 in these cells were 8 nM and 20 nM respectively. These results could indicate the ability of β-lactams as CA-4 analogues to inhibit tumour invasion and angiogenesis which are characteristic of tumour growth and metastasis. These β-lactam compounds may provide potential development leads for this subset of aggressive breast cancers. Compound **7s** was also evaluated in the leukemia cell lines HL-60 and K562 and was found to be extremely potent with IC_{50} values of 17 nM and 26 nM respectively, comparing favourable with CA-4 [IC_{50} values of 4 nM (HL-60) and 4 nM (K562)].

The novel compounds **7h**, **7s**, **7t**, **17b** and **17c** were selected for further investigation based on analysis of their drug-like properties (Lipinski) from a Tier-1 profiling screen, together with predictions of blood brain barrier partition, permeability, plasma protein binding, metabolic stability and human intestinal absorption properties which confirmed that these compounds are moderately lipophilic-hydrophilic drugs and are suitable candidates for further investigation (Tables S1 and S2, Supporting information).

2.3.2. Evaluation of β-Lactams in the NCI60 Cell Line Screen

A series of the more potent compounds **7h**, **7s**, **7t**, **17b** and **17c** were evaluated in the National Cancer Institute (NCI)/Division of Cancer Treatment and Diagnosis (DCTD)/Developmental Therapeutics Program (DTP) [70], in which the activity of each compound was determined using approximately 60 different cancer cell lines of diverse tumor origins. The results are summarized in Tables S3–S5, Supplementary Information. The compounds were tested for inhibition of growth (GI_{50}) and cytotoxicity (LC_{50}) in the NCI panel of cancer cell lines and showed excellent broad-spectrum antiproliferative activity against tumor cell lines derived from leukemia, non-small-cell lung cancer, colon cancer, CNS cancer, melanoma, ovarian cancer, renal cancer, breast cancer and prostate cancer [71] using the sulforhodamine B (SRB) protein assay [72], (Tables S3–S5 Supplementary Information). The NCI results confirmed our in-house evaluations in MCF-7 cells with GI_{50} values for compounds **7h, 7s, 7t, 17b** and **17c** of 30.6, <10, <10, 39.4 and 25.1 nM respectively.

Compound **7s**, the most potent compound in our panel, demonstrated a mean GI_{50} value of 23 nM across all NCI cell lines tested. The GI_{50} values for **7s** were in the sub-micromolar range for each of the cell lines investigated, except for two cell lines (melanoma cell line UACC-257 and the breast cancer cell line T-47D). For compound **7s** the GI_{50} values obtained were below 10 nM for 28 of the cell lines investigated and below 40 nM in all but eight of the panel cell lines tested. Activity was demonstrated for compound **7s** against all of the non-small cell lung (GI_{50} value 85.5 - <10 nM), colon (GI_{50} value 429 - <10 nM), CNS (GI_{50} value 40.5 - <10 nM), ovarian (GI_{50} value 45.3 - <10 nM), prostate (GI_{50} value <10 nM) and renal (GI_{50} value 40.2 - <10 nM) cancer cell lines tested. The mean GI_{50} values over the full 60 cell line panel for compounds **7h, 7t** and **17c** of 52, 48 and 73 nM respectively (see Supplementary Information, Table S5) compares very favourably with the GI_{50} value for CA-4 of 99 nM.

LC_{50} values for compound **7s** were greater than 100 μM in all but three cell lines tested indicating minimal toxicity and the potential use of this compound for a wide range of therapeutic applications (Tables S3–S5 Supplementary Information). A similar result was obtained for compound **7h** with LC_{50} values > 100 μM in all cell lines tested.

The NCI COMPARE algorithm allows a comparison of the activities of β-lactams **7h** and **7s** with compounds of a known mechanism of antiproliferative action in the NCI Standard Agents Database. Compounds **7h** and **7s** showed high correlation to tubulin targeting agents such as maytansine, rhizoxin and the clinically important anticancer drugs vincristine and vinblastine, (see Supplementary Information, Tables S6 and S7).

2.3.3. Evaluation of Toxicity of 7s in Normal Murine Mammary Epithelial Cells

The cytotoxic effect of a selected number of 3-vinyl-β-lactams in MCF-7 cells at 10 μM concentration was initially determined in the lactate dehydrogenase (LDH) assay [73]. The 3-vinyl-β-lactams **7d, 7h, 7i, 7q, 7r** and **7u** resulted in low cytotoxicity with 7.2%, 2.4%, 8.5%, 4.5%, 4.5% and 3.5% cell death respectively while compounds **7s** and **7t** displayed increased cytotoxicity of 16.1% and 25% cell death in this assay. The 3-(1-hydroxyl-1-methylethyl) and 3-(1-hydroxy-1-phenylallyl) substituted compounds **10d** and **10f** resulted in 9.8% and 7.6% cell death respectively while cell death of 8.4% was obtained for the 3-ethylidene compound **12**. CA-4 was used as the positive control in this assay and resulted in 11.8% cell death at 10 μM concentration.

The cytotoxicity of the most potent compound **7s** on non-tumourigenic cell line HEK-293 (normal human embryonic kidney) was also investigated. We demonstrated an IC_{50} value greater than 5 μM in HEK-293T cells for **7s**. Cell viability of HEK-293T cells was significantly higher than MCF-7 cells at 10, 1 and 0.5 μM concentrations of compound **7s** (Figure 4A), demonstrating the lack of cellular toxicity of the compounds in these non-cancerous cells.

Further toxicity studies were carried out on the most potent compound β-lactam **7s** in primary cells (mouse mammary healthy epithelial cells) at two different cell concentrations (25,000 and 50,000 cells/mL), with CA4 as a positive control. The cells were harvested from mid- to late-pregnant CD-1 mice and were cultured as previously reported [74,75]. Both CA-4 [76] and **7s** were not cytotoxic at concentrations up to 10 μM in the NCI cell line panel (See Tables S8 and S9 Supplementary Information). The IC_{50} values for both compounds **7s** and CA-4 evaluated in normal murine mammary epithelial cells was greater than 10 μM which indicated a minimal toxicity for these compounds (Figure 4B). At both 25,000 cells/mL and 50,000 cells/mL and a concentration of 10 μM, CA-4 was lethal to the highest percentage of cells. The percentage of viable murine mammary epithelial cells at the IC_{50} value of each compound in MCF-7 cells (see Table 3) was calculated in order to give an estimation of the toxicity at this value. At 50,000 cells/mL, over 90% of cells were viable after 72 h for compound **7s**, (Figure 4B). At 25,000 cells/mL, the percentage of cells remaining viable after treatment with compound **7s** for 72 h was 93%, compared to 74% for CA-4. (Supplementary Information Tables S8 and S9).

These results indicate a favourable toxicity profile for **7s** in comparison to CA4. This provides further evidence, in addition to the NCI60 LC_{50} values for **7s**, that the β-lactam compound developed in this study is minimally toxic to cells that are not proliferating.

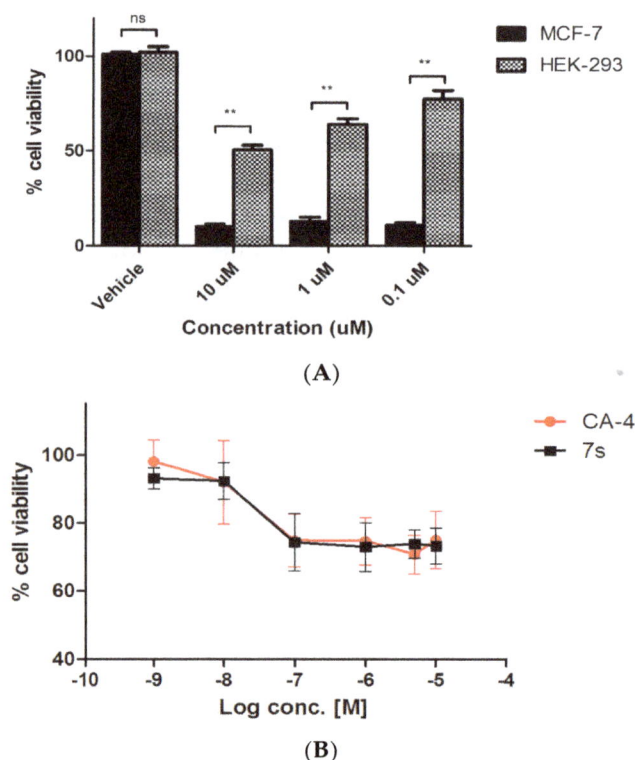

(A)

(B)

Figure 4. (**A**) Antiproliferative activity of β-lactam **7s** in tumorigenic MCF-7 cells and non-tumourigenic HEK-293T cells. Values represent the mean for two independent experiments. Statistical analysis was performed using a non-paired two-tailed t-test (ns, not significant; **, $p < 0.01$). (**B**) Cell viability for compound **7s** and CA-4 in murine mammary epithelial cells. Mouse mammary epithelial cells were harvested from mid- to late- pregnant CD-1 mice and cultured. The isolated mammary epithelial cells were seeded at 50,000 cells/mL. After 24 h, they were treated with 2 μL volumes of test compound which had been pre-prepared as stock solutions in ethanol to furnish the concentration range of study, 1 nM–100 μM, and re-incubated for a further 72 h. Control wells contained the equivalent volume of the vehicle ethanol (1%, v/v). The cytotoxicity was assessed using alamar blue dye.

2.3.4. Effect of β-Lactam 7s on Cell Cycle and Apoptosis

It is well recognised that tubulin destabilizing agents arrest the cell cycle in the G_2/M phase due to cytoskeleton disruption and microtubule depolymeriztion. The effects of β-lactam **7s** on cell cycle events and induction of apoptosis in MCF-7 cells were next explored. Initial analysis by flow cytometry of propidium iodide stained MCF-7 cells showed G_2M arrest at 24 h by compound **7s** [64% (10 nM) and 82% (100 nM)] (Figure 5C). A time dependent increase in the percentage of apoptotic cells (sub-G_0G_1) after 72 h (14% and 26% respectively for 10 nM and 100 nM concentration) was also evident compared to the vehicle control (6% at 72 h), (Figure 5A), with a corresponding decrease of cells in the G_0–G_1 phase of the cell cycle, (Figure 5C). The positive control CA-4 (100 nM) showed 52% of cells in G_2M arrest at 48 h, and 9.4% in the sub-G_0G_1 population.

To characterize the mode of cell death induced by **7s** in MCF-7 cells, analysis of apoptosis was performed using propidium iodide (PI), which stains DNA and enters only dead cells, and annexin-V, which binds selectively to phosphatidyl serine (Figure 6). Dual staining for annexin-V and PI facilitates discrimination between live cells (annexin-V-/PI-), early apoptotic cells (annexin-V+/PI-), late apoptotic cells (annexin-V+/PI+) and necrotic cells (annexin-V-/PI+). Each concentration induced an accumulation of annexin-V positive cells when compared to the vehicle control (5%), Figure 6.

About 13.6% of cells were found to be apoptotic (annexin-V positive) when treated with compound **7s** at 10 nM for 72 h. With an increase in concentration of **7s**, 31.9% of cells were found to be apoptotic at 100 nM. The positive control CA-4 (50 nM) resulted in 34.6% apoptotic cells. The observed effect of compound **7s** on cell cycle resulting in G_2M arrest followed by apoptosis is typical of tubulin targeting compounds. However, we have previously reported that prolonged exposure of colon cancer cells CT-26, CaCo-2 and HT-29 to our structurally related 3-aryl-β-lactams induced autophagy [77]; it is possible that autophagy may be the cell death mechanism in the present case, because of the level of apoptosis observed.

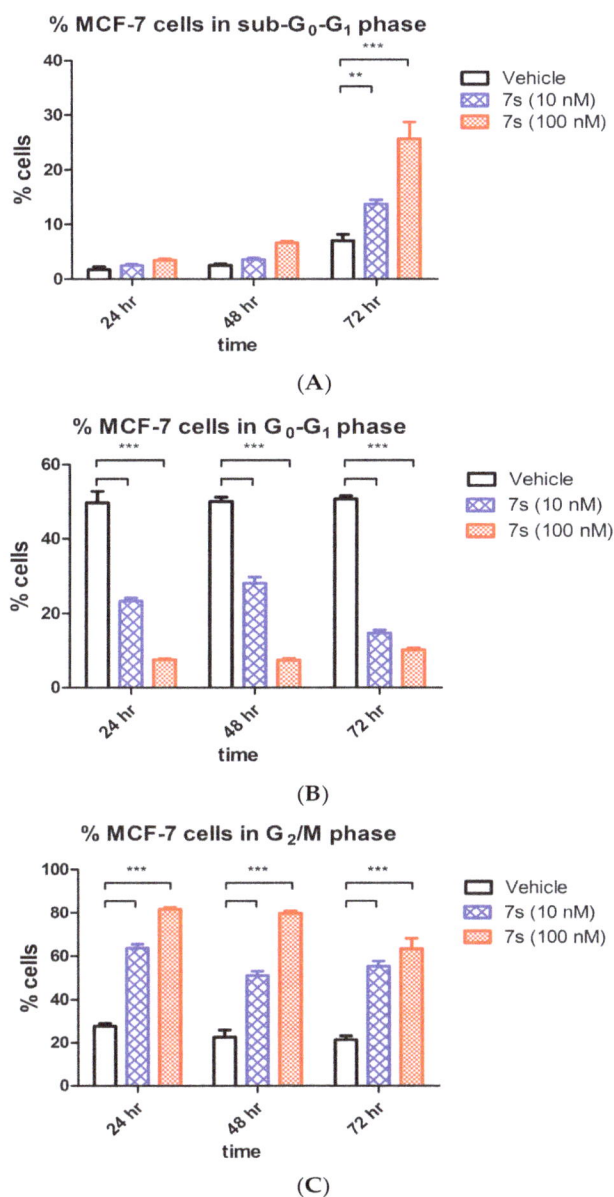

(A)

(B)

(C)

Figure 5. Effect of compound **7s** on the cell cycle and apoptosis in MCF-7 cells. Cells were treated with either vehicle [0.1% ethanol (*v/v*)], **7s** (10 nM and 100 nM) for 24 h, 48 h and 72 h. Cells were then fixed, stained with PI, and analyzed by flow cytometry. Cell cycle analysis was performed on histograms of gated counts per DNA area (FL2-A). The number of cells with (**A**) <2N (sub-G_1), (**B**) 2N(G_0G_1), and (**C**) 4N (G_2/M) DNA content was determined with CellQuest software. Values represent the mean ± SEM for three independent experiments. Statistical analysis was performed using two-way ANOVA (**, $p < 0.01$; ***, $p < 0.001$).

(A)

(B)

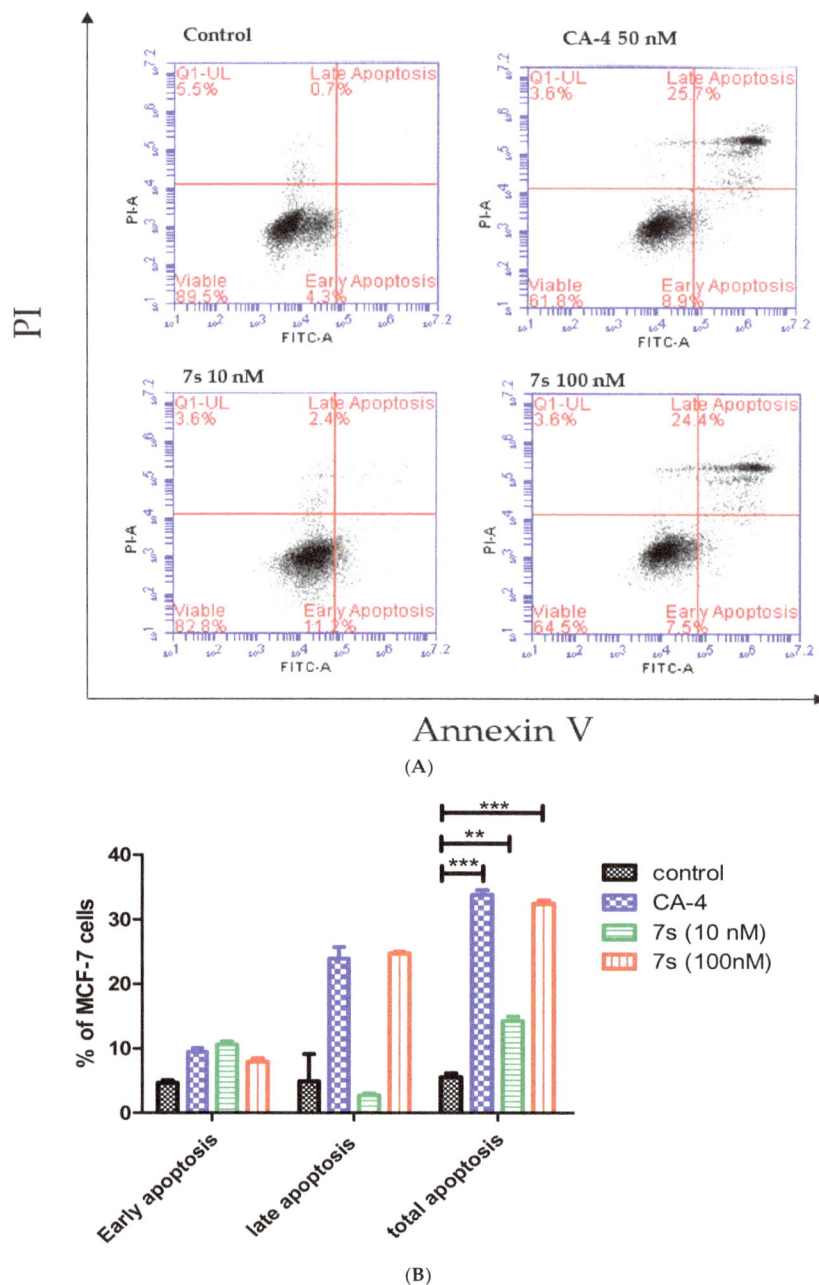

Figure 6. Compound **7s** potently induces apoptosis in MCF-7 cells (Annexin V/PI FACS). (**A**) Effect of compound 7s and CA-4 on apoptosis in MCF-7 cells analysed by flow cytometry after double staining of the cells with Annexin-V-FITC and PI. MCF-7 cells treated with 10 and 100 nM of compound 7s or 50 nM of CA-4 for 72 h and collected and processed for analysis. (**B**) Quantitative analysis of apoptosis. Values represent the mean ± SEM for three independent experiments. Statistical analysis was performed using two-way ANOVA (**, $p < 0.01$; ***, $p < 0.001$).

2.3.5. Tubulin Polymerization Studies

The effect of selected β-lactam CA-4 compounds (**7h, 7i, 7s, 7t**) which demonstrated the most potent antiproliferative effects in vitro was assessed on the assembly of purified bovine tubulin. CA-4 which effectively inhibits the assembly of tubulin was used as a positive control, while paclitaxel was used to demonstrate effective tubulin polymerization. Tubulin polymerization was determined for compounds **7h, 7i** and **7t** at 10 μM for 30 min and compound **7s** at 1, 5 and 10 μM for 60 min by measuring the increase in absorbance at 340 nm, (Figure 7A,B) [78]. The degree of light scattering by microtubules is proportional to their degree of polymerization. For the paclitaxel control the v_{max} was found to be 89.4 mOD/min. The v_{max} value provides a sensitive indication of the tubulin/ligand interactions for the tubulin polymerization. The most potent antiproliferative compound **7s** (10 μM) demonstrated a significant 8.7-fold reduction in v_{max} value while exposure to CA-4 (10 μM) brings about a 5.28-fold reduction in the v_{max} value. Compound **7s** compares very favourably to CA-4 in this respect. These effects are in good agreement with the antiproliferative data recorded for both CA-4 (IC_{50} = 4.2 nM) and **7s** (IC_{50} = 8 nM) in the MCF-7 cell line. The v_{max} value for compounds **7h**, **7i** and **7t** was determined as 3.43, 3.84 and 0.92 mOD/min respectively, together with the fold-reduction in the v_{max} values of 2.45, 2.19 and 9.15 respectively for the tubulin polymerization with reference to ethanol control. These results confirm that the molecular target of these antiproliferative 3-vinyl-β-lactams is tubulin and that they are microtubule-destabilising agents.

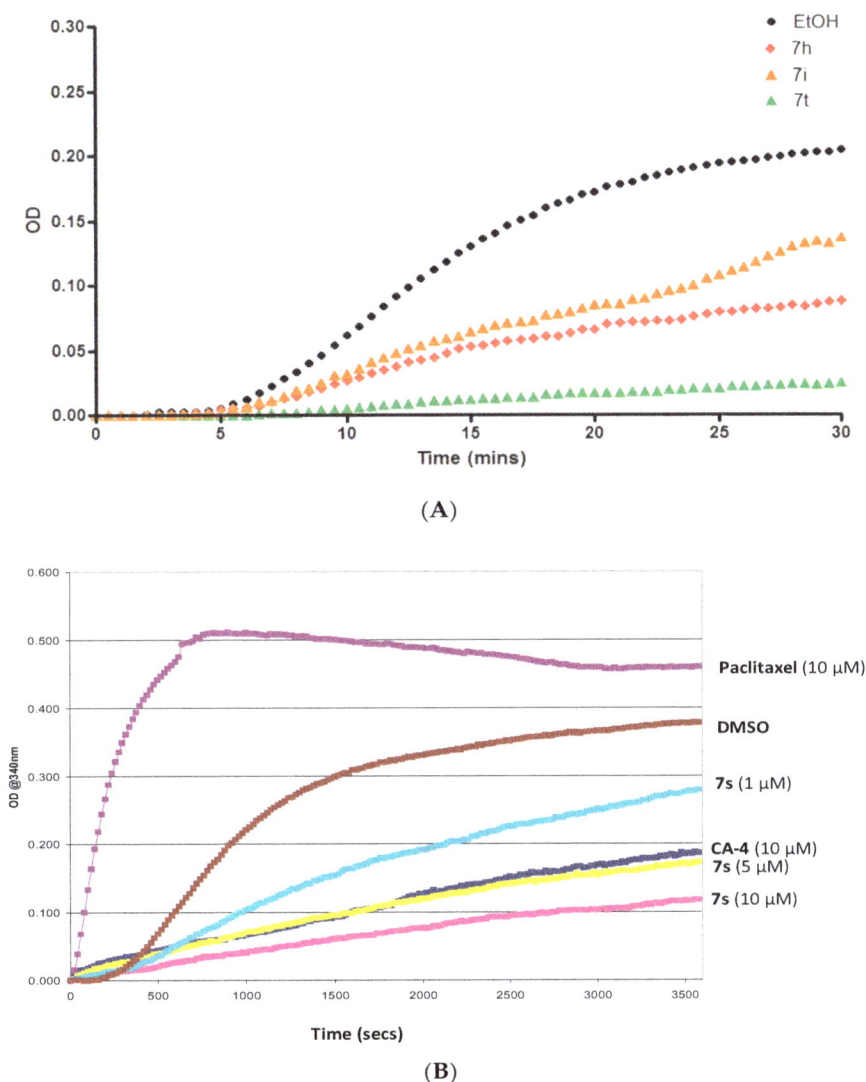

(A)

(B)

Figure 7. (A) Effect of compounds **7h**, **7i**, **7t** on tubulin polymerization in vitro. (B) Tubulin polymerization assay for compound **7s** at 10 μM, 5μM and 1μM. Paclitaxel (10 μM) and CA4 (10 μM) were used as references while ethanol (1% *v/v*) was used as a vehicle control. Purified bovine tubulin and GTP were mixed in a 96-well plate. The polymerization reaction was initated by warming the solution from 4 °C to 37 °C. The effect on tubulin assembly was monitored in a Spectramax 340PC spectrophotometer at 340 nm at 30 s intervals for 60 min at 37 °C. DMSO. Fold inhibition of tubulin polymerization was calculated using the V_{max} value for each reaction. The results represent the mean for three separate experiments.

The dose-dependent effect of **7s** on tubulin polymerization is illustrated in Figure 7. Exposure of the tubulin to 10 μM, 5 μM and 1 μM of **7s** resulted in a dose-dependent fold reduction of v_{max} of 8.70, 7.31 and 2.61 respectively while the IC_{50} value for **7s** for the inhibition of polymerization was calculated to be 1.37 μM, Figure 7. Taken together, these results demonstrate that for these novel β-lactam containing CA4 analogues, antiproliferative activity against the MCF-7 cell line and the inhibition of tubulin polymerization are closely related. It has also been shown that the most potent antiproliferative compound synthesised (**7s**) inhibits tubulin polymerization to a greater extent than CA-4.

2.3.6. Immunofluorescence Microscopy

Alterations in the microtubule network induced by β-lactam **7s** in MCF-7 cells were investigated using immunofluorescence and confocal microscopy (Figure 8). A well organised microtubular network was observed in MCF-7 control cells when stained with α-tubulin mAb (Figure 8) and in untreated cells (data not shown). Formation of microtubule bundles and pseudo asters was demonstrated for cells when exposed to paclitaxel (a microtubule-stabilising agent), Figure 8 [79]. A complete loss of microtubule formation was induced in cells exposed to CA-4 or β-lactam **7s** for 16 h. This effect is consistent with depolymerised microtubules. Following treatment with CA-4 or β-lactam **7s**, MCF-7 cells were observed to contain multiple micronuclei. Mitotic catastrophe resulting from premature or inappropriate entry of cells into mitosis is a type of programmed cell death in response to DNA damage, and is characterised by multinucleated cells [80]. CA-4 induced mitotic catastrophe has also been reported in non-small cell lung cancer cells [81,82], human endothelial cells (HUVEC) [83], human lung carcinoma cells (H460) [83] and human breast cancer cells (MCF-7) [84]. Taken together with the effects demonstrated above in Section 2.3.5 on the inhibition of polymerisation of isolated tubulin, the confocal imaging results confirm that β-lactam **7s** is targeting tubulin.

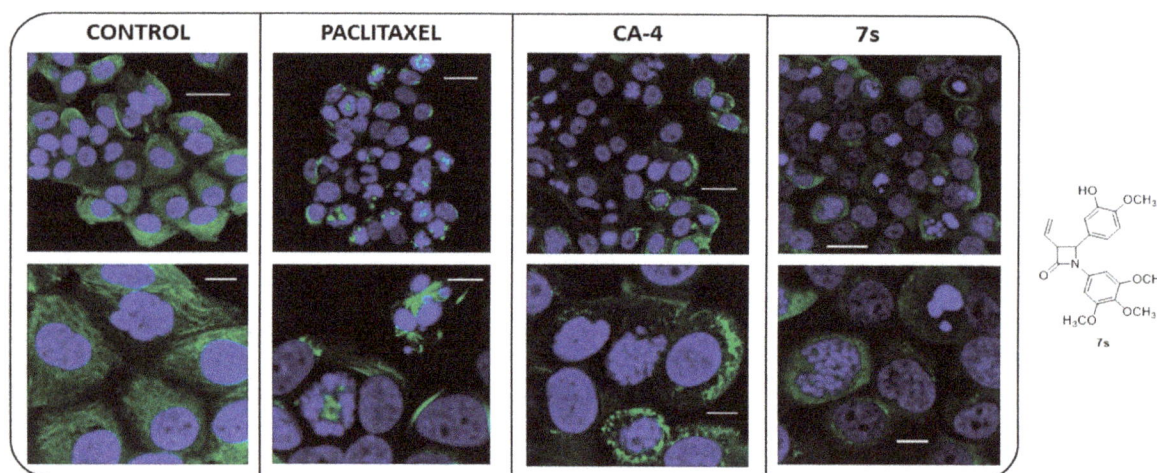

Figure 8. CA-4 and β-lactam (**7s**) depolymerise the microtubule network of MCF-7 cells. MCF-7 cells were treated with vehicle control [1% ethanol (*v/v*)], paclitaxel (1 μM), CA-4 (100 nM) or **7s** (*trans* isomer, 100 nM) for 16 h. Cells were fixed in 4% paraformaldehyde and stained with mouse monoclonal anti-α-tubulin-FITC antibody (clone DM1A) (green), Alexa Fluor 488 dye and counterstained with DAPI (blue). Images were captured by Leica SP8 confocal microscopy with Leica application suite X software. Representative confocal micrographs of three separate experiments are shown. Scale bar: 30 μM (top images); 10 μM (bottom images).

2.3.7. Interaction of β-Lactam 7s with Colchicine Binding Site of Tubulin

The binding of the lead compound **7s** to the colchicine binding site of tubulin was confirmed in a whole cell-based assay. *N,N'*-ethylene-bis(iodoacetamide) (EBI) is an alkylating agent that cross-links cysteine residues 239 and 354 in the colchicine-binding site of tubulin to form the β-tubulin-EBI adduct that migrates faster than β-tubulin [85,86], and is detected by Western blotting. However, when the

MCF-7 cells are pre-treated with colchicine or a colchicine-site ligand such as CA-4, the formation of the β-tubulin-EBI adduct is prevented. The MCF-7 cells were initially treated with selected β-lactam **7s** (10 μM) or CA- 4 for 2 h, then followed by addition of EBI for a further 1.5 h (Figure 9). The presence of the β-tubulin-EBI adduct was demonstrated for the control samples (no drug) at a lower position on the gel, indicating that EBI has cross-linked Cys239 and Cys354 on β-tubulin. When the cells are treated with β-lactam **7s** and CA-4, the EBI adduct formation is inhibited, indicating that **7s** is interacting with tubulin at the colchicine site of tubulin.

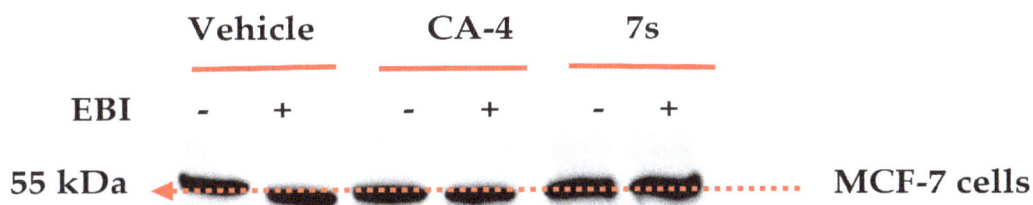

Figure 9. Colchicine binding assay: Effect of compound **7s** on the inhibition of the bisthioalkylation of Cys239 and Cys354 of β-tubulin by N,N'-ethylene-bis(iodoacetamide) (EBI) in MCF-7 cells. MCF-7 cells were treated with vehicle control [ethanol 0.1% (v/v)], **CA-4** and **7s** (10 μM) for 2 h; selected samples were then treated with EBI (100 μM) for an additional 1.5 h. Cells were harvested, lysed and analysed using sedimentation and Western blotting for β-tubulin and β-tubulin-EBI adduct.

2.4. Molecular Modelling Studies

The 3-vinyl-β-lactam compound **7s** represents the most potent compound synthesised in the study with IC_{50} value of 8 nM in MCF-7 breast cancer cells. The tubulin binding and immunofluorescence studies of 3-vinyl-β-lactam **7s** have demonstrated that the colchicine binding site of tubulin is the target for the compound. Flexible alignment of compound **7s** with CA-4 resulted in a good degree of overlap between the trimethoxyphenyl rings (Ring A) and the phenolic hydroxyl group of ring B (Figure 10A). The energy minimised structure of compound **7s** demonstrates the inter-atomic distances of the oxygens of the methoxy groups of ring A and ring B as 9.17 Å, which is similar to that calculated for CA-4 (9.27 Å).

The X-ray structure of CA-4 co-crystallised with tubulin has been determined suggesting that *cis*-CA-4 inhibits tubulin polymerization by preventing the transition from curved to straight tubulin [49]. The X-ray structure of *cis* and *trans* stereoisomers of a 3-methyl-1,4-diarylazetidinone [87] co-crystallised with tubulin was reported by Zhou et al. [37,38]. In the present study the potential interaction of our novel synthesised 3-vinyl-β-lactams with the colchicine binding site of tubulin, a series of docking calculations using MOE 2018.0101 [88] was undertaken on both the 3*S*/4*R* and 3*R*/4*S* enantiomers of the β–lactams **7s** and **7t** using the tubulin co-crystallised with DAMA-colchicine X-ray crystal structure (PDB entry 1SA0) [5]. Only results for the 3*S*/4*R* studies will be discussed as these stereoisomers were more highly ranked than the 3*R*/4*S* enantiomer and this is also supported by the crystallographic evidence [37,38]. The 3*S*/4*R* enantiomers of the hydroxyl **7s** and amino **7t** substituted analogues overlay their B-rings on the C-ring of DAMA-colchicine, collocate the trimethoxyphenyl substituents, overlap the 3-hydroxyl/amino groups on the DAMA-colchicine carbonyl oxygen atom and form HBA interactions with Lys β352 as shown in Figure 10B and 10C. The 3,4,5-trimethoxyphenyl groups of all analogues are able to make favourable van der Waals contacts within the lower subpocket delineated by Val β318 and Cys β241. The β-lactam carbonyl oxygen atom can make an HBA interaction with the backbone amine of Asp β251 for both analogues. For both compounds, the *trans* geometry at C3/C4 facilitates a more favourable interaction of rings A and B with the residues of the β-tubulin colchicine binding site. Protein-ligand interactions for **7s** are illustrated in Figure 11. The enantioselective synthesis of **7s** and **7t** are in progress which will provide the optimum configuration of these compounds to be determined for biological activity.

7s

2a (CA-4)

(A)

(B)

(C)

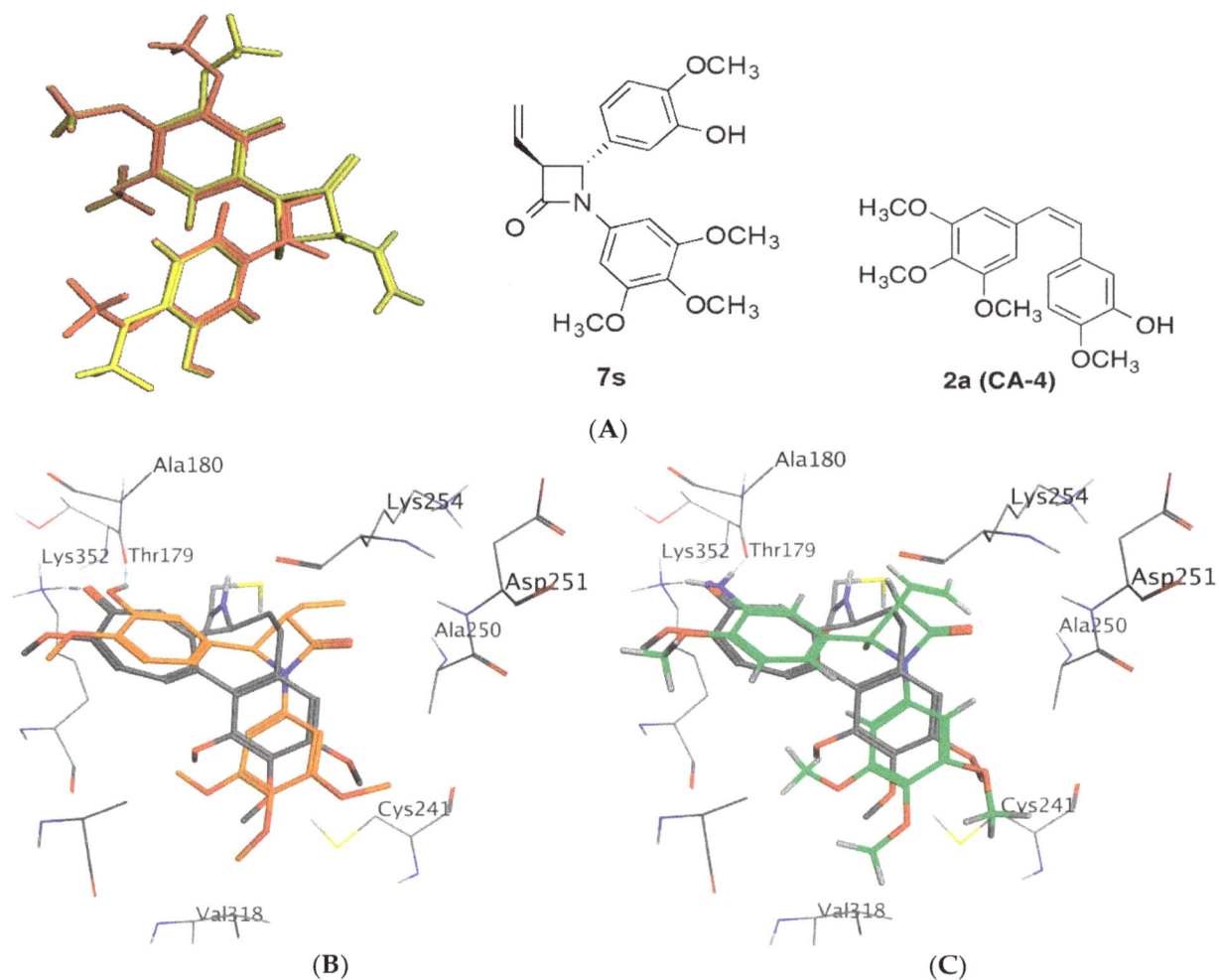

Figure 10. (**A**): Flexible alignment of **7s** (yellow) and CA-4 (**2a**)(red). (**B,C**): Overlay of the X-ray structure of tubulin cocrystallised with DAMA-colchicine (PDB entry 1SA0) on the best ranked docked poses of the 3S/4R enantiomers of (**B**) **7s** and (**C**) **7r**. The B-ring substituted analogues both overlap well on the C-ring of DAMA-colchicine. Ligands are rendered as tube and amino acids as line. Tubulin amino acids and DAMA-colchicine are coloured by atom type, **7s** orange and **7t** green. The atoms are coloured by element type, carbon = grey, hydrogen = white, oxygen = red, nitrogen = blue, sulphur = yellow. Key amino acid residues are labelled and multiple residues are hidden to enable a clearer view.

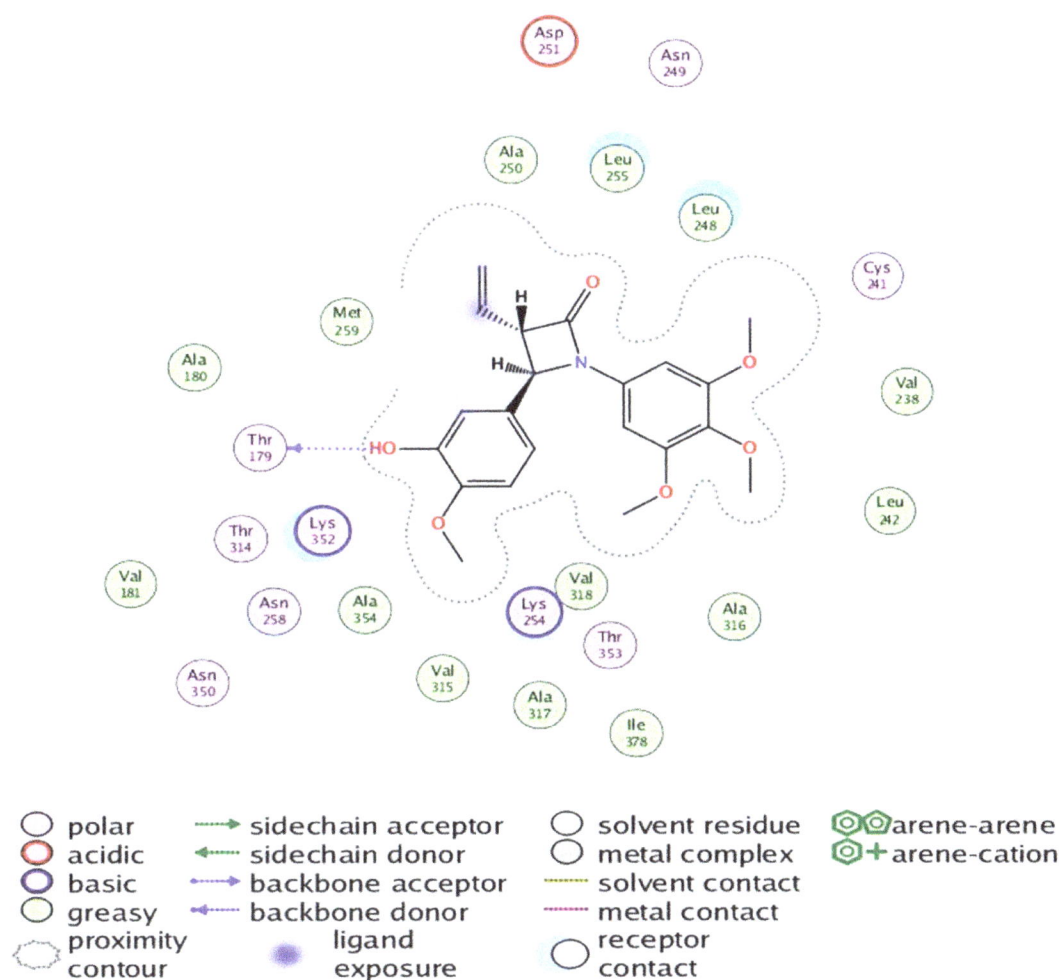

Figure 11. Protein-ligand interactions for the 3-vinyl-β-lactam compound (**7s**). 2D representation of the ligand−protein interactions of **7s** with the colchicine-binding site rendered using LigX module of MOE.

3. Conclusions

We have developed an interesting series of 3-vinylazetidinones which selectively modulate the activity of the tubulin protein, resulting in significant cytotoxicity to cancer cells and minimum cytotoxic effects to normal cells. Molecular modelling studies indicated that these compounds could interact with the colchicine binding site of tubulin, and consequently disrupt tubulin polymerization. X-Ray crystallographic studies confirmed that the torsional angle between Ring A and Ring B of the β-lactam was similar to CA-4 and was important in maintaining antiproliferative and tubulin disrupting activity. Biochemical evaluation of these compounds coupled with a molecular modeling study contributes to our understanding of the attributes of the 3-vinylazetidinones such as **7s** and **7t** that result in exceptional antiproliferative activity and dose-dependent microtubule assembly inhibition. Analysis of DNA content by flow cytometry demonstrated that the cells were arrested in the G_2/M phase; induction of apoptosis was confirmed by an increase in the sub-G_0G_1 population, which was confirmed by Annexin-V staining. Immunofluorescence staining with α-tubulin antibodies in MCF-7 cells demonstrated disorder and fragmentation of the microtubule network and disruption of mitotic spindle formation. The phosphate prodrugs **17a–c** were found to retain antitumour potency. The potent antiproliferative activity of the 3-vinylazetidinones **7s** and **7t** in breast cancer cells MCF-7 and notably in the triple negative MDA-MB-231 cell line reported in the present study compare very favourably with examples from the related series of 3-arylazetidinone compounds previously reported by our research group [45]. Vinyl substitution at C-3 of these azetidinones also results potent tubulin destabilizing effects in these derivatives of combretastatin A-4.

In summary, these novel 3-vinyl-β-lactam analogues of CA-4 which we now report show potent antiproliferative effects in preliminary in vitro investigations on MCF-7 and MDA-MB231 breast cancer cells. Further studies to establish the long-term effect of these compounds on cancer cell growth, migration and the potential vascular disrupting effects of these molecules are ongoing.

4. Experimental Section

4.1. Chemistry

All reagents were commercially available and were used without further purification unless otherwise indicated. Tetrahydrofuran (THF) was distilled immediately prior to use from Na/Benzophenone under a slight positive pressure of nitrogen, toluene was dried by distillation from sodium and stored on activated molecular sieves (4Å) and dichloromethane was dried by distillation from calcium hydride prior to use. Uncorrected melting points were measured on a Gallenkamp SMP 11 melting point apparatus. Infra-red (IR) spectra were recorded as thin film on NaCl plates, or as potassium bromide discs on a Perkin Elmer FT-IR Spectum 100 spectrometer, (PerkinElmer Inc., 940 Winter Street, Waltham, MA, USA). ^{1}H and ^{13}C nuclear magnetic resonance (NMR) spectra were recorded at 27 °C on a Brucker Avance DPX 400 spectrometer (Bruker, 40 Manning Road, Billerica, MA, USA), (400.13 MHz, ^{1}H; 100.61 MHz, ^{13}C) at 20 °C in either CDCl$_3$ (internal standard tetramethylsilane TMS) or CD$_3$OD by Dr. John O'Brien and Dr. Manuel Ruether in the School of Chemistry, Trinity College Dublin. For CDCl$_3$, ^{1}H-NMR spectra were assigned relative to the TMS peak at δ 0.00 ppm and ^{13}C-NMR spectra were assigned relative to the middle CDCl$_3$ triplet at δ 77.00 ppm. For CD$_3$OD, ^{1}H and ^{13}C-NMR spectra were assigned relative to the centre peaks of the CD$_3$OD multiplets at δ 3.30 and 49.00 ppm respectively. Electrospray ionisation mass spectrometry (ESI-MS) was performed in the positive ion mode on a liquid chromatography time-of-flight (TOF) mass spectrometer (Micromass LCT, Waters Ltd., Manchester, UK) equipped with electrospray ionization (ES) interface operated in the positive ion mode at the High Resolution Mass Spectrometry Laboratory by Mr. Brian Talbot in the School of Pharmacy and Pharmaceutical Sciences, Trinity College Dublin and Dr. Martin Feeney in the School of Chemistry, Trinity College Dublin. Mass measurement accuracies of < ±5 ppm were obtained. Low resolution mass spectra (LRMS) were acquired on a Hewlett-Packard 5973 MSD GC-MS system in electron impact (EI) mode, (Hewlett-Packard, 6280 America Center, San Jose, CA, USA). R$_f$ values are quoted for thin layer chromatography on silica gel Merck F-254 plates, unless otherwise stated, (Merck, 2000 Galloping Hill Road, Kenilworth, NJ, USA). Flash column chromatography was carried out on Merck Kieselgel 60 (particle size 0.040–0.063 mm). Chromatographic separations were also carried out on Biotage SP4 instrument, (Biotage AB, Box 8, Uppsala, Sweden). All products isolated were homogenous on TLC. Analytical high-performance liquid chromatography (HPLC) to determine the purity of the final compounds was performed using a Waters 2487 Dual Wavelength Absorbance detector, a Waters 1525 binary HPLC pump, a Waters In-Line Degasser AF and a Waters 717plus Autosampler, (Waters, 34 Maple St, Milford, MA, USA). The column used was a Varian Pursuit XRs C18 reverse phase 150 × 4.6 mm chromatography column (Agilent Technologies, 5301 Stevens Creek Blvd, Santa Clara, CA, USA). Samples were detected using a wavelength of 254 nm. Imines **5a** [87], **5b** [89], **5c** [46], **5d** [46], **5e** [84], **5f** [90], **5g** [91], **5h** [45], **5i** [84], **5m** [46], **5n** [84], **5o** [45], **5p** [45], **5q** [46], **5r** [46], **5s** [53], **6a** [92], **6b** [93], **6c** [94], **6f** [45], **6g** [95], **6h** [96], **6i** [45], **6j** [97], **6k** [96] were prepared as previously reported (See Supplementary Information).

4.1.1. 3-(tert-Butyldimethylsilyloxy)-4-methoxybenzaldehyde

To a solution of 3-hydroxy-4-methoxybenzaldehyde (20 mmol) and *tert*-butyl-dimethylsilylchloride (24 mmol) in dry CH$_2$Cl$_2$ (60 mL) under a nitrogen atmosphere, 1,8-diazabicyclo[5.4.0]undec-7-ene (DBU) (32 mmol) was added dropwise via syringe. The resulting mixture was stirred at room temperature under a nitrogen atmosphere until reaction was complete on thin layer chromatography. The solution was then diluted with CH$_2$Cl$_2$ (80 mL) and washed successively with water (60 mL), 0.1M HCl (60 mL) and saturated aqueous NaHCO$_3$ (60 mL), retaining the organic layer each time, before drying over anhydrous Na_2SO_4. The solvent was removed under reduced pressure to yield the protected benzaldehyde, yield 82% [45]. IR (NaCl, film) ν_{max}: 1692 (C=O) cm^{-1}. ^{1}H NMR (400 MHz, CDCl$_3$): δ 0.19 (s, 6H), 1.02 (s, 9H), 3.91 (s, 3H), 6.97 (d, J = 8.56 Hz, 1H), 7.38 (d, J = 2.00 Hz, 1H), 7.48–7.51 (m, 1H), 9.84 (s, 1H). ^{13}C NMR (100 MHz, CDCl$_3$): δ -5.07, 17.97, 25.19 (OTBDMS), 55.13, 110.71, 119.63, 125.82, 129.75, 145.12, 156.16, 190.48. HRMS: found 266.1349 (M$^+$); $C_{14}H_{22}O_3Si$ requires 266.1338.

4.1.2. General Method I: Preparation of Imines 5a–5s, 6a–6k

The appropriately substituted benzaldehyde (10 mmol) and corresponding substituted aniline (10 mmol) were heated reflux in ethanol (40 mL) for 4 h with a catalytic amount of concentrated sulphuric acid. The volume of reaction was then reduced to approximately 10 mL in vacuo. The Schiff base precipitated from solution upon standing at room temperature overnight. The solid product obtained was filtered and purified by recrystallisation from ethanol.

(E)-1-(4-Butoxyphenyl)-N-(3,4,5-trimethoxyphenyl)methanimine (5j)

Preparation as described above from 4-butoxybenzaldehyde and 3,4,5-trimethoxyaniline. The product was obtained as pale yellow solid, yield 67%, Mp: 107–108 °C. IR (KBr) ν_{max}: 1607 (C=N) cm^{-1}. ^{1}H NMR (400 MHz, CDCl$_3$): δ 1.01 (t, J = 7.26Hz, 3H), 1.51–1.56 (m, 2H), 1.79–1.84 (m, 2H), 3.88 (s, 3H), 3.92 (s, 6H), 4.06 (t, J = 6.48 Hz, 2H), 6.42 (br s, 2H), 7.00 (d, J = 8.52 Hz, 2H), 7.87 (br s, 2H), 8.41 (s, 1H). ^{13}C NMR (100 MHz, CDCl$_3$): δ 13.87, 19.24, 31.22, 56.13, 61.04, 67.93, 98.11, 114.76, 128.57, 130.65, 136.12, 148.17, 153.56, 159.24, 162.09. HRMS: found 344.1859 (M$^+$+H); $C_{20}H_{26}NO_4$ requires 344.1862.

(E)-1-(4-Phenoxyphenyl)-N-(3,4,5-trimethoxyphenyl)methanimine (5k)

Preparation as described above from 4-phenoxybenzaldehyde and 3,4,5-trimethoxyaniline. The product was obtained as pale yellow solid, yield 74%, Mp 86–88 °C. IR (KBr) ν_{max}: 1631 (C=N) cm^{-1}. ^{1}H NMR (400 MHz, CDCl$_3$): δ 3.88 (s, 3H), 3.92 (s, 6H), 6.51 (s, 2H), 7.08–7.10 (m, 5H), 7.39–7.41 (m, 2H), 7.89 (d, J = 7.52 Hz, 2H), 8.45 (s, 1H). ^{13}C NMR (100 MHz, CDCl$_3$): δ 55.68, 60.58, 97.68, 117.80, 119.34, 123.78, 124.51, 129.53, 130.10, 135.83, 147.48, 153.12, 155.57, 158.32, 160.06. HRMS: found 364.1534 (M$^+$+H); $C_{22}H_{22}NO_4$ requires 364.1549.

(E)-1-(4-(Benzyloxy)phenyl)-N-(3,4,5-trimethoxyphenyl)methanimine (5l)

Preparation as described above from 4-(benzyloxy)benzaldehyde and 3,4,5-trimethoxyaniline. The product was obtained as colourless solid, yield 79%, Mp 113–115 °C. IR (KBr) ν_{max}: 1623 (C=N) cm^{-1}. ^{1}H NMR (400 MHz, CDCl$_3$): δ 3.88 (s, 3H), 3.92 (s, 6H), 5.17 (s, 2H), 6.51 (s, 2H), 7.09 (d, J = 7.84 Hz, 2H), 7.41–7.46 (m, 5H), 7.89 (d, J = 7.84 Hz, 2H), 8.42 (s, 1H). ^{13}C NMR (100 MHz, CDCl$_3$): δ 55.67, 60.58, 69.66, 97.65, 114.69, 127.90, 127.06, 127.75, 128.23, 128.30, 128.66, 130.16, 135.97, 147.19, 153.10, 158.63, 161.07. HRMS: found 378.1713 (M$^+$+H); $C_{23}H_{24}NO_4$ requires 378.1705.

(E)-N-(4-Nitrophenyl)-1-(3,4,5-trimethoxyphenyl)methanimine (6d)

Preparation as described above from 3,4,5-trimethoxybenzaldehyde and 4-nitroaniline. The product was obtained as yellow solid, yield 72%, Mp 161–162 °C. IR (KBr) ν_{max}: 1627 (C=N) cm^{-1}. ^{1}H NMR (400 MHz, CDCl$_3$): δ 3.96 (s, 3H), 3.97 (s, 6H), 7.20 (s, 2H), 7.27 (d, J = 8.52 Hz, 2H), 8.28 (d, J = 9.04 Hz, 2H), 8.34 (s, 1H). ^{13}C NMR (100 MHz, CDCl$_3$): δ 55.82, 55.85, 60.62, 105.93, 120.86, 124.62, 130.12, 141.48, 144.97, 153.12, 155.56, 161.70. HRMS: found 317.1135 (M$^+$+H); $C_{16}H_{17}N_2O_5$ requires 317.1137.

(E)-N-(4-(tert-Butyl)phenyl)-1-(3,4,5-trimethoxyphenyl)methanimine (6e)

Preparation as described above from 3,4,5-trimethoxybenzaldehyde and 4-(tert-butyl)aniline. The product was obtained as red solid, yield 100%, Mp 81–82 °C. IR (KBr) ν_{max}: 1623 (C=N) cm^{-1}. ^{1}H NMR (400 MHz, CDCl$_3$): δ 1.37 (s, 9H), 3.94 (s, 3H), 3.97 (s, 6H), 7.15–7.21 (m, 4H), 7.44 (d, J = 8.52 Hz,

2H), 8.40 (s, 1H). ^{13}C NMR (100 MHz, CDCl$_3$): δ 30.98, 34.07, 55.82, 60.55, 105.29, 120.10, 125.61, 131.31, 140.41, 148.59, 148.70, 153.05, 158.78. HRMS: found 328.1899 (M$^+$+H); C$_{20}$H$_{26}$NO$_3$ requires 328.1913.

4.1.3. General method II: Preparation of 2-azetidinones 7a–7u, 8a–8k

To a stirring, refluxing solution of the imine (5 mmol) and triethylamine (6 mmol) in anhydrous dichloromethane (40 mL), a solution of crotonyl chloride (6 mmol) in anhydrous dichloromethane (10 mL) was injected dropwise through a rubber septum over 45 min under nitrogen. The reaction was heated at reflux for 5 h and stirred at room temperature overnight, continuously under nitrogen. The reaction mixture coled and washed with water (2 × 100 mL), with the organic layer being retained each time. The reaction was dried over anhydrous sodium sulfate and the solvent was then removed under reduced pressure. The crude product was purified by flash chromatography over silica gel (eluent: *n*-hexane: ethyl acetate, 4:1).

4-(4-Fluorophenyl)-1-(3,4,5-trimethoxyphenyl)-3-vinylazetidin-2-one (7a)

Preparation as described above from crotonyl chloride and (4-fluorobenzylidene)-3,4,5-trimethoxyphenylamine (5a). The product was obtained as yellow solid, yield 36%, Mp 147–149 °C. IR (KBr) ν$_{max}$: 1749 (C=O) cm^{-1}. ^{1}H NMR (400 MHz, CDCl$_3$): δ 3.73 (s, 6H), 3.74–3.75 (m, 1H), 3.78 (s, 3H), 4.78 (d, J = 2.52 Hz, 1H), 5.35–5.43 (m, 2H), 5.99–6.08 (m, 1H), 6.53 (s, 2H), 7.09–7.13 (m, 2H), 7.36–7.38 (m, 2H). ^{13}C NMR (100 MHz, CDCl$_3$): δ 55.57, 60.51, 60.51, 63.51, 94.20, 115.76, 115.97, 119.74, 127.18, 127.25, 129.81, 132.63, 133.16, 134.09, 153.10, 161.10, 164.56. HRMS: found 356.1303 (M$^+$-H); C$_{20}$H$_{19}$FNO$_4$ requires 356.1298.

4-(4-Chlorophenyl)-1-(3,4,5-trimethoxyphenyl)-3-vinylazetidin-2-one (7b)

Preparation as described above from crotonyl chloride and (4-chlorobenzylidene)-(3,4,5-trimethoxyphenyl)amine (5b) to afford the product as a yellow solid, yield 30%, Mp 104 °C. IR (KBr) ν$_{max}$: 1754 (C=O) cm^{-1}. ^{1}H NMR (400 MHz, CDCl$_3$): δ 3.70–3.71 (m, 1H), 3.72 (s, 6H), 3.77 (s, 3H), 4.77 (d, J = 2.48 Hz, 1H), 5.33–5.41 (m, 2H), 5.97–6.06 (m, 1H), 6.51 (s, 2H), 7.32 (d, J = 6.52 Hz, 2H), 7.38 (d, J = 8.56 Hz, 2H). ^{13}C NMR (100 MHz, CDCl$_3$): δ 56.06, 60.88, 60.95, 63.93, 94.64, 120.30, 127.28, 129.50, 130.19, 133.55, 134.54, 134.59, 135.89, 153.58, 164.89. HRMS: found 372.1017 (M$^+$-H); C$_{20}$H$_{19}$^{35}ClNO$_4$ requires 372.1003.

4-(4-Bromophenyl)-1-(3,4,5-trimethoxyphenyl)-3-vinylazetidin-2-one (7c)

Preparation as described above from crotonyl chloride and (4-bromobenzylidene)-3,4,5-trimethoxyphenylamine (5c) to afford the product as a brown oil, yield 48%. IR (NaCl) ν$_{max}$: 1751 (C=O) cm^{-1}. ^{1}H NMR (400 MHz, CDCl$_3$): δ 3.71–3.72 (m, 1H), 3.74 (s, 6H), 3.79 (s, 3H), 4.76 (d, J = 2.52 Hz, 1H), 5.35–5.43 (m, 2H), 5.99–6.08 (m, 1H), 6.53 (s, 2H), 7.27 (d, J = 8.52 Hz, 2H), 7.55 (d, J = 8.52 Hz, 2H). ^{13}C NMR (100 MHz, CDCl$_3$): δ 55.63, 60.50, 60.52, 63.43, 94.19, 119.88, 122.19, 127.08, 129.69, 132.01, 133.06, 135.95, 139.98, 153.13, 164.42. HRMS: found 418.0643 (M$^+$+H); C$_{20}$H$_{21}$^{79}BrNO$_4$ requires 418.0654.

4-(4-Nitrophenyl)-1-(3,4,5-trimethoxyphenyl)-3-vinylazetidin-2-one (7d)

Preparation as described above from crotonyl chloride and (4-nitrobenzylidene)-3,4,5-trimethoxyphenylamine (5d) to afford the product as a brown solid, yield 28%, Mp 132–133 °C. IR (KBr) ν$_{max}$: 1754 (C=O) cm^{-1}. ^{1}H NMR (400 MHz, CDCl$_3$): δ 3.73 (s, 6H), 3.75–3.76 (m, 1H), 3.78 (s, 3H), 4.92 (d, J = 2.48 Hz, 1H), 5.39–5.45 (m, 2H), 6.01–6.06 (m, 1H), 6.50 (s, 2H), 7.56 (d, J = 9.04 Hz, 2H), 8.28 (d, J = 9.04 Hz, 2H). ^{13}C NMR (100 MHz, CDCl$_3$): δ 55.68, 60.03, 60.52, 63.53, 94.16, 120.46, 124.14, 126.26, 129.24, 132.75, 134.44, 144.28, 147.61, 153.27, 163.83. HRMS: found 385.1389 (M$^+$+H); C$_{20}$H$_{21}$N$_2$O$_6$ requires 385.1400.

4-(4-Dimethylaminophenyl)-1-(3,4,5-trimethoxyphenyl)-3-vinylazetidin-2-one (**7e**)

Preparation as described above from crotonyl chloride and (4-(dimethylamino)benzylidene)-3,4,5-trimethoxyphenylamine (**5e**) to afford the product as a brown oil, yield 61%. IR (NaCl) ν_{max}: 1746 (C=O) cm^{-1}. ^{1}H NMR (400 MHz, CDCl$_3$): δ 2.98 (s, 6H), 3.73 (s, 6H), 3.77 (s, 3H), 3.78–3.92 (m, 1H), 4.70 (d, J = 2.00 Hz, 1H), 5.30–5.40 (m, 2H), 5.99–6.08 (m, 1H), 6.60 (s, 2H), 6.74 (d, J = 8.04 Hz, 2H), 7.27 (d, J = 9.04 Hz, 2H). ^{13}C NMR (100 MHz, CDCl$_3$): δ 40.01, 55.55, 60.49, 61.27, 63.30, 94.27, 112.20, 119.15, 126.67, 130.38, 133.58, 134.62, 137.93, 147.60, 152.95, 165.25. HRMS: found 381.1819 (M$^+$-H); C$_{22}$H$_{25}$N$_2$O$_4$ requires 381.1814.

4-Phenyl-1-(3,4,5-trimethoxyphenyl)-3-vinylazetidin-2-one (**7f**)

Preparation as described above from crotonyl chloride and benzylidene-(3,4,5-trimethoxyphenyl) amine (**5f**) to afford the product as a yellow solid, yield 29%, Mp 109–111 °C. IR (KBr) ν_{max}: 1750 (C=O) cm^{-1}. ^{1}H NMR (400 MHz, CDCl$_3$): δ 3.72 (s, 6H), 3.78 (s, 3H), 3.80–3.81 (m, 1H), 4.79 (d, J = 2.52 Hz, 1H), 5.35–5.43 (m, 2H), 6.01–6.06 (m, 1H), 6.56 (s, 2H), 7.39–7.41 (m, 5H). ^{13}C NMR (100 MHz, CDCl$_3$): δ 55.54, 60.51, 61.22, 63.35, 94.22, 119.57, 125.44, 125.53, 128.31, 128.80, 130.02, 133.34, 133.97, 136.85, 153.04, 164.75. HRMS: found 338.1383 (M$^+$-H); C$_{20}$H$_{20}$NO$_4$ requires 338.1392.

4-p-Tolyl-1-(3,4,5-trimethoxyphenyl)-3-vinylazetidin-2-one (**7g**)

Preparation as described above from crotonyl chloride and (4-methylbenzylidene)-(3,4,5-trimethoxyphenyl)amine (**5g**) to afford the product as a yellow solid, yield 35%, Mp 106–107 °C. IR (KBr) ν_{max}: 1746 (C=O) cm^{-1}. ^{1}H NMR (400 MHz, CDCl$_3$): δ 2.37 (s, 3H), 3.72 (s, 6H), 3.75 (m, 1H), 3.77 (s, 3H), 4.76 (d, J = 2.04 Hz, 1H), 5.32–5.41 (m, 2H), 5.99–6.08 (m, 1H), 6.56 (s, 2H), 7.21 (d, J = 8.00 Hz, 2H), 7.28 (d, J = 8.00 Hz, 2H). ^{13}C NMR (100 MHz, CDCl$_3$): δ 20.76, 55.54, 60.49, 61.07, 63.39, 94.22, 119.44, 125.48, 129.45, 130.11, 133.40, 133.78, 133.92, 138.18, 153.01, 164.87. HRMS: found 354.1706 (M$^+$+H); C$_{21}$H$_{24}$NO$_4$ requires 354.1705.

4-(4-Methoxyphenyl)-1-(3,4,5-trimethoxyphenyl)-3-vinylazetidin-2-one (**7h**)

Preparation as described above from crotonyl chloride and (4-methoxybenzylidene)-3,4,5-trimethoxyphenylamine (**5h**) to afford the product as a brown oil, yield 34% [98]. IR (NaCl) ν_{max}: 1747 (C=O) cm^{-1}. ^{1}H NMR (400 MHz, CDCl$_3$): δ 3.64 (s, 6H), 3.67–3.68 (m, 1H), 3.69 (s, 3H), 3.72 (s, 3H), 4.70 (d, J = 2.00 Hz, 1H), 5.22–5.32 (m, 2H), 5.91–6.00 (m, 1H), 6.51 (s, 2H), 6.85 (d, J = 8.52 Hz, 2H), 7.26 (d, J = 8.52 Hz, 2H). ^{13}C NMR (100 MHz, CDCl$_3$): δ 55.37, 56.03, 60.97, 61.37, 63.92, 94.70, 114.61, 119.90, 127.31, 129.14, 130.58, 133.86, 133.93, 153.48, 159.90, 165.39. HRMS: found 370.1658 (M$^+$+H); C$_{21}$H$_{24}$NO$_5$ requires 370.1654.

4-(4-Ethoxyphenyl)-1-(3,4,5-trimethoxyphenyl)-3-vinylazetidin-2-one (**7i**)

Preparation as described above from crotonyl chloride and (4-ethoxybenzylidene)-(3,4,5-trimethoxyphenyl)amine (**5i**) to afford a colourless solid, yield 33%, Mp 92–93 °C. [98] IR (KBr) ν_{max}: 1749 (C=O) cm^{-1}. ^{1}H NMR (400 MHz, CDCl$_3$): δ 1.43 (t, J = 6.84 Hz, 3H), 3.73 (s, 6H), 3.75–3.76 (m, 1H), 3.78 (s, 3H), 4.05 (q, J = 6.86 Hz, 2H), 4.73 (d, J = 2.48 Hz, 1H), 5.33–5.42 (m, 2H), 6.00–6.08 (m, 1H), 6.57 (s, 2H), 6.93 (d, J = 8.80 Hz, 2H), 7.31 (d, J = 8.80 Hz, 2H). ^{13}C NMR (100 MHz, CDCl$_3$): δ 14.33, 55.55, 60.50, 60.94, 63.11, 63.43, 94.22, 114.65, 119.40, 126.83, 128.49, 130.14, 133.42, 133.90, 153.01, 158.81, 164.94 (C=O). HRMS: found 384.1819 (M$^+$+H); C$_{22}$H$_{26}$NO$_5$ requires 384.1811.

4-(4-Butoxyphenyl)-1-(3,4,5-trimethoxyphenyl)-3-vinylazetidin-2-one (**7j**)

Preparation as described above from crotonyl chloride and (4-butoxybenzylidene)-3,4,5-trimethoxyphenylamine (**5j**) to afford a yellow solid, yield 40%, Mp 100–102 °C. IR (KBr) ν_{max}: 1749 (C=O) cm^{-1}. ^{1}H NMR (400 MHz, CDCl$_3$): δ 0.98 (t, J = 7.32 Hz, 3H), 1.45–1.54 (m, 2H), 1.74–1.81 (m, 2H), 3.72 (s, 6H), 3.73-3.74 (m, 1H), 3.77 (s, 3H), 3.97 (t, J = 6.84 Hz, 2H), 4.73 (d, J = 1.96 Hz,

1H), 5.31–5.40 (m, 2H), 6.00–6.05 (m, 1H), 6.56 (s, 2H), 6.92 (d, J = 7.84 Hz, 2H), 7.30 (d, J = 8.80 Hz, 2H). ^{13}C NMR (100 MHz, CDCl$_3$): δ 13.39, 18.77, 30.78, 55.53, 60.48, 60.93, 63.43, 67.33, 94.22, 114.66, 119.36, 126.80, 128.40, 130.15, 133.42, 133.89, 153.00, 159.03, 164.93. HRMS: found 412.2129 (M$^+$+H); C$_{24}$H$_{30}$NO$_5$ requires 412.2124.

4-(4-Phenoxyphenyl)-1-(3,4,5-trimethoxyphenyl)-3-vinylazetidin-2-one (7k)

Preparation as described above from crotonyl chloride and (4-phenoxylbenzylidene)-(3,4,5-trimethoxyphenyl)amine (5k) to afford a pale yellow solid, yield 37%, Mp 128–130 °C. IR (KBr) ν_{max}: 1749 (C=O) cm^{-1}. ^{1}H NMR (400 MHz, CDCl$_3$): δ 3.75 (s, 6H), 3.77–3.78 (m, 1H), 3.79 (s, 3H), 4.78 (d, J = 2.52 Hz, 1H), 5.35–5.44 (m, 2H), 6.01–6.10 (m, 1H), 6.57 (s, 2H), 7.02–7.05 (m, 4H), 7.14–7.17 (m, 1H), 7.35–7.39 (m, 4H). ^{13}C NMR (100 MHz, CDCl$_3$): δ 55.58, 60.52, 60.77, 63.42, 94.26, 118.73, 118.77, 119.58, 123.37, 127.03, 129.44, 130.00, 131.27, 133.29, 134.18, 153.07, 156.09, 157.40, 164.74. HRMS: found 454.1610 (M$^+$+Na); C$_{26}$H$_{25}$NO$_5$Na requires 454.1630.

4-(4-Benzyloxyphenyl)-1-(3,4,5-trimethoxyphenyl)-3-vinylazetidin-2-one (7l)

Preparation as described above from crotonyl chloride and (4-benzyloxybenzylidene)-3,4,5-trimethoxyphenylamine (5l) to afford a cream solid, yield 37%, Mp 148–149 °C. IR (KBr) ν_{max}: 1746 (C=O) cm^{-1}. ^{1}H NMR (400 MHz, CDCl$_3$): δ 3.72 (s, 6H), 3.75–3.76 (m, 1H), 3.78 (s, 3H), 4.74 (d, J = 2.52 Hz, 1H), 5.09 (s, 2H), 5.33–5.42 (m, 2H), 5.99–6.08 (m, 1H), 6.56 (s, 2H), 7.02 (d, J = 8.56 Hz, 2H), 7.31–7.46 (m, 7H). ^{13}C NMR (100 MHz, CDCl$_3$): δ 56.03, 60.97, 61.36, 63.89, 70.08, 94.69, 115.57, 119.92, 127.36, 127.48, 128.14, 128.67, 129.44, 130.58, 133.86, 136.61, 139.50, 153.49, 159.05, 165.37. HRMS: found 468.1774 (M$^+$+Na); C$_{27}$H$_{27}$NO$_5$Na requires 468.1787.

4-Naphthalen-1-yl-1-(3,4,5-trimethoxyphenyl)-3-vinylazetidin-2-one (7m)

Preparation as described above from crotonyl chloride and naphthalen-1-ylmethylene-(3,4,5-trimethoxyphenyl)amine (5m) to afford the product as a yellow solid, yield 34%, Mp 121–122 °C. IR (KBr) ν_{max}: 1754 (C=O) cm^{-1}. ^{1}H NMR (400 MHz, CDCl$_3$): δ 3.71 (s, 6H), 3.76–3.78 (m, 1H), 3.82 (s, 3H), 5.44–5.49 (m, 2H), 5.60 (d, J = 2.00 Hz, 1H), 6.22–6.31 (m, 1H), 6.67 (s, 2H), 7.44–8.04 (m, 7H). ^{13}C NMR (100 MHz, CDCl$_3$): δ 55.69, 58.42, 60.54, 63.11, 94.49, 120.72, 122.29, 125.10, 125.74, 126.28, 127.86, 128.22, 128.75, 129.96, 130.67, 132.21, 133.45, 133.62, 134.13, 153.19, 164.82. HRMS: found 390.1715 (M$^+$+H); C$_{24}$H$_{24}$NO$_4$ requires 390.1705.

4-Naphthalen-2-yl-1-(3,4,5-trimethoxyphenyl)-3-vinylazetidin-2-one (7n)

Preparation as described above from crotonyl chloride and naphthalen-2-ylmethylene-(3,4,5-trimethoxyphenyl)amine (5n) to afford the product as a yellow solid, yield 30%, Mp 145–146 °C. IR (KBr) ν_{max}: 1749 (C=O) cm^{-1}. ^{1}H NMR (400 MHz, CDCl$_3$): δ 3.69 (s, 6H), 3.77 (s, 3H), 3.84–3.87 (m, 1H), 4.97 (d, J = 2.52 Hz, 1H), 5.37–5.45 (m, 2H), 6.06–6.12 (m, 1H), 6.62 (s, 2H), 7.47–7.92 (m, 7H). ^{13}C NMR (100 MHz, CDCl$_3$): δ 55.58, 60.50, 61.38, 63.44, 94.25, 119.71, 122.47, 124.97, 126.13, 126.34, 127.39, 127.42, 129.01, 130.00, 132.86, 132.94, 133.45, 134.05, 134.33, 153.08, 164.80. HRMS: found 390.1714 (M$^+$+H); C$_{24}$H$_{24}$NO$_4$ requires 390.1705.

4-(4-Methoxy-3-nitrophenyl)-1-(3,4,5-trimethoxyphenyl)-3-vinylazetidin-2-one (7p)

Preparation as described above from crotonyl chloride and (4-methoxy-3-nitrobenzylidene)-(3,4,5-trimethoxyphenyl)amine (5p) to afford a brown oil, yield 14%. IR (NaCl) ν_{max}: 1754 (C=O) cm^{-1}. ^{1}H NMR (400 MHz, CDCl$_3$): δ 3.75 (s, 6H), 3.78 (s, 3H), 3.85–3.86 (m, 1H), 3.99 (s, 3H), 4.80 (d, J = 2.00 Hz, 1H), 5.37–5.43 (m, 2H), 5.98–6.07 (m, 1H), 6.52 (s, 2H), 7.14–7.16 (m, 1H), 7.54–7.57 (m, 1H), 7.90 (br s, 1H). ^{13}C NMR (100 MHz, CDCl$_3$): δ 55.61, 56.27, 59.66, 60.52, 63.43, 94.23, 114.14, 120.19, 123.18, 129.23, 129.38, 130.74, 132.80, 134.36, 138.76, 152.65, 153.23, 164.19. HRMS: found 437.1326 (M$^+$+Na); C$_{21}$H$_{22}$N$_2$O$_7$Na requires 437.1325.

4-[4-Oxo-1-(3,4,5-trimethoxyphenyl)-3-vinyl-azetidin-2-yl]benzonitrile (7q)

Preparation as described above from 4-[(3,4,5-trimethoxyphenylimino)methyl]benzonitrile (5q) and *trans*-crotonyl chloride to afford the product as a colourless oil (31%). IR ν_{max} 1756.1(CO), 2312.0 (CN) cm^{-1}. ^{1}H NMR (400 MHz, CDCl$_3$): δ 3.76 (s, br, 10H), 4.86 (d, J = 2.52 Hz, 1H), 5.40 (m, 2H), 5.90–6.08 (m, 1H), 6.48 (s, 2H), 7.49 (d, 2H), 7.71 (d, 2H). HRMS: Found: 387.1335 (M$^+$+Na); C$_{21}$H$_{20}$N$_2$O$_4$Na requires 387.1321.

4-(4-Methylsulfanylphenyl)-1-(3,4,5-trimethoxyphenyl)-3-vinylazetidin-2-one (7r)

Preparation as described above from crotonyl chloride and *N*-(3,4,5-trimethoxybenzylidene)-4-methylsulfanylphenylamine (5r), yield 17%, brown oil [98]. IR (NaCl ν max): 1744 (C=O) cm^{-1}. ^{1}H NMR (400 MHz, CDCl$_3$): δ 2.48 (s, 3H), 3.72–3.76 (m, 10H, OMe), 4.75 (d, J = 2.33Hz, 1H), 5.31–5.40 (m, 2H), 5.98–6.05 (m, 1H), 6.54 (s, 2H), 7.25–7.31 (m, 4H). ^{13}C NMR (100 MHz, CDCl$_3$): δ15.55, 55.88, 55.61, 60.77, 60.47, 63.39, 94.23, 119.59, 125.98, 126.09, 129.96, 133.25, 133.49, 139.00, 141.19, 153.05, 164.70. HRMS: found 408.1230 (M$^+$+Na); C$_{21}$H$_{23}$NO$_4$SNa, requires 408.1245.

1-(3,5-Dimethoxyphenyl)-4-(4-methoxyphenyl)-3-vinylazetidin-2-one (7u)

Preparation as described above from imine 5s and crotonyl chloride to afford the product as brown oil; Yield: 17%, IR ν_{max}: 1748.72 cm^{-1} (C=O, β- lactam). δ ^{1}H NMR (400 MHz, CDCl$_3$): 3.69 (s, 7 H), 3.79 (s, 3 H), 4.68 (s, 1 H), 5.27–5.39 (m, 2 H), 5.94–6.06 (m, 1 H), 6.15 (s, 1 H), 6.48 (s, 2 H), 6.89 (d, J = 7.93 Hz, 2 H), 7.27 (d, J = 8.54 Hz, 2 H). ^{13}C NMR (100 MHz, CDCl$_3$): δ 55.31, 55.49, 61.24, 63.97, 95.66, 96.27, 114.58, 119.77, 127.14, 129.16, 130.54, 139.23, 159.79, 161.06, 165.63. HRMS: found 340.1540 (M$^+$ + H); C$_{20}$H$_{22}$NO$_4$ requires 340.1549.

4-(3,4,5-Trimethoxyphenyl)-1-(4-fluorophenyl)-3-vinylazetidin-2-one (8a)

Preparation as described above from crotonyl chloride and *N*-(3,4,5-trimethoxybenzylidene)-4-fluorophenylamine (6a) as a yellow oil, yield 18%. IR (NaCl) ν_{max}: 1751 (C=O) cm^{-1}. ^{1}H NMR (400 MHz, CDCl$_3$): δ 3.77–3.79 (m, 1H), 3.83 (s, 6H), 3.86 (s, 3H), 4.71 (d, J = 2.48 Hz, 1H), 5.35–5.43 (m, 2H), 6.00–6.09 (m, 1H), 6.54 (s, 2H), 6.96–7.00 (m, 2H), 7.29–7.32 (m, 2H). ^{13}C NMR (100 MHz, CDCl$_3$): δ 55.76, 60.43, 61.39, 63.73, 101.99, 115.34, 115.57, 117.98, 118.06, 119.84, 129.87, 132.18, 133.36, 137.63, 153.54, 159.88, 164.74. HRMS: found 358.1454 (M$^+$+H); C$_{20}$H$_{21}$FNO$_4$ requires 358.1455.

4-(3,4,5-Trimethoxyphenyl)-1-(4-chlorophenyl)-3-vinylazetidin-2-one (8b)

Preparation as described above from crotonyl chloride and *N*-(3,4,5-trimethoxybenzylidene)-4-chlorophenylamine (6b) as a yellow solid, yield 32%, Mp 131–133 °C. IR (KBr) ν_{max}: 1753 (C=O) cm^{-1}. ^{1}H NMR (400 MHz, CDCl$_3$): δ 3.78–3.79 (m, 1H), 3.83 (s, 6H), 3.87 (s, 3H), 4.71 (d, J = 1.00 Hz, 1H), 5.36–5.43 (m, 2H), 6.02–6.08 (m, 1H), 6.54 (s, 2H), 7.24 (d, J = 5.88 Hz, 2H), 7.28 (d, J = 5.88 Hz, 2H). ^{13}C NMR (100 MHz, CDCl$_3$): δ 56.11, 60.70, 61.67, 64.09, 102.43, 118.11, 120.10, 129.04, 130.08, 130.24, 132.33, 135.94, 138.15, 153.91, 165.18. HRMS: found 396.0966 (M$^+$+Na); C$_{20}$H$_{20}$^{35}ClNO$_4$Na requires 396.0979.

4-(3,4,5-Trimethoxyphenyl)-1-(4-bromophenyl)-3-vinylazetidin-2-one (8c)

Preparation as described above from crotonyl chloride and *N*-(3,4,5-trimethoxy benzylidene)-4-bromophenylamine (6c) as a colourless solid, yield 32%, Mp 120–122 °C. IR (KBr) ν_{max}: 1754 (C=O) cm^{-1}. ^{1}H NMR (400 MHz, CDCl$_3$): δ 3.77–3.79 (m, 1H), 3.83 (s, 6H), 3.86 (s, 3H), 4.71 (d, J = 2.48 Hz, 1H), 5.36–5.44 (m, 2H), 6.00–6.07 (m, 1H), 6.53 (s, 2H), 7.22 (d, J = 8.56 Hz, 2H), 7.40 (d, J = 8.52 Hz, 2H). ^{13}C NMR (100 MHz, CDCl$_3$): δ 55.79, 60.43, 61.33, 63.82, 101.97, 116.38, 118.16, 119.93, 129.72, 131.67, 132.00, 136.05, 137.70, 153.58, 164.96. HRMS: found 440.0466 (M$^+$+Na); C$_{20}$H$_{20}$^{79}BrNO$_4$Na requires 440.0473.

4-(3,4,5-Trimethoxyphenyl)-1-(4-nitrophenyl)-3-vinylazetidin-2-one (8d)

Preparation as described above from crotonyl chloride and N-(3,4,5-trimethoxybenzylidene)-4-nitrophenylamine (6d) as a yellow oil, yield 42%. IR (NaCl) ν_{max}: 1762 (C=O) cm^{-1}. ^{1}H NMR (400 MHz, CDCl$_3$): δ 3.85 (s, 6H), 3.87 (s, 3H), 3.89–3.91 (m, 1H), 4.81 (d, J = 2.52 Hz, 1H), 5.40–5.47 (m, 2H), 6.01–6.10 (m, 1H), 6.54 (s, 2H), 7.45 (d, J = 9.04 Hz, 2H), 8.19 (d, J = 9.04 Hz, 2H). ^{13}C NMR (100 MHz, CDCl$_3$): δ 55.83, 60.45, 61.77, 64.16, 101.95, 116.45, 120.38, 124.85, 129.10, 131.32, 137.97, 142.11, 143.00, 153.73, 165.55. HRMS: found 383.1234 (M$^+$-H); C$_{20}$H$_{19}$N$_2$O$_6$ requires 383.1243.

4-(3,4,5-Trimethoxyphenyl)-1-(4-tert-butylphenyl)-3-vinylazetidin-2-one (8e)

Preparation as described above from crotonyl chloride and N-(3,4,5-trimethoxybenzylidene)-4-*tert*-butylphenylamine (6e) as a yellow solid, yield 22%, Mp 172–174 °C. IR (KBr) ν_{max}: 1746 (C=O) cm^{-1}. ^{1}H NMR (400 MHz, CDCl$_3$): δ 1.29 (s, 9H), 3.76–3.78 (m, 1H), 3.84 (s, 6H), 3.87 (s, 3H), 4.69 (d, J = 2.48 Hz, 1H), 5.33–5.42 (m, 2H), 6.98–6.07 (m, 1H), 6.58 (s, 2H), 7.27 (d, J = 9.04 Hz, 2H), 7.31 (d, J = 9.04 Hz, 2H). ^{13}C NMR (100 MHz, CDCl$_3$): δ 30.86, 33.96, 55.78, 60.43, 61.25, 63.56, 102.13, 116.27, 119.58, 125.45, 130.15, 132.77, 134.69, 137.51, 146.63, 153.45, 164.84. HRMS: found 396.2182 (M$^+$+H); C$_{24}$H$_{30}$NO$_4$ requires 396.2175.

4-(3,4,5-Trimethoxyphenyl)-1-phenyl-3-vinylazetidin-2-one (8f)

Preparation as described above from crotonyl chloride and N-(3,4,5-trimethoxybenzylidene)phenylamine (6f) as a colourless solid, yield 34%, Mp 150–151 °C. IR (KBr) ν_{max}: 1752 (C=O) cm^{-1}. ^{1}H NMR (400 MHz, CDCl$_3$): δ 3.77–3.79 (m, 1H), 3.83 (s, 6H), 3.86 (s, 3H), 4.74 (d, J = 2.48 Hz, 1H), 5.35–5.44 (m, 2H), 6.01–6.10 (m, 1H), 6.56 (s, 2H), 7.07–7.11 (m, 1H), 7.27–7.33 (m, 4H). ^{13}C NMR (100 MHz, CDCl$_3$): δ 55.76, 60.43, 61.19, 63.57, 102.01, 116.60, 119.72, 123.67, 128.65, 130.02, 132.54, 137.12, 137.53, 153.49, 165.02. HRMS: found 362.1371 (M$^+$+Na); C$_{20}$H$_{21}$NO$_4$Na requires 362.1368.

4-(3,4,5-Trimethoxyphenyl)-1-p-tolyl-3-vinylazetidin-2-one (8g)

Preparation as described above from crotonyl chloride and N-(3,4,5-trimethoxybenzylidene)-4-methylphenylamine (6g) as a yellow oil, yield 16%. IR (NaCl) ν_{max}: 1749 (C=O) cm^{-1}. ^{1}H NMR (400 MHz, CDCl$_3$): δ 2.30 (s, 3H), 3.75–3.77 (m, 1H), 3.83 (s, 6H), 3.86 (s, 3H), 4.71 (d, J = 2.48 Hz, 1H), 5.34–5.43 (m, 2H), 6.00–6.09 (m, 1H), 6.55 (s, 2H), 7.09 (d, J = 8.04 Hz, 2H), 7.23 (d, J = 8.56 Hz, 2H). ^{13}C NMR (100 MHz, CDCl$_3$): δ 20.48, 55.75, 60.42, 61.16, 63.54, 102.03, 116.54, 119.62, 129.12, 130.15, 132.66, 133.29, 134.69, 137.48, 153.45, 164.76. HRMS: found 376.1534 (M$^+$+Na); C$_{21}$H$_{23}$NO$_4$Na requires 376.1525.

4-(3,4,5-Trimethoxyphenyl)-1-(4-ethylphenyl)-3-vinylazetidin-2-one (8h)

Preparation as described above from crotonyl chloride and N-(3,4,5-trimethoxybenzylidene)-4-ethylphenylamine (6h) as yellow crystals, yield 15%, Mp 110–112 °C. IR (KBr) ν_{max}: 1749 (C=O) cm^{-1}. ^{1}H NMR (400 MHz, CDCl$_3$): δ 1.21 (t, J = 7.48 Hz, 3H), 2.57–2.63 (q, J = 7.52 Hz, 2H), 3.75–3.78 (m, 1H), 3.84 (s, 6H), 3.87 (s, 3H), 4.71 (d, J = 2.52 Hz, 1H), 5.34–5.43 (m, 2H), 6.00–6.09 (m, 1H), 6.57 (s, 2H), 7.12 (d, J = 8.76 Hz, 2H), 7.25–7.29 (m, 2H). ^{13}C NMR (100 MHz, CDCl$_3$): δ 15.62, 28.34, 56.23, 60.89, 61.67, 64.00, 102.54, 117.07, 120.07, 128.42, 130.63, 133.18, 135.37, 137.98, 140.20, 153.93, 165.25. HRMS: found 390.1666 (M$^+$+Na). C$_{22}$H$_{25}$NO$_4$Na requires 390.1681.

4-(3,4,5-Trimethoxyphenyl)-1-(4-methoxyphenyl)-3-vinylazetidin-2-one (8i)

Preparation as described above from crotonyl chloride and N-(3,4,5-trimethoxybenzylidene)-4-methoxyphenylamine (6i) as a yellow oil, yield 18%. IR (NaCl) ν_{max}: 1744 (C=O) cm^{-1}. ^{1}H NMR (400 MHz, CDCl$_3$): δ 3.78 (s, 3H), 3.80–3.82 (m, 1H), 3.83 (s, 6H), 3.86 (s, 3H), 4.69 (d, J = 2.48 Hz, 1H), 5.34–5.43 (m, 2H), 6.03–6.05 (m, 1H), 6.55 (s, 2H), 6.83 (d, J = 9.00 Hz, 2H), 7.28 (d, J = 9.00 Hz, 2H). ^{13}C NMR (100 MHz, CDCl$_3$): δ 54.99, 55.75, 60.42, 61.30, 63.59, 102.06, 113.85, 117.92, 119.62, 130.20,

130.68, 132.62, 137.49, 153.46, 155.67, 164.44. HRMS: found 392.1479 (M$^+$+Na); C$_{21}$H$_{23}$NO$_5$Na requires 392.1474.

N-(4-(2-(3,4,5-Trimethoxyphenyl)-4-oxo-3-vinylazetidin-1-yl)phenyl)acetamide (8j)

Preparation as described above from crotonyl chloride and N-((E)-4-(3,4,5-trimethoxybenzylideneamino) phenyl)acetamide (6j) as a colourless solid, yield 14%, Mp 223–224 °C. IR (KBr) v_{max}: 1742 (C=O) 1689 (C=O) cm^{-1}. ^{1}H NMR (400 MHz, CDCl$_3$): δ 2.16 (s, 3H), 3.76–3.78 (m, 1H), 3.82 (s, 6H), 3.86 (s, 3H), 4.71 (d, J = 2.52 Hz, 1H), 5.34–5.42 (m, 2H), 6.00–6.09 (m, 1H), 6.54 (s, 2H), 7.27 (d, J = 8.56 Hz, 2H), 7.43 (d, J = 8.56 Hz, 2H), 7.49 (s, 1H). ^{13}C NMR (100 MHz, CDCl$_3$): δ 23.99, 55.75, 60.43, 61.26, 63.63, 102.04, 117.16, 119.80, 120.27, 129.99, 132.36, 133.41, 133.70, 137.52, 153.49, 164.76, 167.92. HRMS: found 419.1579 (M$^+$+Na); C$_{22}$H$_{24}$N$_2$O$_5$Na requires 419.1583.

1-(4-(Methylthio)phenyl)-4-(3,4,5-trimethoxyphenyl)-3-vinylazetidin-2-one (8k)

Preparation as described above from crotonyl chloride and N-(3,4,5-trimethoxybenzylidene) -4-thiomethylphenylamine (6k) as a colourless solid, yield 41%, Mp 104–106 °C. IR (NaCl, film) v_{max}: 1748.72 cm^{-1} (C=O, β-lactam). ^{1}H NMR (400 MHz, CDCl$_3$): δ ppm 2.41 (s, 3 H), 3.73 (d, J = 7.93, 1.22 Hz, 1 H), 3.77–3.85 (m, 9 H), 4.67 (d, J = 2.44 Hz, 1 H), 5.30–5.40 (m, 2 H), 5.98 (d, J = 10.07, 7.63 Hz, 1 H), 6.50 (s, 2 H), 7.13–7.18 (m, 2 H), 7.23 (d, J = 7.32 Hz, 2 H). ^{13}C NMR (100 MHz, CDCl$_3$): δ ppm 16.50, 56.21, 60.83, 61.70, 64.07, 102.52, 117.59, 120.12, 127.90, 130.40, 132.77, 133.52, 135.16, 153.95, 165.19. HRMS: found 408.1255 (M$^+$+Na); C$_{21}$H$_{23}$NNaO$_4$S requires 408.1246.

4.1.4. 4-[3-Hydroxy-4-methoxyphenyl]-1-(3,4,5-trimethoxyphenyl)-3-vinylazetidin-2-one (7s)

To a stirring, refluxing solution of the TBDMS protected imine 5o (5 mmol) and triethylamine (6 mmol) in anhydrous dichloromethane (40 mL), a solution of crotonyl chloride (6 mmol) in anhydrous dichloromethane (10 mL) was added over 45 min under nitrogen. The reaction was kept at reflux for 5 h and then at room temperature overnight (16 h), until the starting material had disappeared as monitored by TLC in (1:1 n-hexane: ethyl acetate). The reaction mixture was washed with water (2 × 100 mL). The combined organic extract was dried over anhydrous Na$_2$SO$_4$ before the solvent was removed under reduced pressure. The crude product was purified by flash chromatography over silica gel (eluant: n-hexane: ethyl acetate, 4:1) to afford the β-lactam 7o as an oil. To a stirring solution of the protected β-lactam 7o (5 mmol) under N$_2$ and 0 °C in dry THF was added dropwise 1.5 equivalents of 1.0 M tert-butylammonium fluoride (t-BAF) solution in hexanes (5 mmol). The resulting solution was left to stir at 0 °C until reaction was complete as monitored by TLC. The reaction mixture was diluted with ethyl acetate (75 mL) and washed with 0.1M HCl (100 mL). The aqueous layer was further extracted with ethyl acetate (2 × 25 mL). All organic layers were combined and washed with water (100 mL) and saturated brine (100 mL) before being dried over anhydrous sodium sulphate. The solvent was removed under reduced pressure to yield the phenol which was further purified by flash chromatography over silica gel (eluent: n-hexane: ethyl acetate, 4:1) to afford the product as a yellow oil, yield 20%. IR (NaCl, film) v_{max}: 3367 (OH), 1749 (C=O, β-lactam), 1587, 1501, 1235, 1127 cm^{-1}. ^{1}H NMR (400 MHz, CDCl$_3$): δ 3.74 (s, 6H), 3.74–3.75 (m, 1H), 3.78 (s, 3H), 3.91 (s, 3H), 4.69 (d, J = 2.52 Hz, 1H), 5.32–5.40 (m, 2H), 5.77 (br s, 1H), 5.98–6.05 (m, 1H), 6.57 (s, 2H), 6.87–6.96 (m, 3H). ^{13}C NMR (100 MHz, CDCl$_3$): δ 55.56, 55.58, 60.50, 60.86, 63.38, 94.24, 110.50, 111.54, 117.30, 119.44, 129.90, 130.08, 133.38, 133.91, 145.82, 146.36, 153.01, 164.86. HRMS: found 408.1434 (M$^+$+Na); C$_{21}$H$_{23}$NO$_6$Na requires 408.1423.

4.1.5. 4-(3-Amino-4-methoxyphenyl)-1-(3,4,5-trimethoxyphenyl)-3-vinylazetidin-2-one (7t)

To a flask containing the 4-(4-methoxy-3-nitrophenyl)-1-(3,4,5-trimethoxyphenyl)-3-vinylazetidin-2 -one (7p) (0.25 mmol) and zinc powder 10 μm (2.5 mmol) was added 15 mL of acetic acid at room temperature under N$_2$ and reaction left to stir for 7 days. The reaction was filtered through a celite pad and the filtrate collected. Solvent was removed under reduced pressure and purified by flash chromatography over silica gel (elutent: ethyl acetate: n-hexane, 1:1) to yield the title compound as a brown solid, yield 43%, Mp 100–101 °C. IR (KBr) v_{max}: 3370 (NH$_2$), 1747 (C=O) cm^{-1}. ^{1}H NMR (400 MHz, CDCl$_3$): δ 3.75 (s, 6H), 3.79 (s, 3H), 3.87–3.88 (m, 1H), 3.88 (s, 3H), 4.65 (d, J = 2.52 Hz, 1H), 5.31–5.41 (m, 2H), 5.98–6.07 (m, 1H), 6.60 (s, 2H), 6.72–6.78 (m, 3H). ^{13}C NMR (100 MHz, CDCl$_3$): δ 55.11, 55.58, 60.50, 61.15, 63.35, 94.23, 109.93, 111.06, 115.86, 119.29, 129.26, 130.25, 133.53, 134.01, 136.50, 147.09, 152.99, 165.07. HRMS: found 407.1597(M$^+$+Na); C$_{21}$H$_{24}$N$_2$O$_5$Na requires 407.1583.

4.1.6. 4-(4-Methoxyphenyl)-1-(3,4,5-trimethoxyphenyl)azetidin-2-one (9a)

Zinc powder (9 mmol) was activated using trimethylchlorosilane (0.5 mmol) in anhydrous benzene (1 mL) by heating for 15 min at 40 °C and followed by 5 min at 100 °C in a microwave. After cooling, the imine 5h (2 mmol) and ethyl bromoacetate (2.4 mmol) were added to the reaction vessel and the mixture was placed in the microwave for 30 min at 100 °C. The reaction mixture was filtered through Celite to remove the zinc catalyst and then diluted with dichloromethane. This solution was washed with saturated ammonium chloride solution (20 mL) and 25% ammonium hydroxide (20 mL) and then with dilute HCl (40 mL), followed by water (40 mL). The organic phase was dried over anhydrous sodium sulphate and the solvent was removed under reduced pressure. The crude product was purified by flash column chromatography over silica gel (eluent: n-hexane: ethyl acetate, 2:1) to afford the product as a yellow solid, 39%, 267 mg, Mp 60–62 °C [87]. Purity (HPLC): 99.6%. IR (KBr) v_{max}: 2938, 1747 (C=O), 1603, 1507, 1246, 1126 cm^{-1}. ^{1}H NMR (400 MHz, CDCl$_3$): δ 2.96 (dd, J = 15.20, 2.50 Hz, 1H), 3.55 (dd, J = 15.18, 5.86 Hz, 1H), 3.73 (s, 6H), 3.77 (s, 3H), 3.83 (s, 3H), 4.94 (dd, J = 5.84, 2.36 Hz, 1H), 6.56 (s, 2H), 6.93 (d, J = 8.76 Hz, 2H), 7.34 (d, J = 8.76 Hz). ^{13}C NMR (100 MHz, CDCl$_3$): δ 46.49, 53.66, 54.88, 55.54, 60.49, 93.98, 114.09, 126.84, 129.53, 133.62, 133.93, 152.99, 159.34, 164.16. HRMS: found 344.1506 (M$^+$+H); C$_{19}$H$_{22}$NO$_5$ requires 344.1498.

4.1.7. 4-(3-Hydroxy-4-methoxyphenyl)-1-(3,4,5-trimethoxyphenyl)-azetidin-2-one (9c)

(i) Zinc powder (458 mg, 7 mmol (method A) or 21 mmol (method B)) and chlorotrimethylsilane (0.32 mL, 2.5 mmol) were refluxed for 3 min in anhydrous benzene (10 mL) under N$_2$ and then allowed to cool. To the cooled stirring solution, the appropriately substituted imine (5o) (5 mmol) and ethylbromoacetate (0.66 mL, 6 mmol) were added and refluxed for 7 h. The reaction was cooled to 0 °C and poured onto NH$_4$Cl (sat), (10 mL) and 30% NH$_4$OH (10 mL). The resulting solution was extracted with DCM (2 × 20 mL) and the organic layer further washed with 0.1N HCl (20 mL) and water (20 mL) before being dried over Na$_2$SO$_4$, filtered and the solvent removed under reduced pressure to afford the protected product (9b), yield 37%, 876 mg (method A), 77%, 1.823 g (method B) as a pale brown resin which was used immediately in the following reaction. IR (NaCl $_v$max): 1749 (C=O) cm^{-1}. ^{1}H NMR (400 MHz, CDCl$_3$): δ 0.07 (s, 3H, OTBDMS), δ0.09 (s, 3H), 2.91–2.95 (dd, J = 2.47 Hz, 15.04, 1H), 3.48–3.53 (dd, J = 5.52 Hz, 15.55 Hz, 1H), 3.71 (s, 6H), 3.76 (s, 3H), 3.80 (s, 3H), 4.86–4.88 (dd, J = 2.52 Hz, 5.52, 1H), 6.54 (s, 2H), 6.83–6.94 (m, 3H). ^{13}C NMR (100 MHz, CDCl$_3$): −5.19, −5.17, 17.98, 25.02, 46.41, 53.59, 55.03, 60.46, 55.49, 94.04, 111.82, 117.99, 119.05, 129.98, 133.57, 133.74, 145.15, 150.74, 152.95, 164.14. (ii) To a stirring solution of the silyl ether β-lactam (9b) (4 mmol) in dry THF (30 mL) was added a solution of 1.0M tBAF in hexanes (4 mL, 4 mmol) under N$_2$ at 0 °C. The reaction mixture was stirred for a further 90 min. Reaction was diluted with ethyl acetate (150 mL) and washed with 0.1M HCl (200 mL). The aqueous layer was further extracted with ethyl acetate (2 × 50 mL). All the organic layers were collected and washed with water (200 mL) and saturated brine (200 mL) before being dried over Na$_2$SO$_4$. Solvent was removed under reduced pressure and the phenol was isolated by flash chromatography over silica gel (eluent: n-hexane: ethyl actetate, 1:1) to afford the desired product, yield 73%, 1.05 g, as a yellow solid, Mp 78–80 °C [87]. IR (NaCl $_v$max): 1741 cm^{-1}, 3443 cm^{-1}, 2937 cm^{-1}. ^{1}H NMR (400 MHz, CDCl$_3$): δ2.88–2.93 (dd, J = 2.48 Hz, 15.06 Hz, 1H), 3.45–3.50 (dd, J = 5.52 Hz, 15.56Hz, 1H), 3.67 (s, 6H), 3.72 (s, 3H), 3.84 (s, 3H), 4.84–4.86 (dd, J = 2.52 Hz, 5.52 Hz, 1H), 6.14 (s, 1H), 6.53 (s, 2H), 6.81–6.93 (m, 3H). ^{13}C NMR (100 MHz, CDCl$_3$): δ 46.27, 53.68, 60.44,

55.52, 94.04, 110.57, 111.63, 117.36, 130.61, 133.56, 133.75, 145.90, 146.48, 152.94, 164.27. HRMS: Found 382.1251 (M$^+$+Na); C$_{19}$H$_{21}$NO$_6$Na requires 382.1267.

4.1.8. 3-(1-Hydroxyethyl)-4-(3-hydroxy-4-methoxyphenyl)-1-(3,4,5-trimethoxyphenyl) azetidin-2-one (10a)

To a solution of the TBDMS protected 3-unsubstituted β-lactam (9b) (125 mg, 0.264 mmol) in dry THF (3 mL) under N$_2$ at −78 °C (dry ice and acetone) was added 2.0 M LDA solution (0.264 mL, 0.528 mmol). The resulting solution was left to stir for 5 min before a solution of acetaldehyde (49 mg, 0.396 mmol) in dry THF (1.5 mL) was added. The reaction was left to stir for 30 min at −78 °C, then poured onto saturated NaCl solution (25 mL). The resulting solution was extracted with ethyl acetate (50 mL) and the solvent was dried over Na$_2$SO$_4$ before being removed under reduced pressure. Preliminary purification was achieved by passage through a short pad (5 cm) of silica (eluent: DCM) to yield the OTBDMS protected ether 10i as an oil. To a stirring solution of the OTBDMS protected ether 10i (2 mmol) in dry THF (10 mL) was added a solution of 1.0 M TBAF in hexanes (2 mL, 2 mmol) under N$_2$ at 0 °C. The reaction mixture was stirred for a further 90 min then diluted with ethyl acetate (75 mL) and washed with 0.1 M HCl (100 mL). The aqueous layer was further extracted with ethyl acetate (2 × 25 mL). All the organic extracts were collected and washed with H$_2$O (100 mL), and saturated brine (100 mL) before being dried over Na$_2$SO$_4$ and solvent was removed under reduced pressure. Purification was carried out by chromatography using a Biotage SP1 chromatography system using a +12M column and detection set at 280 nM and a fraction volume of 12 mL. A gradient elution of 2% ethyl acetate in n-hexane to 100% ethyl acetate over 15 column volumes was used. The desired product was obtained as a brown oil, 36 mg, yield 17% [99] IR (NaCl γmax): 1738 (C=O), 3427 (OH) cm^{-1}. ^{1}H NMR (400 MHz, CDCl$_3$): δ1.33 (d, J = 6.28 Hz, 1H), 1.40 (d, J = 6.52 Hz, 2H), 2.58 (br s, 1H), 3.14 (m, 1H), 3.72 (s, 6H), 3.76 (s, 3H), 3.89 (s, 3H), 4.24 (q, J = 6.04 Hz, 0.66H), 4.36 (q, J = 5.76 Hz, 0.33H), 4.77 (d, J = 2.28 Hz, 0.6H), 4.99 (d, J = 2.28, 0.4H), 5.95 (s, 0.6H), 5.96 (s, 0.4H), 6.54 (s, 2H), 6.83–7.01 (m, 3H). ^{13}C NMR (100 MHz, CDCl$_3$): δ 21.34, 21.52, 55.99, 56.06, 57.64 57.68, 56.68, 60.93, 64.94, 66.05, 66.10, 94.70, 94.75, 111.05, 112.16, 112.22, 117.88, 130.50, 130.97, 133.67, 134.32, 146.25, 146.32, 146.88, 153.43, δ165.89, 166.06. HRMS: Found 426.1540 (M$^+$+Na); C$_{21}$H$_{25}$NO$_7$Na requires 426.1529.

4.1.9. 3-((E)-1-Hydroxybut-2-enyl)-1-(3,4,5-trimethoxyphenyl)-4-(4-methoxyphenyl) azetidin-2-one (10b)

Following the procedure described above for compound 10a, using the β-lactam 9a and crotonaldehyde, the product was obtained as a colourless solid, 82 mg, yield 25%, Mp 143–144 °C. IR (KBr) ν_{max}: 3455 (OH), 1745 (C=O), 1591, 1502, 1248, 1127 cm^{-1}. ^{1}H NMR (400 MHz, CDCl$_3$): δ 1.73–1.77 (m, 2H), 3.25–3.28 (m, 1H), 3.73 (s, 6H), 3.77 (s, 3H), 3.83 (s, 3H), 4.69–4.72 (m, 1H), 4.83 (d, J = 2.52 Hz, 1H), 5.57–5.62 (m, 1H), 5.80–5.88 (m, 1H), 6.56 (s, 2H), 6.91–6.94 (m, 2H), 7.28–7.32 (m, 2H). ^{13}C NMR (100 MHz, CDCl$_3$): δ 17.28, 54.86, 55.52, 55.90, 60.49, 64.70, 68.68, 94.25, 114.06, 114.11, 126.96, 127.81, 129.27, 129.37, 129.75, 133.31, 152.97, 159.16, 165.00. HRMS: found 436.1740 (M$^+$+Na); C$_{23}$H$_{27}$NO$_6$Na requires 436.1736.

4.1.10. 3-(1-Hydroxybut-2-enyl)-4-(3-hydroxy-4-methoxyphenyl)-1-(3,4,5-trimethoxyphenyl) azetidin-2-one (10c)

Following the procedure described above for compound 10a, using the β-lactam (9b) and crotonaldehyde, the title compound was obtained as a brown oil, 73 mg, yield 32%. IR (NaCl γmax): 1732 (C=O), 3427 (OH) cm^{-1}. ^{1}H NMR (400 MHz, CDCl$_3$): δ1.72 (d, J = 7.0 Hz, 1.8H), 1.74 (d, J = 1.0Hz, 1.2H), 2.50 (br, s, 1 H), 3.24 (m, 1H), 3.73–3.79 (overlapping singlets, 9H), 3.89 (s, 3H), 4.51 (t, J = 6.53Hz, 0.4H), 4.67 (t, J = 6.80 Hz, 0.6H), 4.76 (d, J = 2.48 Hz, 0.4H), 4.96 (d, J = 2.0 Hz, 0.6H), 5.78–5.85 (m, 2H). ^{13}C NMR (100 MHz, CDCl$_3$): δ17.25, 55.53, 55.84, 64.38, 60.47, 64.65, 68.42, 70.60, 94.26, 110.50, 111.75, 111.82, 117.42, 117.48, 127.62, 129.22, 129.78, 130.47, 133.25, 133.27, 146.17, 146.32, 152.93, 165.21. HRMS: Found 452.1707 (M$^+$+Na); C$_{23}$H$_{27}$NO$_7$Na requires 452.1685.

4.1.11. 4-(3-Hydroxy-4-methoxyphenyl)-3-(1-hydroxy-1-methylethyl)-1-(3,4,5-trimethoxy-phenyl) azetidin-2-one (10d)

Following the procedure described above for compound **10a**, using the β-lactam (**9b**) and acetone, the title compound was obtained as a brown oil, 51 mg, yield 23%. IR (NaCl ν max): 1732 (C=O), 3429 (OH) cm^{-1}. ^{1}H NMR (400 MHz, CDCl$_3$): δ1.35 (s, 3H), 1.48 (s, 3H), 1.91 (br, s, 1H), 3.13 (d, J = 2.52 Hz, 1H), 3.72 (s, 6H), 3.76 (s, 3H), 3.89 (s, 3H), 4.89 (d, J = 2.52 Hz, 1H), 5.90 (br, s, 1H), 6.56 (s, 2H), 6.83–6.96 (m, 3H). ^{13}C NMR (100 MHz, CDCl$_3$): δ 27.36, 27.62, 55.50, 55.53, 56.73, 60.47, 69.50, 94.27, 110.57, 111.78, 117.48, 130.51, 133.18, 133.79, 145.80, 146.25, 152.93, 165.29. HRMS: found 440.1671 (M$^+$+Na); C$_{22}$H$_{27}$NO$_7$Na requires 440.1685.

4.1.12. 3-((E)-1-Hydroxy-3-phenylallyl)-1-(3,4,5-trimethoxyphenyl)-4-(4-methoxyphenyl) azetidin-2-one (10e)

Following the procedure described above for compound **10a**, using the β-lactam **9a** and cinnamaldehyde, the product was obtained as a brown oil, 88 mg, yield 23%. IR (NaCl, film) ν$_{max}$: 3456 (OH), 1746 (C=O), 1579, 1503, 1266, 1123 cm^{-1}. ^{1}H NMR (400 MHz, CDCl$_3$): δ 3.38–3.39 (m, 1H), 3.73 (s, 6H), 3.78 (s, 3H), 3.82 (s, 3H), 4.53–4.56 (m, 1H), 4.78 (br s, 1H), 6.26–6.33 (m, 1H), 6.57 (s, 2H), 6.71–6.80 (m, 1H), 6.89–7.35 (m, 9H). HRMS: found 498.1885 (M$^+$+Na); C$_{28}$H$_{29}$NO$_6$Na requires 498.1893.

4.1.13. 4-(3-Hydroxy-4-methoxy-phenyl)-3-(1-hydroxy-3-phenyl-allyl)-1-(3,4,5-trimethoxy-phenyl) -azetidin-2-one (10f)

Following the procedure described above for compound **10a**, using 3-unsubstituted β-lactam (**9b**) and cinnamaldehyde, the title compound was obtained as a brown oil, 99 mg, yield 38%. IR (NaCl ν max): 1732 (C=O) 3418 (OH) cm^{-1}. ^{1}H NMR (400 MHz, CDCl$_3$): δ3.21 (br, s, 1H), 3.34 (dd, J = 2.55 Hz, 5.63 Hz, 0.53H), 3.37 (dd, J = 2.55 Hz, 5.62 Hz, 0.57H), 3.69 (s, 6H), 3.76 (s, 3H), 3.85 (s, 3H), 4.75 (dd, J = 6.13 Hz, 12.40 Hz, 0.43H), 4.86 (d, J = 2.45 Hz, 0.43H), 4.91 (dd, J = 3.82 Hz, 7.63 Hz, 0.57H), 5.03 (d, J = 2.45 Hz, 0.53H), 5.81–5.98 (m, 1H), 6.24 (dd, J = 5.54 Hz, 16.28 Hz, 0.57H), 6.41 (dd, J = 5.54 Hz, 16.28 Hz, 0.43H), 6.58 (s, 2H), 6.72–6.96 (m, 3H), 7.35–7.39 (m, 5H). ^{13}C NMR (100 MHz, CDCl$_3$): 53.32, 55.84, 56.17, 60.75, 57.35, 57.41, 64.81, 68.41, 70.77, 94.81, 94.86, 95.12, 110.61, 110.95, 110.98, 117.84, 117.91, 126.37, 126.61, 128.03, 128.46, 129.49, 130.33, 131.45, 133.12, 134.48, 136.20, 146.16, 146.61, 148.29, 153.29, 153.31, 165.48, 165.48. HRMS: found 514.1826 (M$^+$+Na); C$_{28}$H$_{29}$NO$_7$Na requires 514.1842.

4.1.14. 4-(3-Hydroxy-4-methoxyphenyl)-3-(1-hydroxyallyl)-1-(3,4,5-trimethoxy phenyl) azetidin-2-one (10g)

Following the procedure described above for compound **10a**, using 3-unsubstituted β-lactam (**9b**) and acrolein, the title compound was obtained as a brown oil, 48 mg, yield 22%. IR (NaCl ν max): 1732 (C=O), 3428 (OH) cm^{-1}. ^{1}H NMR (400 MHz, CDCl$_3$): δ 1.78 (br, s, 1H), 2.42 (br, s, 1H), 3.24–3.30 (m, 1H), 3.73 (s, 6H), 3.77 (s, 3H), 3.91 (s, 3H), 6.60 (t, J = 6.4 Hz, 6.6 Hz, 0.58H), 4.74 (dd, J = 6.4 Hz, 6.5 Hz, 0.32H), 4.80 (d, J = 2.3 Hz, 0.58H), 4.96 (d, J = 2.7 Hz, 0.32H), 5.28–5.44 (m, 2H), 5.78 (br, s, 1H), 5.90–5.98 (m, 0.32H), 6.02–6.10 (m, 0.68H), 6.56 (s, 2H), 6.84–7.28 (m, 3H). ^{13}C NMR (100 MHz, CDCl$_3$): δ 55.53, 55.55, 55.62, 60.48, 56.85, 63.99, 68.28, 70.76, 94.34, 110.47, 110.52, 111.74 111.81, 115.56, 117.47, 117.51, 129.93, 130.20, 133.20, 136.59, 136.80, 145.79, 146.14, 146.33, 152.96, 164.89. HRMS: found 438.1547 (M$^+$+Na); C$_{22}$H$_{25}$NO$_7$Na requires 438.1529.

4.1.15. 4-(3-Hydroxy-4-methoxy-phenyl)-3-(1-hydroxy-1-methylallyl)-1-(3,4,5-trimethoxy-phenyl) -azetidin-2-one (10h)

Following the procedure described above for compound **10a**, using 3-unsubstituted β-lactam (**9b**) and 3-buten-2-one, the title compound was obtained as a brown oil, 41mg, yield 18%. IR (NaCl ν max): 1734 (C=O), 3433 (OH) cm^{-1}. ^{1}H NMR (400 MHz, CDCl$_3$): δ1.46 (s, 1.53H), 1.56 (s, 1.34H), 1.8 (br, s, 1H), 3.17 (d, J = 2.40 Hz, 0.45H), 3.25 (d, J = 2.42 Hz, 0.42H), 3.71 (s, 6H), 3.76 (s, 3H), 3.88 (s, 3H), 4.81 (d, J = 2.40 Hz, 0.47H), 4.86 (d, J = 2.41 Hz, 0.44H), 5.17–5.23 (m, 1H), 5.31–5.42 (m, 1H), 5.81–6.81 (m,

1H), 5.81–5.83 (overlapping singlets, 1H), 6.54 (s, 2H), 6.83–6.96 (m, 3H). ^{13}C NMR (100 MHz, CDCl$_3$): δ 26.06, 26.19, 53.00, 56.01, 60.46, 55.51, 55.54, 67.47, 68.46, 71.70, 71.76, 94.28, 110.46, 110.54, 111.84, 111.92, 117.51, 117.60, 130.35, 133.17, 133.81, 140.73, 141.39, 141.46, 145.66, 146.13, 152.94, 164.45, δ164.91. HRMS: found 452.1691 (M$^+$Na); C$_{23}$H$_{27}$NO$_7$Na requires 452.1685.

4.1.16. 3-Acetyl-4-(3-hydroxy-4-methoxyphenyl)-1-(3,4,5-trimethoxyphenyl)azetidin-2-one (11)

Method A: To a stirring solution of pyridinium chlorochromate (132 mg, 0.57 mmol) in dry DCM (2 mL) under N$_2$ at room temperature was added quickly a solution of the silyl protected β-lactam (10i) (195 mg, 0.38 mmol). The reaction was stirred at room temperature for 18 h and then diluted with diethyl ether (25 mL) and the resulting suspension allowed to settle and the diethyl ether layer decanted off. The remaining solid was washed and decanted twice with two further 25 mL portions of diethylether. The organic extracts were combined and dried over MgSO$_4$, filtered, and the solvent removed under reduced pressure. The *t*BDMS ether was removed by treatment with tBAF as previously described, to afford the title compound as an oil, 7%, 11mg. **Method B:** The 3-unsubstituted β-lactam (9b) (378 mg, 0.80 mmol) was dissolved in THF (7 mL) in a dry flask flushed with N$_2$ and cooled to −78 °C. To this stirring solution LDA (1.0 M solution, 0.8 mL, 0.8 mmol) was added all at once and the reaction left to stir for 5 min prior to the dropwise addition of acetyl chloride (0.085 mL, 1.2 mmol), in THF (2 mL). The reaction mixture was allowed to stir at −78 °C for 30 min then stirred at room temperature for 5 min before being poured into saturated brine (50 mL). The brine solution was extracted with ethyl acetate (2 × 50 mL), the organic layers combined, dried over MgSO$_4$, filtered, and the solvent removed under reduced pressure. Purification by flash column chromatography over silica gel (eluent: *n*-hexane: ethyl acetate, 1:1) followed by removal of the TBDMS ether by treatment with tBAF as previously described afforded the title compound as an oil, 35 mg, yield 11%. IR (NaCl ν max): 1731 (C=O), 1739, (C=O) 3434 (OH) cm^{-1}. ^{1}H NMR (400 MHz, CDCl$_3$): δ1.99 (s, 3H), 3.73 (s, 6H), 3.75 (s, 3H), 3.81 (s, 3H), 4.23 (d, J = 1.98 Hz, 1H), 5.12 (d, J = 1.99 Hz, 1H), 6.08 (s, 2H), 6.37–6.57 (m, 3H). ^{13}C NMR (100 MHz, CDCl$_3$): δ 23.14, 53.93, 55.71, 60.87, 65.03, 61.71, 93.81, 111.21, 113.02, 118.21, 130.98, 131.02, 134.27, 147.12, 147.34, 153.27, 164.45, 181.23. HRMS: found 402.1463 (M$^+$+H); C$_{21}$H$_{24}$NO$_7$ requires 402.1553.

4.1.17. 3-Ethylidene-4-(3-hydroxy-4-methoxy-phenyl)-1-(3,4,5-trimethoxy-phenyl)-azetidin-2-one (12)

To a solution of the silyl ether protected β-lactam 10i (1 mmol) in DCM (10 mL), stirring at 0 °C under N$_2$, was added PPh$_3$ (1 mmol) and DEAD (1.2 mmol). Stirring at 0 °C was continued for a further 3 min before the reaction was allowed to warm to room temperature. Diethyl ether (30 mL) was added to the reaction mixture to precipitate the triphenylphosphine oxide side product which was removed by filtration. The filtrate was collected and evaporated to dryness under reduced pressure to afford the product. Separation of the *E/Z* isomers was carried out on a Biotage SP1 system using a gradient elution from 2% ethyl acetate in hexanes to 100% ethyl acetate over 20 column volumes, and detection at 280 nm. The product was obtained as a colourless resin, [99], [100], 87 mg, yield 52%. IR (NaCl ν max): 1738 (C=O), 2935 (CH), 3327 (OH) cm^{-1}. ^{1}H NMR (400 MHz, CDCl$_3$): *E isomer*, δ 1.62 (d, J = 4.40 Hz, 3H), 3.76 (s, 6H), 3.78 (s, 3H), 3.92 (s, 3H), 5.32 (s, 1H), 5.68, s, 1H), 6.32 (m, 1H), 6.61 (s, 2H), 6.86 (d, J = 8.2 Hz, 1H), 7.03 (d, J = 1.96 Hz, 1H), 6.99 (m, 1H). *Z isomer*, δ 2.05 (d, J = 4.16 Hz, 3H), 3.76 (s, 6H), 3.79 (s, 3H), 3.92 (s, 3H), 5.19 (s, 1H), 5.65–5.66 (m, 2H), 6.63 (s, 2H), 6.85–6.90 (m, 3H). ^{13}C NMR (100 MHz, CDCl$_3$): *E isomer* δ 13.26, 55.80, 55.88, 60.76, 62.72, 94.47, 110.68, 113.04, 118.87, 123.32, 129.72, 133.94, 134.20, 142.32, 146.04, 146.74, 153.33, 161.19. *Z isomer* δ 14.30, 55.81, 55.82, 60.81, 62.80, 94.57, 110.61, 112.73, 118.48, 126.89, 130.37, 133.93, 134.15, 141.71, 146.11, 146.72, 153.38, 161.79. HRMS: found 408.1411(M$^+$+Na); C$_{21}$H$_{23}$NO$_6$Na requires 408.1423.

4.1.18. 3-(1,2-Dihydroxyethyl)-4-(3-hydroxy-4-methoxyphenyl)-1-(3,4,5-trimethoxyphenyl) azetidin-2-one (13)

To a solution of the silyl ether protected azetidin-2-one (7o) (156 mg, 0.312 mmol) in pyridine (0.5 mL) stirring under N_2 at room temperature was added osmium tetroxide, OsO_4 (80 mg, 0.312 mmol). The reaction darkened in colour and became hot to the touch upon completion of the addition. The flask was immersed in ice-water for 60 s, then left to stir at room temperature under N_2 for 22 h. A solution of $Na_2(SO_3)_2$ (1.343 g, 6.8 mmol) in a 1:4 mixture of pyridine/water (20 mL) was added and the reaction was stirred at room temperature for a further 7 h. The reaction mixture was extracted with warm ethyl acetate (100 mL). The organic layer was collected and washed with 0.1M HCl (100 mL), saturated $NaHCO_3$ (100 mL), and water (100 mL). The organic layer was collected and dried over $MgSO_4$, filtered and the solvent removed under reduced pressure. The product was purified by passage through a short silica column (5 cm) and eluted with DCM. The tBDMS group was cleaved by treatment with tBAF as described above, to afford the product as a colourless resin, yield 39%, 51 mg. IR (NaCl ν max): 1727 (C=O), 3454 (OH) cm^{-1}. ^{1}H NMR (400 MHz, CDCl$_3$): δ 2.72 (br s, 1H, OH), 3.16 (dd, 0.72H, J = 2.42 Hz, 5.55 Hz), 3.19 (dd, 0.29H, J = 2.46 Hz, 4.56 Hz), 3.60-3.67 (m, 8H), 3.74 (s, 3H), 3.83 (s, 3H), 4.10 (dd, J = 4.05 Hz, 0.26H), 4.19 (dd, J = 5.50 Hz, 0.75H), 4.25 (br s, 0.5H), 4.90 (d, J = 2.37 Hz, 0.31H), 5.00 (d, J = 2.36 Hz, 0.69H), 6.25 (br, s, 0.30H), 6.46 (br, s, 0.70H), 6.53 (s, 2H), 6.77–6.94 (m, 3H). ^{13}C NMR (100 MHz, CDCl$_3$): δ 55.79, 55.85, 56.80, 56.97, 60.73, 62.18, 64.46, 64.76, 68.54, 69.30, 94.92, 111.06, 111.11, 112.23, 112.43, 117.76, 117.90, 129.92, 130.29, 133.17, 133.33, 146.07, 146.22, 146.85, 146.98, 153.27, 165.76, 165.96. HRMS: found 442.1490 (M$^+$+Na); C$_{21}$H$_{25}$NO$_8$Na requires 442.1478.

4.1.19. (1-((2-Methoxy-5-(4-oxo-1-(3,4,5-trimethoxyphenyl)-3-vinylazetidin-2-yl)phenyl)-amino)-1 -oxopropan-2-yl) carbamaic acid 9H-fluoren-9-ylmethyl ester (14)

To a stirred solution of β-lactam 7t (4.76 mmol) in anhydrous DMF (30 mL) were added DCC (5.7 mmol), Fmoc-protected alanine (5.6 mmol) and HOBt.H$_2$O (7.3 mmol) at room temperature. The mixture was stirred for 24 h, then ethyl acetate (50 mL) was added and the reaction mixture was filtered. The DMF was removed by washing with water (5 × 50 mL). The organic solvent was removed under reduced pressure, and the product was isolated by flash column chromatography over silica gel (eluent: dichloromethane: methanol gradient) as a brown oil, yield, 58%, 173 mg. IR (NaCl, film) ν_{max}: 3323 (NH), 1723 (C=O), 1640 (C=O), 1598 cm^{-1}. H NMR (400 MHz, CDCl$_3$): δ 1.52 (br s, 3H), 3.74 (s, 6H), 3.77 (s, 4H), 3.83 (s, 3H), 4.25 (t, J = 6.78 Hz, 1H), 4.45–4.47 (m, 3H), 4.76 (br s, 1H), 5.31–5.34 (m, 1H), 5.37–5.41 (m, 1H), 5.98–6.07 (m, 1H), 6.59 (s, 2H), 6.86–7.79 (m, 11H), 8.39–8.44 (br s, 1H), 8.50 (s, 1H). ^{13}C NMR (100 MHz, CDCl$_3$): δ 20.62, 46.63, 55.47, 55.64, 60.49, 59.96, 60.93, 63.32, 66.83, 94.30, 110.15, 117.70, 119.50, 120.58, 124.52, 126.64, 127.35, 128.39, 128.80, 128.84, 129.31, 130.03, 133.38, 133.91, 137.63, 140.85, 143.22, 153.03, 164.91, 169.98, 170.76. HRMS: Found 700.2632 (M$^+$+Na); C$_{39}$H$_{39}$N$_3$O$_8$Na requires 700.2635.

4.1.20. 2-Amino-N-(2-methoxy-5-(1-(3,4,5-trimethoxyphenyl)-4-oxo-3-vinylazetidin-2-yl)phenyl) propanamide (15)

To amino acid amide 14 (1.56 mmol) in methanol (10 mL)/CH$_2$Cl$_2$ (10 mL) was added 2N NaOH (3.4 mmol) at room temperature and the mixture was stirred for 24 h. Saturated aq. NaHCO$_3$ was added and the mixture was extracted with CH$_2$Cl$_2$ three times. The organic solution was dried and evaporated. The product was dissolved diethyl ether and extracted with 2N HCl (5 × 50 mL). 2N NaOH was added to the HCl mixture solution and the mixture was washed with diethyl ether (5 × 50 mL). The organic solution was dried and the solvent was removed under reduced pressure to afford the product as an off-yellow oil, yield 57%. IR (NaCl) ν_{max}: 3307 cm^{-1} (NH$_2$), 1741 (C=O), 1679 (C=O) cm^{-1}. ^{1}H NMR (400 MHz, CDCl$_3$): δ 1.61–1.64 (m, 3H), 3.76 (s, 9H), 3.68–3.69 (m, 1H), 3.78 (br s, 1H), 3.79 (s, 3H), 5.40 (br s, 1H), 6.33–6.35 (m, 1H), 6.65 (s, 2H), 6.83–6.90 (m, 2H), 7.08–7.20 (m, 3H). ^{13}C NMR (100 MHz, CDCl$_3$): δ 21.65, 51.69, 55.87, 55.90, 60.92, 62.95, 65.87, 94.47, 109.81, 119.33, 121.61,

123.70, 127.72, 133.57, 133.69, 134.14, 148.34, 153.45, 161.44, 167.06. HRMS: found 456.2137 (M^++H); $C_{24}H_{30}N_3O_6$ requires 456.2135.

4.1.21. General procedure III: Preparation of dibenzyl phosphates **16a**, **16b**

To a solution of phenol **7s**, **9a** (17 mmol) in acetonitrile (100 mL cooled to 0 °C) was added carbon tetrachloride (85 mmol). The resulting solution was stirred for 10 min prior to adding diisopropylethylamine (35 mmol) and dimethylaminopyridine (1.7 mmol). The dibenzyl phosphite (24.5 mmol) was then added dropwise to the mixture. When the reaction was complete, 0.5M KH_2PO_4 (aq) was added and the reaction mixture was allowed to warm to room temperature. An ethyl acetate extract (3 × 50 mL) was washed with saturated sodium chloride (aqueous, 100 mL) followed by water (100 mL) and dried using anhydrous sodium sulfate. The organic solvent was removed under reduced pressure and the product was isolated by flash column chromatography over silica gel (*n*-hexane: ethyl acetate gradient).

2-Methoxy-5-(1-(3,4,5-trimethoxyphenyl)-4-oxoazetidin-2-yl)phenyl dibenzyl phosphate (**16a**)

Preparation as described in the general method above from β-lactam **9a**. Yield: 60%, 507 mg, brown oil. IR (NaCl, film) ν_{max}: 2940, 1730 (C=O, β-lactam), 1507, 1300 (P=O), 1235, 1127 cm^{-1}. ^{1}H NMR (400 MHz, CDCl$_3$): δ 2.90 (dd, J = 15.08 Hz, 2.52 Hz, 1H), 3.50 (dd, J = 15.56 Hz, 5.52 Hz, 1H), 3.76 (s, 6H), 3.76 (s, 3H), 3.81 (s, 3H), 4.84 (dd, J = 5.04 Hz, 2.52 Hz, 1H), 5.15–5.18 (m, 4H), 6.53 (s, 2H), 6.93–7.23 (m, 3H), 7.31–7.36 (m, 10H). ^{13}C NMR (100 MHz, CDCl$_3$): δ 46.44, 53.23, 55.54, 55.61, 60.47, 69.44, 69.48, 69.54, 93.97, 112.77, 119.36, 122.59, 127.43, 127.47, 128.14, 128.16, 130.14, 133.47, 133.89, 135.10, 139.47, 139.54, 150.35, 153.06, 163.87. HRMS: found 642.1838 (M^++Na); $C_{33}H_{34}NO_9PNa$ requires 642.1869.

2-Methoxy-5-(1-(3,4,5-trimethoxyphenyl)-4-oxo-3-vinylazetidin-2-yl)phenyl dibenzyl phosphate (**16b**)

Preparation as described in the general method above from β-lactam **7s**. Yield: 61%, 502 mg, brown oil. IR (NaCl, film) ν_{max}: 2946, 1749 (C=O, β-lactam), 1502, 1300 (P=O), 1240, 1127 cm^{-1}. ^{1}H NMR (400 MHz, CDCl$_3$): δ 3.70 (br s, 1H), 3.71 (s, 6H), 3.76 (s, 3H), 3.82 (s, 3H), 4.65 (d, J = 2.00 Hz, 1H), 5.14–5.18 (m, 4H), 5.33–5.40 (m, 2H), 5.97–6.02 (m, 1H), 6.53 (s, 2H), 6.94–7.20 (m, 3H), 7.28–7.35 (m, 10H). ^{13}C NMR (100 MHz, CDCl$_3$): δ 55.56, 55.61, 60.43, 60.48, 63.29, 69.48, 69.50, 94.19, 112.79, 119.27, 119.62, 122.75, 127.41, 127.49, 128.15, 128.22, 129.29, 129.85, 133.22, 134.00, 135.07, 135.12, 139.57, 150.52, 153.07, 164.69. HRMS: found 668.2017 (M^++Na); $C_{35}H_{36}NO_9PNa$ requires 668.2025.

4.1.22. Phosphoric acid 2-methoxy-5-[4-oxo-1-(3,4,5-trimethoxyphenyl)azetidin-2-yl]phenyl ester dimethyl ester (**16c**)

A solution of β-lactam phenol **7s** (280 mg, 0.64 mmol), acetonitrile (5 mL) and carbon tetrachloride (0.62 mL, 0.64 mmol) was cooled to −10 °C and stirred under a nitrogen atmosphere for ten minutes. Diisopropyl ethylamine (1.28 mmol) and dimethylaminopyridine (0.06 mmol) were added. After one minute, dimethyl phosphite (0.96 mmol) was added over three minutes. The mixture was stirred for a further 3 h allowing the reaction to come to ambient temperature slowly. The reaction was terminated via the addition of 0.5 M potassium dihydrogen phosphate. The mixture was extracted with ethyl acetate. The organic phases were combined and evaporated to dryness under reduced pressure. The residue was purified by flash chromatography on silica gel to afford the product (155 mg, 52%). IR (KBr) ν_{max}: 3437.4, 2960.9, 1752.1, 1603.4, 1509.2, 1466.2, 1281.4, 1239.3, 1185.6, 1130.0, 1052.1, 999.4, 855.8. ^{1}H-NMR (400 MHz, CDCl$_3$): δ 2.94 (dd, 1H, J = 2.8 Hz, 15.3 Hz), 3.52 (dd, 1H, J = 5.5 Hz, 15.3 Hz), 3.72 (s, 6H), 3.74 (s, 3H), 3.82–3.87 (m, 9H, OCH$_3$), 4.92 (m, 1H), 6.52 (s, 2H), 6.95–6.96 (m, 1H), 7.16–7.18 (m, 1H), 7.29–7.30 (m, 1H). ^{13}C NMR (100 MHz, CDCl$_3$): δ 46.80, 53.61, 54.91, 54.97, 55.98, 56.05, 60.83, 94.40, 113.29, 119.61, 119.64, 123.21, 130.61, 133.84, 134.23, 139.81, 139.89, 150.72, 150.76, 153.43, 164.37. HRMS: Found 468.1425 (M^++H), $C_{21}H_{27}NO_9P$ requires 468.1423.

4.1.23. Phosphoric acid diethyl ester 2-methoxy-5-[4-oxo-1-(3,4,5-trimethoxyphenyl)azetidin-2-yl]phenyl ester (16d)

Preparation as described above for β-lactam **16c** using diethyl phosphite (0.96 mmol). Yield 250 mg, 79%. IR (KBr) ν_{max}: 3487.5, 2988.0, 1756.3, 1603.4, 1586.6, 1507.1, 1451.5, 1292.0, 1238.7, 1127.0, 1035.6, 1000.2, 988.1, 823.1. ^{1}H-NMR (400 MHz, CDCl$_3$): δ 1.29 (t, 6H), 2.90 (dd, 1H, J = 2.5 Hz, 15.3 Hz), 3.49 (dd, 1H, J = 5.8 Hz, 15.3 Hz), 3.69 (s, 6H), 3.71 (s, 3H), 3.83 (s, 3H), 4.03–4.07 (m, 4H), 6.50 (s, 2H), 6.92 (m, 1H), 7.12–7.15 (m, 1H), 7.29–7.30 (m, 1H). ^{13}C NMR (100 MHz, CDCl$_3$): δ: 15.96, 16.03, 46.84, 53.65, 56.00, 60.84, 63.45, 63.50, 94.38, 113.17, 119.49, 119.51, 123.07, 130.53, 133.88, 134.24, 140.06, 140.13, 150.80, 150.85, 153.45, 164.36. HRMS: Found 496.1734 (M$^+$+H); C$_{23}$H$_{31}$NO$_9$P requires 496.1736.

4.1.24. 2-Methoxy-5-(1-(3,4,5-trimethoxyphenyl)-4-oxoazetidin-2-yl)phenyl dihydrogen phosphate (17a)

Dibenzyl phosphate ester (**16a**) (0.27 mmol) was dissolved in dry dichloromethane (5 mL) under nitrogen at 0 °C. Bromotrimethylsilane (0.59 mmol) was added to the reaction mixture and allowed to stir for 45 min. Sodium thiosulfate solution (10%, 5 mL) was added to the reaction and stirring was continued for 5 min. The aqueous phase was extracted with ethyl acetate (3 × 25 mL). The combined organic phases were concentrated under reduced pressure and the crude product was purified by flash chromatography on silica gel (eluent: n-hexane: ethyl acetate, 1:1) to afford the product as a brown solid. Yield: 91%, 289 mg, Mp 207–209 °C. Purity (HPLC): 100.0%. IR (KBr) ν_{max}: 3497 (OH), 1730 (C=O, β-lactam), 1303 (P=O), 1237, 1128 cm^{-1}. ^{1}H NMR (400 MHz, DMSO-d_6): δ 2.91 (dd, J = 15.04 Hz, 2.52 Hz, 1H), 3.51 (dd, J = 15.64 Hz, 5.52 Hz, 1H), 3.58 (s, 3H), 3.64 (s, 6H), 3.74 (s, 3H), 5.08 (br s, 1H), 6.52 (s, 2H), 7.03–7.48 (m, 3H). ^{13}C NMR (100 MHz, DMSO-d_6): δ 45.88, 52.92, 55.64, 55.72, 60.06, 94.30, 113.02, 118.96, 121.91, 130.08, 130.71, 133.53, 133.68, 150.19, 153.09, 164.47. HRMS: found 438.0947 (M-H)$^-$; C$_{19}$H$_{21}$NO$_9$P requires 438.0954

4.1.25. 2-Methoxy-5-(1-(3,4,5-trimethoxyphenyl)-4-oxo-3-vinylazetidin-2-yl)phenyl dihydrogen phosphate (17b)

Following the preparation described above for compound **16a**, using dibenzyl phosphate ester (**16b**) (0.27 mmol) and bromotrimethylsilane (0.59 mmol). Purification by flash chromatography on silica gel (eluent: n-hexane: ethyl acetate, 1:1) afforded the product as a yellow oil, yield 63%. IR (NaCl) ν_{max}: 3483 (OH), 1749 (C=O), 1307 (P=O) cm^{-1}. ^{1}H NMR (400 MHz, CDCl$_3$): δ 3.70 (s, 6H), 3.76 (s, 3H), 3.79 (s, 3H), 4.68–4.70 (m, 1H), 5.14 (br s, 1H), 5.28–5.38 (m, 2H), 5.94–6.00 (m, 1H), 6.51 (s, 2H), 6.91–7.35 (m, 3H). ^{13}C NMR (100 MHz, CDCl$_3$): δ 55.49, 55.58, 60.43, 60.50, 63.07, 94.31, 112.69, 119.18, 119.55, 122.70, 129.81, 133.08, 133.99, 134.67, 135.23, 150.52, 153.02, 165.14. HRMS: found 488.1106 (M$^+$+Na); C$_{21}$H$_{24}$NO$_9$PNa requires 488.1086.

4.1.26. 5-(3-Ethyl-1-(3,4,5-trimethoxyphenyl)-4-oxoazetidin-2-yl)-2-methoxyphenyl dihydrogen phosphate (17c)

The dibenzylphosphate ester protected compound **16b** (2 mmol) was dissolved in ethanol: ethyl acetate (50 mL; 1:1 mixture) and hydrogenated over 1.2 g of 10% palladium on carbon until complete on TLC, typically less than 3 h. The catalyst was filtered, the solvent was removed under reduced pressure and the product was isolated by flash column chromatography over silica gel (eluent: n-hexane: ethyl acetate gradient) to afford the product as a brown oil, 140 mg, 98%. Purity (HPLC): 100%. IR (NaCl, film) ν_{max}: 3483 (OH), 1742 (C=O), 1272 (P=O), 1236, 1126 cm^{-1}. ^{1}H NMR (400 MHz, CDCl$_3$): δ 0.97 (br s, 3H), 1.76–1.83 (m, 2H), 3.09 (s, 1H), 3.66 (s, 6H), 3.71 (s, 6H), 4.56 (br s, 1H), 6.51 (s, 2H), 6.82–7.38 (m, 3H). ^{13}C NMR (100 MHz, CDCl$_3$): δ 13.74, 20.62, 55.47, 55.55, 59.67, 59.99, 60.39, 94.33, 112.48, 118.69, 122.27, 130.12, 133.16, 133.86, 135.64, 150.06, 152.97, 168.22. HRMS: found 490.1239 (M$^+$+Na); C$_{21}$H$_{26}$NO$_9$PNa requires 490.1243.

4.2. Biochemical Evaluation

All biochemical assays were performed in triplicate on at least three independent occasions for the determination of mean values reported.

4.2.1. Cell Culture

The human breast carcinoma cell line MCF-7, was purchased from the European Collection of Animal Cell Cultures (ECACC) and was cultured in Eagle's minimum essential medium with 10% fetal bovine serum, 2 mM L-glutamine and 100 µg/mL penicillin/streptomycin. The medium was supplemented with 1% non-essential amino acids. The human breast carcinoma cell line MDA-MB-231 was purchased from the European Collection of Animal Cell Cultures (ECACC). MDA-MB-231 cells were maintained in Dulbecco's modified Eagle's medium (DMEM) supplemeted with 10% (v/v) fetal bovine serum, 2 mM L-glutamine and 100 µg/mL penicillin/streptomycin (complete medium). All media contained 100 U/mL penicillin and 100 µg/mL streptomycin. Triple negative breast cancer Hs578T cells and its invasive variant Hs578Ts(i)$_8$ were obtained as a kind gift from Dr. Susan McDonnell, School of Chemical and Bioprocess Engineering, University College Dublin and were cultured in Dulbecco's Modified Eagle's Media (DMEM) with GlutaMAX^{TM}-I, with the same supplement as for MDA-MB-231 cells in the absence of non-essential amino acids. HEK-293T normal epithelial embryonic kidney cells were cultured in Dulbecco's Modified Eagle's Medium (DMEM) with GlutaMAX^{TM}-I in the absence of non-essential amino acids. K562 and HL-60 cells were originally obtained from the European Collection of Cell Cultures (Salisbury, UK).The K562 cells were derived from a patient in the blast crisis stage of CML HL-60 cells were derive from a patient with acute myeloid leukaemia. Cells were cultured in RPMI-1640 Glutamax medium supplemented with 10% FCS media, and 100 µg/mL penicillin/streptomycin. Cells were maintained at 37 °C in 5% CO_2 in a humidified incubator. All cells were sub-cultured three times/week (adherent cells by trypsinisation).

4.2.2. Cell Viability Assay

Cells were seeded at a density of 5×10^3 cells/well (MCF-7), in triplicate in 96-well plates. After 24 h, cells were then treated with either medium alone, vehicle [1% ethanol (v/v)] or with serial dilutions of CA-4 or β-lactam analogue. Cell viability for MCF-7 and MDA-MB-231 was analysed using the Alamar Blue assay (Invitrogen Corp, Thermo Fisher Scientific, 168 Third Avenue, Waltham, MA, USA) according to the manufacturer's instructions. After 72 h, Alamar Blue [10% (v/v)] was added to each well and plates were incubated for 3–5 h at 37 °C in the dark. Fluorescence was read using a 96-well fluorimeter with excitation at 530 nm and emission at 590 nm. Results were expressed as percentage viability relative to vehicle control (100%). Dose response curves were plotted and IC$_{50}$ values (concentration of drug resulting in 50% reduction in cell survival) were obtained using the commercial software package Prism (GraphPad Software, Inc., 2365 Northside, Suite 560, San Diego, CA, USA). Experiments were performed in triplicate on at least three separate occasions.

4.2.3. Lactate Dehydrogenase Assay for Cytotoxicity

Cytotoxicity was determined using the CytoTox 96 non-radioactive cytotoxicity assay (Promega Corporation; 2800 Woods Hollow Road, Madison, WI, USA) [101] following the manufacturer's protocol. Briefly, MCF-7 cells were seeded in 96-well plates, incubated for 24 hr and then treated with test compounds (**7d, 7h, 7i, 7q, 7r, 7u, 7t, 10d, 10f, 12**) as described in the cell viability assay above. After 72 h, 20 µL of 'lysis solution (10X)' was added to control wells and the plate was incubated for a further 1 hr to ensure 100% death. 50 µL of supernatant was carefully removed from each well and transferred to a new 96-well plate. 50 µL of reconstituted 'substrate mix' was added and the plate was placed in the dark at room temperature for 30 min. After this period, 50 µL of 'stop solution' was added to each well and the absorbance was read at a wavelength of 490 nm using a Dynatech MR5000 plate reader. The percentage cell death at 10 µM was calculated.

4.2.4. Cytotoxicity Assay

As previously reported [45,74,75] mammary glands from 14–18 day pregnant CD-1 mice were used as source and primary mammary epithelial cell cultures were prepared from these. The isolated mammary epithelial cells were seeded at two concentrations (25,000 cells/mL and 50,000 cells/mL). Initially a third concentration of 100,000 cells/mL was also used, but this proved to be too high to give meaningful results. After 24 h, the cells were treated with 2 μL volumes of test compound **7s** which had been pre-prepared as stock solutions in ethanol to furnish the concentration range of study, 1 nM–100 μM, and re-incubated for a further 72 h. Control wells contained the equivalent volume of the vehicle ethanol (1% v/v). The cytotoxicity was assessed using alamar blue dye.

4.2.5. Cell Cycle Analysis

MCF-7 cells (adherent and detached) were treated with the appropriate concentration of compound **7s** and incubated for the designated time. Cells were collected, trypsinised and centrifuged at 800× g for 15 min. Cells were washed twice with ice-cold PBS and fixed in ice-cold 70% ethanol overnight at −20 °C. Fixed cells were centrifuged at 800× g for 15 min and stained with 50 μg/mL of PI, containing 50 μg/mL of DNase-free RNase A, at 37 °C for 30 min. The DNA content of cells (10,000 cells/experimental group) was analysed by flow cytometer at 488 nm using a FACSCalibur flow cytometer (BD Biosciences, 2350 Qume Dr, San Jose, CA, USA) all data were recorded and analysed using the CellQuest™ software, (BD Biosciences, 2350 Qume Dr, San Jose, CA, USA)

4.2.6. Annexin V/PI Apoptotic Assay

Apoptotic cell death was detected by flow cytometry using Annexin V and propidium iodide (PI). MCF-7 Cells were seeded in 6 well plated at density of 1×10^5 cells/mL and treated with either vehicle (0.1% (v/v) EtOH), CA-4 or β-lactam compound **7s** at different concentrations for selected time. Cells were then harvested and prepared for flow cytometric analysis. Cells were washed in 1X binding buffer (20X binding buffer: 0.1M HEPES, pH 7.4; 1.4 M NaCl; 25 mM $CaCl_2$ diluted in dH_2O) and incubated in the dark for 30 min on ice in Annexin V-containing binding buffer [1:100]. Cells were then washed once in binding buffer and then re-suspended in PI-containing binding buffer [1:1000]. Samples were analysed immediately using the BD accuri flow cytometer (BD Biosciences, 2350 Qume Dr, San Jose, CA, USA) and prism software for analysis the data (GraphPad Software, Inc., 2365 Northside Dr., Suite 560, San Diego, CA, USA). Four populations are produced during the assay Annexin V and PI negative (Q4, healthy cells), Annexin V positive and PI negative (Q3, early apoptosis), Annexin V and PI positive (Q2, late apoptosis) and Annexin V negative and PI positive (Q1, necrosis). Paclitaxel was used as a positive control for cell death

4.2.7. Tubulin Polymerization Assay

The assembly of purified bovine tubulin was monitored using a kit, BK006, purchased from Cytoskeleton Inc., 1830 S Acoma St, Denver, CO, 80223, USA. [78]. The assay was carried out in accordance with the manufacturer's instructions in the tubulin polymerisation assay kit manual using the standard assay conditions. The values reported represent the average values from two independent assays. Purified (>99%) bovine brain tubulin (3 mg/mL) in a buffer consisting of 80 mM PIPES (pH 6.9), 0.5 mM EGTA, 2 mM $MgCl_2$, 1 mM GTP and 10% glycerol was incubated at 37 °C in the presence of either vehicle (2% (v/v) ddH_2O) or compounds **7h, 7i, 7s, 7t** (initially 10 μM in EtOH); CA-4 and Paclitaxel were used as controls. Light is scattered proportionally to the concentration of polymerised microtubules in the assay. Therefore, tubulin assembly was monitored turbidimetrically at 340 nm at 37 °C in a Spectramax 340 PC spectrophotometer (Molecular Devices, 3860 N 1st St, San Jose, CA, USA). The absorbance was measured at 30 s intervals for 60 min.

4.2.8. Colchicine-Binding Site Assay

MCF-7 cells were seeded at a density of 5×10^4 cells/well in 6-well plates and incubated overnight. Cells were treated with vehicle control [ethanol (0.1% v/v)] or compound **7s** (10 µM) for 2 h. After this time, selected wells were treated with N,N'-ethylene-bis(iodoacetamide)(EBI) (100 µM) (Santa Cruz Biotechnology Inc. 10410 Finnell Street, Dallas, Texas, USA) for 1.5 h. Following treatment, cells were twice washed with ice-cold PBS and lysed by addition of Laemmli buffer. Samples were separated by SDS-PAGE, trasnsferred to polyvinylidene difluoride membranes and probed with β-tubulin antibodies (Sigma-Aldrich, 2033 Westport Center Dr, St. Louis, MO, USA) [85].

4.2.9. Immunofluorescence Microscopy

Confocal microscopy was used to study the effects of drug treatment on MCF-7 cytoskeleton. For immunofluorescence, MCF-7 cells were seeded at 1×10^5 cells/mL on eight chamber glass slides (BD Biosciences, 2350 Qume Dr, San Jose, CA, USA). Cells were either untreated or treated with vehicle [1% ethanol (v/v)], paclitaxel (1 µM), combretastatin A-4 (100 nM) or compound **7s** (100 nM) for 16 h. Following treatment cells were gently washed in PBS, fixed for 20 min with 4% paraformaldehyde in PBS and permeabilised in 0.5% Triton X-100. Following washes in PBS containing 0.1% Tween (PBST), cells were blocked in 5% bovine serum albumin diluted in PBST. Cells were then incubated with mouse monoclonal anti-α-tubulin−FITC antibody (clone DM1A) (Sigma-Aldrich, 2033 Westport Center Dr, St. Louis, MO, USA) (1:100) for 2 h at room temperature. Following washes in PBST, cells were incubated with Alexa Fluor 488 dye (1:450) for 1 h at room temperature. Following washes in PBST, the cells were mounted in Ultra Cruz Mounting Media (Santa Cruz Biotechnology Inc., 10410 Finnell Street, Dallas, TX, USA) containing 4,6-diamino-2-phenolindol dihydrochloride (DAPI). Images were captured by Leica SP8 confocal microscopy with Leica application suite X software (Leica Microsystems CMS GmbH Am Friedensplatz 3 D-68165 Mannheim, Germany). All images in each experiment were collected on the same day using identical parameters. Experiments were performed on three independent occasions.

4.3. Stability Study of Compounds 7s, 17b and 17c

Analytical high-performance liquid chromatography (HPLC) stability studies were performed using a Symmetry® column (C$_{18}$, 5 µm, 4.6 × 150 mm), a Waters 2487 Dual Wavelength Absorbance detector, a Waters 1525 binary HPLC pump and a Waters 717 plus Autosampler (Waters Corporation, 34 Maple St, Milford, MA, USA). Samples were detected at wavelength of 254 nm. All samples were analysed using acetonitrile (80%) and water (20%) as the mobile phase over 10 min and a flow rate of 1 mL/min. Stock solutions were prepared by dissolving 5 mg of compound **7s**, **17b** and **17c** in 10 mL of mobile phase. Phosphate buffers at the desired pH values (4, 7.4 and 9) were prepared in accordance with the British Pharmacopoeia monograph 2015. 30 µL of stock solution was diluted with 1 mL of appropriate buffer, shaken and injected immediately. Samples were withdrawn and analysed at time intervals of $t = 0$ min, 5 min, 30 min, 60 min, 90 min, 120 min, 24 h and 48 h. **Plasma stability studies**: 360 µL stock solution of compounds **7s**, **17b** and **17c** were transferred to buffered plasma (plasma: buffer = 1:9, 4 mL in total) at 37 °C in screw cap container. Immediately a 250 µL aliquot was withdrawn and added to the Eppendorf tube containing 500 µL ZnSO$_4$.7H$_2$O solution (2% w/v ZnSO$_4$ solution in acetonitrile: water, 1:1). The samples were then centrifuged at 10,000 rpm for 3 min and filtered through a 0.2-micron filter and injected according to the HPLC conditions listed above. Further samples were taken in the same manner every 1 h thereafter up to 6 h. A final sample was taken after 24 h. **Whole blood stability studies**. A 360 µL aliquot of stock solution of compounds **17b** and **17c** in acetonitrile was added in whole blood (4 mL, treated with 2% sodium citrate) at 37 °C and 300 µL aliquots were withdrawn at approptiate intervals. Samples were transferred to 1.5 mL Eppenddorf tubes containing 1 mL of ZnSO$_4$. 7H$_2$O solution (2% w/v ZnSO$_4$ solution in acetonitrile: water, 1:1), vortexed and then centrifuged for 5 min at 14,000 rpm. The sample filtered through a 0.2-micron filter and injected according to the HPLC conditions listed above.

4.4. X-Ray Crystallography

Data for samples **6k, 7h** and **8i, 8k** were collected on a Bruker APEX DUO and Bruker D8 Quest ECO respectively using Cu Kα (λ = 1.54178 Å; **7h**) and Mo Kα radiation (λ = 0.71073 Å; **6k, 8i, 8k**), (Bruker, 40 Manning Road, Billerica, MA, USA) Each sample was mounted on a Mitegen cryoloop and data collected at 100(2) K (Oxford Cobra and Cryostream cryosystems, Oxford Cryosystems, 3 Blenheim Office Park, Long Hanborough, Oxford OX29 8LN, UK). Bruker APEX [102] software was used to collect and reduce data and determine the space group. The structures were solved using direct methods (XS) [103] or intrinsic phasing (XT) [104] and refined with least squares minimization (XL) [105] in Olex2 [106]. Absorption corrections were applied using SADABS 2014 [107]. Data for sample **8h** were collected on a Rigaku Saturn 724 at 150(2) K (X-Stream), (Rigaku, Tokyo, Tōkyō Prefecture, JP 151-0051) and CrystalClear [108,109] was used for cell refinement and data reduction and absorption corrections. Bruker APEX software as well as XT, XL were used to determine the space group, solve and refine the structure in Olex2 [106]. Crystal data, details of data collections and refinement are given in Table 1. CCDC 1820354-1820359 contains the supplementary crystallographic data for this paper. These data can be obtained free of charge from The Cambridge Crystallographic Data Centre (www.ccdc.cam.ac.uk/data_request/cif).

All non-hydrogen atoms were refined anisotropically. Hydrogen atoms were assigned to calculated positions using a riding model with appropriately fixed isotropic thermal parameters. Some structures have multiple independent molecules in the asymmetric unit: **7h** has 4 independent molecules with chirality C3: R, C4: S, C30: R, C31: S, C57: S, C58: R, C84: S and C85: R; **8i** has 2 independent molecules with chirality: C3: R, C4: S, C30: R and C3: S.

4.5. Computational Procedure: Molecular Docking Study

For ligand preparation, all compounds were built using ChemBioDraw 13.0, (PerkinElmer Inc., 940 Winter Street, Waltham, MA 02451, USA) saved as mol files and opened in MOE (Molecular Operating Environment (MOE) Version 2015.10, Chemical Computing Group Inc., 1010 Sherbrooke St W, Montreal, QC, Canada). For the receptor preparation, the PDB entry1SA0 was downloaded from the Protein Data Bank PDB [5]. A UniProt Align analysis confirmed a 100% sequence identity between human and bovine beta tubulin. All waters were retained in both isoforms. Addition and optimisation of hydrogen positions for these waters was carried out using MOE 2015.10 ensuring all other atom positions remained fixed [110]. For both enantiomers of each compound, MMFF94x partial charges were calculated and each was minimised to a gradient of 0.001 kcal/mol/Å. Default parameters were used for docking except that 500 poses were sampled for each enantiomer and the top 50 docked poses were retained for subsequent analysis. The crystal structure was prepared using QuickPrep (minimised to a gradient of 0.001 kcal/mol/Å), Protonate 3D, Residue pKa and Partial Charges protocols in MOE 2016 with the MMFF94x force field.

Author Contributions: S.W. synthesised and characterised compounds in the studies according to Schemes 1, 2 and 4 performed cell studies and generated data in Tables 3–5, performed the HPLC analytical study and the stability study. and performed data analysis and interpreted data. A.M.M. synthesised and characterised some molecules in Schemes 1 and 2, performed cell studies and generated the the data for Figures 4–6 and 9. T.F.G. synthesised compounds in Schemes 1–4, characterised these compounds, performed the cell studies and generated data in Tables 3–5 and Figure 7, and performed HPLC analytical and stability studies. N.M.O. performed biochemical experiments and generated the data in Figure 8. D.F. performed the molecular modelling studies in Figures 10 and 11. S.M.N. performed biochemical experiments and generated data in Figure 7. X-Ray Crystallographic structures were determined by B.T. (Figure 2A,B and Figure 3A,B), and T.M. (Figure 3C), Tables 1 and 2. N.O.K. synthesised compounds in Scheme 4. D.M.Z. assisted with the design of the biochemical studies. M.J.M. designed the studies, wrote drafts of the manuscript and submitted the manuscript.

Acknowledgments: We thank Gavin McManus for assistance with confocal microscopy and Orla Woods for assistance with biochemical experiments. We thank Orla Bergin, UCD Conway Institute and School of Biomolecular and Biomedical Science, University College Dublin, Belfield, Dublin4, Ireland, Triple negative breast cancer Hs578T cells and its invasive variant Hs578Ts(i)8 were obtained as a kind gift from Susan McDonnell, School of Chemical and Bioprocess Engineering, University College Dublin. The Trinity Biomedical Sciences Institute (TBSI) is supported by a capital infrastructure investment from Cycle 5 of the Irish Higher Education Authority's Programme for Research in Third Level Institutions (PRTLI). DF thanks the software vendors for their continuing support of academic research efforts, in particular the contributions of the Chemical Computing Group, Biovia and OpenEye Scientific. The support and provisions of Dell Ireland, the Trinity Centre for High Performance Computing (TCHPC) and the Irish Centre for High-End Computing (ICHEC) are also gratefully acknowledged.

Abbreviations

The following abbreviations are used in this manuscript:

CA-4	Combretastatin A-4
DBU	1,8-Diazabicyclo[5.4.0]undec-7-ene
DCC	*N,N'*-Dicyclohexyl carbodiimide
DCM	Dichloromethane
DCTD	Division of Cancer Treatment and Diagnosis
DEAD	Diethyl azodicarboxylate
DIPEA	*N,N*-diisopropylethylamine
DMAP	4-Dimethylaminopyridine
DMF	*N,N*-Dimethylformamide
DTP	Development Therapeutics Program
Et_3N	Triethylamine
EBI	*N,N'*-Ethylene-bis(iodoacetamide)
ESI	Electrospray ionisation
FMOC	Fluorenylmethyloxycarbonyl
HPLC	High-performance liquid chromatography
HRMS	High Resolution Mass Spectrometry
IC	Inhibitory concentration
IR	Infrared
MIC	Minimum inhibitory concentration
MTD	Maximum tolerated dose
MS	Mass spectrometry
NCI	National Cancer Institute
NIH	National Institute of Health
NMR	Nuclear Magnetic Resonance
PBS	Phosphate-buffered saline
SAR	Structure-activity relationship
SERM	Selective Estrogen Receptor Modulator
TBAF	Tetrabutylammonium fluoride
TBDMS	*tert*-Butyldimethylchlorosilane
TEA	Triethylamine
TLC	Thin layer chromatography
TMS	Tetramethylsilane
TMCS	Tetramethylchlorosilane
UV	Ultraviolet
VDA	Vascular disrupting agent

References

1.   Bates, D.; Eastman, A. Microtubule destabilising agents: Far more than just antimitotic anticancer drugs. *Br. J. Clin. Pharmcol.* **2017**, *83*, 255–268. [CrossRef] [PubMed]

2.   Rohena, C.C.; Mooberry, S.L. Recent progress with microtubule stabilizers: New compounds, binding modes and cellular activities. *Nat. Prod. Rep.* **2014**, *31*, 335–355. [CrossRef]

3.   Van Vuuren, R.J.; Visagie, M.H.; Theron, A.E.; Joubert, A.M. Antimitotic drugs in the treatment of cancer. *Cancer Chemother. Pharmcol.* **2015**, *76*, 1101–1112. [CrossRef]

4.   Gigant, B.; Wang, C.; Ravelli, R.B.; Roussi, F.; Steinmetz, M.O.; Curmi, P.A.; Sobel, A.; Knossow, M. Structural basis for the regulation of tubulin by vinblastine. *Nature* **2005**, *435*, 519–522. [CrossRef] [PubMed]

5.   Ravelli, R.B.; Gigant, B.; Curmi, P.A.; Jourdain, I.; Lachkar, S.; Sobel, A.; Knossow, M. Insight into tubulin regulation from a complex with colchicine and a stathmin-like domain. *Nature* **2004**, *428*, 198–202. [CrossRef] [PubMed]

6.   De Filippis, B.; Ammazzalorso, A.; Fantacuzzi, M.; Giampietro, L.; Maccallini, C.; Amoroso, R. Anticancer activity of stilbene-based derivatives. *ChemMedChem* **2017**, *12*, 558–570. [CrossRef] [PubMed]

7.   Tron, G.C.; Pirali, T.; Sorba, G.; Pagliai, F.; Busacca, S.; Genazzani, A.A. Medicinal chemistry of combretastatin a4: Present and future directions. *J. Med. Chem.* **2006**, *49*, 3033–3044. [CrossRef] [PubMed]

8.   Hsieh, H.P.; Liou, J.P.; Mahindroo, N. Pharmaceutical design of antimitotic agents based on combretastatins. *Curr. Pharm. Des.* **2005**, *11*, 1655–1677. [CrossRef]

9.   Tozer, G.M.; Kanthou, C.; Baguley, B.C. Disrupting tumour blood vessels. *Nat. Rev. Cancer* **2005**, *5*, 423–435. [CrossRef]

10.   Kanthou, C.; Greco, O.; Stratford, A.; Cook, I.; Knight, R.; Benzakour, O.; Tozer, G. The tubulin-binding agent combretastatin a-4-phosphate arrests endothelial cells in mitosis and induces mitotic cell death. *Am. J. Pathol.* **2004**, *165*, 1401–1411. [CrossRef]

11.   Rustin, G.J.; Shreeves, G.; Nathan, P.D.; Gaya, A.; Ganesan, T.S.; Wang, D.; Boxall, J.; Poupard, L.; Chaplin, D.J.; Stratford, M.R.; et al. A phase ib trial of ca4p (combretastatin a-4 phosphate), carboplatin, and paclitaxel in patients with advanced cancer. *Br. J. Cancer* **2010**, *102*, 1355–1360. [CrossRef]

12.   Bilenker, J.H.; Flaherty, K.T.; Rosen, M.; Davis, L.; Gallagher, M.; Stevenson, J.P.; Sun, W.; Vaughn, D.; Giantonio, B.; Zimmer, R.; et al. Phase i trial of combretastatin a-4 phosphate with carboplatin. *Clin. Cancer Res.* **2005**, *11*, 1527–1533. [CrossRef] [PubMed]

13.   Liu, P.; Qin, Y.; Wu, L.; Yang, S.; Li, N.; Wang, H.; Xu, H.; Sun, K.; Zhang, S.; Han, X.; et al. A phase i clinical trial assessing the safety and tolerability of combretastatin a4 phosphate injections. *Anticancer Drugs* **2014**, *25*, 462–471. [CrossRef] [PubMed]

14.   Grisham, R.; Ky, B.; Tewari, K.S.; Chaplin, D.J.; Walker, J. Clinical trial experience with ca4p anticancer therapy: Focus on efficacy, cardiovascular adverse events, and hypertension management. *Gynecol. Oncol. Res. Pract.* **2018**, *5*, 1. [CrossRef]

15.   Combretastatin A4 Phosphate in Treating Patients with Advanced Anaplastic Thyroid Cancer. Available online: https://clinicaltrials.Gov/ct2/show/nct00060242 (accessed on 16 January 2019).

16.   Pazofos: Phase IB and Phase II Trial of Pazopanib +/− Fosbretabulin in Advanced Recurrent Ovarian Cancer (pazofos)clinicaltrials.Gov; a Service of the U.S. National Institutes of Health. Available online: https://www.Clinicaltrials.Gov/ct2/show/nct02055690 (accessed on 16 January 2019).

17.   Nathan, P.; Zweifel, M.; Padhani, A.R.; Koh, D.M.; Ng, M.; Collins, D.J.; Harris, A.; Carden, C.; Smythe, J.; Fisher, N.; et al. Phase i trial of combretastatin a4 phosphate (ca4p) in combination with bevacizumab in patients with advanced cancer. *Clin. Cancer Res.* **2012**, *18*, 3428–3439. [CrossRef] [PubMed]

18.   Aboubakr, E.M.; Taye, A.; Aly, O.M.; Gamal-Eldeen, A.M.; El-Moselhy, M.A. Enhanced anticancer effect of combretastatin a-4 phosphate when combined with vincristine in the treatment of hepatocellular carcinoma. *Biomed. Pharmcol.* **2017**, *89*, 36–46. [CrossRef]

19.   Ng, Q.S.; Mandeville, H.; Goh, V.; Alonzi, R.; Milner, J.; Carnell, D.; Meer, K.; Padhani, A.R.; Saunders, M.I.; Hoskin, P.J. Phase ib trial of radiotherapy in combination with combretastatin-a4-phosphate in patients with non-small-cell lung cancer, prostate adenocarcinoma, and squamous cell carcinoma of the head and neck. *Ann. Oncol.* **2012**, *23*, 231–237. [CrossRef] [PubMed]

20.   Siemann, D.W.; Chaplin, D.J.; Walicke, P.A. A review and update of the current status of the vasculature-disabling agent combretastatin-a4 phosphate (ca4p). *Expert Opin. Investig. Drugs* **2009**, *18*, 189–197. [CrossRef] [PubMed]

21. Greene, L.M.; Meegan, M.J.; Zisterer, D.M. Combretastatins: More than just vascular targeting agents? *J. Pharmacol. Exp. Ther.* **2015**, *355*, 212–227. [CrossRef]

22. Pettit, G.R.; Toki, B.; Herald, D.L.; Verdier-Pinard, P.; Boyd, M.R.; Hamel, E.; Pettit, R.K. Antineoplastic agents. 379. Synthesis of phenstatin phosphate. *J. Med. Chem.* **1998**, *41*, 1688–1695. [CrossRef] [PubMed]

23. Lu, Y.; Chen, J.; Xiao, M.; Li, W.; Miller, D.D. An overview of tubulin inhibitors that interact with the colchicine binding site. *Pharm. Res.* **2012**, *29*, 2943–2971. [CrossRef]

24. Pettit, G.R.; Rhodes, M.R.; Herald, D.L.; Hamel, E.; Schmidt, J.M.; Pettit, R.K. Antineoplastic agents. 445. Synthesis and evaluation of structural modifications of (z)- and (e)-combretastatin a-41. *J. Med. Chem.* **2005**, *48*, 4087–4099. [CrossRef]

25. Theeramunkong, S.; Caldarelli, A.; Massarotti, A.; Aprile, S.; Caprioglio, D.; Zaninetti, R.; Teruggi, A.; Pirali, T.; Grosa, G.; Tron, G.C.; et al. Regioselective suzuki coupling of dihaloheteroaromatic compounds as a rapid strategy to synthesize potent rigid combretastatin analogues. *J. Med. Chem.* **2011**, *54*, 4977–4986. [CrossRef]

26. Hadimani, M.B.; Macdonough, M.T.; Ghatak, A.; Strecker, T.E.; Lopez, R.; Sriram, M.; Nguyen, B.L.; Hall, J.J.; Kessler, R.J.; Shirali, A.R.; et al. Synthesis of a 2-aryl-3-aroyl indole salt (oxi8007) resembling combretastatin a-4 with application as a vascular disrupting agent. *J. Nat. Prod.* **2013**, *76*, 1668–1678. [CrossRef]

27. Macdonough, M.T.; Strecker, T.E.; Hamel, E.; Hall, J.J.; Chaplin, D.J.; Trawick, M.L.; Pinney, K.G. Synthesis and biological evaluation of indole-based, anti-cancer agents inspired by the vascular disrupting agent 2-(3′-hydroxy-4′-methoxyphenyl)-3-(3″,4″,5″-trimethoxybenzoyl)-6-methoxyindole (oxi8006). *Bioorg. Med. Chem.* **2013**, *21*, 6831–6843. [CrossRef]

28. Romagnoli, R.; Baraldi, P.G.; Prencipe, F.; Oliva, P.; Baraldi, S.; Tabrizi, M.A.; Lopez-Cara, L.C.; Ferla, S.; Brancale, A.; Hamel, E.; et al. Design and synthesis of potent in vitro and in vivo anticancer agents based on 1-(3′,4′,5′-trimethoxyphenyl)-2-aryl-1h-imidazole. *Sci. Rep.* **2016**, *6*, 26602. [CrossRef]

29. Lee, S.; Kim, J.N.; Lee, H.K.; Yoon, K.S.; Shin, K.D.; Kwon, B.M.; Han, D.C. Biological evaluation of kribb3 analogs as a microtubule polymerization inhibitor. *Bioorg. Med. Chem. Lett.* **2011**, *21*, 977–979. [CrossRef]

30. Odlo, K.; Fournier-Dit-Chabert, J.; Ducki, S.; Gani, O.A.; Sylte, I.; Hansen, T.V. 1,2,3-triazole analogs of combretastatin a-4 as potential microtubule-binding agents. *Bioorg. Med. Chem.* **2010**, *18*, 6874–6885. [CrossRef]

31. Romagnoli, R.; Baraldi, P.G.; Salvador, M.K.; Preti, D.; Aghazadeh Tabrizi, M.; Brancale, A.; Fu, X.H.; Li, J.; Zhang, S.Z.; Hamel, E.; et al. Synthesis and evaluation of 1,5-disubstituted tetrazoles as rigid analogues of combretastatin a-4 with potent antiproliferative and antitumor activity. *J. Med. Chem.* **2012**, *55*, 475–488. [CrossRef]

32. Rasolofonjatovo, E.; Provot, O.; Hamze, A.; Rodrigo, J.; Bignon, J.; Wdzieczak-Bakala, J.; Lenoir, C.; Desravines, D.; Dubois, J.; Brion, J.D.; et al. Design, synthesis and anticancer properties of 5-arylbenzoxepins as conformationally restricted isocombretastatin a-4 analogs. *Eur. J. Med. Chem.* **2013**, *62*, 28–39. [CrossRef]

33. Xu, Q.L.; Qi, H.; Sun, M.L.; Zuo, D.Y.; Jiang, X.W.; Wen, Z.Y.; Wang, Z.W.; Wu, Y.L.; Zhang, W.G. Synthesis and biological evaluation of 3-alkyl-1,5-diaryl-1h-pyrazoles as rigid analogues of combretastatin a-4 with potent antiproliferative activity. *PLoS ONE* **2015**, *10*, e0128710. [CrossRef]

34. Zheng, S.; Zhong, Q.; Mottamal, M.; Zhang, Q.; Zhang, C.; Lemelle, E.; McFerrin, H.; Wang, G. Design, synthesis, and biological evaluation of novel pyridine-bridged analogues of combretastatin-a4 as anticancer agents. *J. Med. Chem.* **2014**, *57*, 3369–3381. [CrossRef]

35. Prota, A.E.; Danel, F.; Bachmann, F.; Bargsten, K.; Buey, R.M.; Pohlmann, J.; Reinelt, S.; Lane, H.; Steinmetz, M.O. The novel microtubule-destabilizing drug bal27862 binds to the colchicine site of tubulin with distinct effects on microtubule organization. *J. Mol. Biol.* **2014**, *426*, 1848–1860. [CrossRef]

36. Rajak, H.; Dewangan, P.K.; Patel, V.; Jain, D.K.; Singh, A.; Veerasamy, R.; Sharma, P.C.; Dixit, A. Design of combretastatin a-4 analogs as tubulin targeted vascular disrupting agent with special emphasis on their cis-restricted isomers. *Curr. Pharm. Des.* **2013**, *19*, 1923–1955. [CrossRef]

37. Zhou, P.; Liu, Y.; Zhou, L.; Zhu, K.; Feng, K.; Zhang, H.; Liang, Y.; Jiang, H.; Luo, C.; Liu, M.; et al. Potent antitumor activities and structure basis of the chiral beta-lactam bridged analogue of combretastatin a-4 binding to tubulin. *J. Med. Chem.* **2016**, *59*, 10329–10334. [CrossRef]

38. Zhou, P.L.; Liang, Y.; Zhang, H.; Jiang, H.; Feng, K.; Xu, P.; Wang, J.; Wang, X.; Ding, K.; Luo, C.; et al. Design, synthesis, biological evaluation and cocrystal structures with tubulin of chiral b-lactam bridged combretastatin a-4 analogues as potent antitumor agents. *Eur. J. Med. Chem.* **2018**, *144*, 817–842. [CrossRef]

39. Galletti, P.; Soldati, R.; Pori, M.; Durso, M.; Tolomelli, A.; Gentilucci, L.; Dattoli, S.D.; Baiula, M.; Spampinato, S.; Giacomini, D. Targeting integrins alphavbeta3 and alpha5beta1 with new beta-lactam derivatives. *Eur. J. Med. Chem.* **2014**, *83*, 284–293. [CrossRef]

40. Geesala, R.; Gangasani, J.K.; Budde, M.; Balasubramanian, S.; Vaidya, J.R.; Das, A. 2-azetidinones: Synthesis and biological evaluation as potential anti-breast cancer agents. *Eur. J. Med. Chem.* **2016**, *124*, 544–558. [CrossRef]

41. Arya, N.; Jagdale, A.Y.; Patil, T.A.; Yeramwar, S.S.; Holikatti, S.S.; Dwivedi, J.; Shishoo, C.J.; Jain, K.S. The chemistry and biological potential of azetidin-2-ones. *Eur. J. Med. Chem.* **2014**, *74*, 619–656. [CrossRef]

42. Fu, D.J.; Fu, L.; Liu, Y.C.; Wang, J.W.; Wang, Y.Q.; Han, B.K.; Li, X.R.; Zhang, C.; Li, F.; Song, J.; et al. Structure-activity relationship studies of beta-lactam-azide analogues as orally active antitumor agents targeting the tubulin colchicine site. *Sci. Rep.* **2017**, *7*, 12788. [CrossRef]

43. Kamath, A.; Ojima, I. Advances in the chemistry of beta-lactam and its medicinal applications. *Tetrahedron* **2012**, *68*, 10640–10664. [CrossRef]

44. O'Boyle, N.M.; Pollock, J.K.; Carr, M.; Knox, A.J.; Nathwani, S.M.; Wang, S.; Caboni, L.; Zisterer, D.M.; Meegan, M.J. Beta-lactam estrogen receptor antagonists and a dual-targeting estrogen receptor/tubulin ligand. *J. Med. Chem.* **2014**, *57*, 9370–9382. [CrossRef]

45. O'Boyle, N.M.; Carr, M.; Greene, L.M.; Bergin, O.; Nathwani, S.M.; McCabe, T.; Lloyd, D.G.; Zisterer, D.M.; Meegan, M.J. Synthesis and evaluation of azetidinone analogues of combretastatin a-4 as tubulin targeting agents. *J. Med. Chem.* **2010**, *53*, 8569–8584. [CrossRef] [PubMed]

46. Greene, T.F.; Wang, S.; Greene, L.M.; Nathwani, S.M.; Pollock, J.K.; Malebari, A.M.; McCabe, T.; Twamley, B.; O'Boyle, N.M.; Zisterer, D.M.; et al. Synthesis and biochemical evaluation of 3-phenoxy-1,4-diarylazetidin -2-ones as tubulin-targeting antitumor agents. *J. Med. Chem.* **2016**, *59*, 90–113. [CrossRef] [PubMed]

47. Nathwani, S.M.; Hughes, L.; Greene, L.M.; Carr, M.; O'Boyle, N.M.; McDonnell, S.; Meegan, M.J.; Zisterer, D.M. Novel cis-restricted beta-lactam combretastatin a-4 analogues display anti-vascular and anti-metastatic properties in vitro. *Oncol. Rep.* **2013**, *29*, 585–594. [CrossRef] [PubMed]

48. Singh, G.S.; Sudheesh, S. Advances in synthesis of monocyclic beta-lactams. *Arkivoc* **2014**, 337–385. [CrossRef]

49. Gaspari, R.; Prota, A.E.; Bargsten, K.; Cavalli, A.; Steinmetz, M.O. Structural basis of cis- and trans-combretastatin binding to tubulin. *Chem* **2017**, *2*, 102–113. [CrossRef]

50. Zamboni, R.; Just, G. Beta-lactams. 7. Synthesis of 3-vinyl and 3-isopropenyl 4-substituted azetidinones. *Can. J. Chem.* **1979**, *57*, 1945–1948. [CrossRef]

51. Neary, A.D.; Burke, C.M.; O'Leary, A.C.; Meegan, M.J. Transformation of 4-acetoxy-3-vinylazetidin-2-ones to 3-(1-hydroxyethyl)azetidin-2-ones and 3-ethylideneazetidin-2-ones: Intermediates for carbapenem antibiotics. *J. Chem. Res.* **2001**, *2001*, 166–169. [CrossRef]

52. Chang, J.Y.; Yang, M.F.; Chang, C.Y.; Chen, C.M.; Kuo, C.C.; Liou, J.P. 2-amino and 2'-aminocombretastatin derivatives as potent antimitotic agents. *J. Med. Chem.* **2006**, *49*, 6412–6415. [CrossRef]

53. Tripodi, F.; Pagliarin, R.; Fumagalli, G.; Bigi, A.; Fusi, P.; Orsini, F.; Frattini, M.; Coccetti, P. Synthesis and biological evaluation of 1,4-diaryl-2-azetidinones as specific anticancer agents: Activation of adenosine monophosphate activated protein kinase and induction of apoptosis. *J. Med. Chem.* **2012**, *55*, 2112–2124. [CrossRef]

54. O'Boyle, N.M.; Greene, L.M.; Bergin, O.; Fichet, J.B.; McCabe, T.; Lloyd, D.G.; Zisterer, D.M.; Meegan, M.J. Synthesis, evaluation and structural studies of antiproliferative tubulin-targeting azetidin-2-ones. *Bioorg. Med. Chem.* **2011**, *19*, 2306–2325. [CrossRef]

55. Mayrhofer, R.; Otto, H.H. Simple preparation of 3-benzylidene-2-azetidinones. *Synthesis* **1980**, *1980*, 247–248. [CrossRef]

56. Kano, S.; Ebata, T.; Funaki, K.; Shibuya, S. New and facile synthesis of 3-alkylideneazetidin-2-ones by reactions of 3-trimethylsilylazetidin-2-one with carbonyl-compounds. *Synthesis* **1978**, *1978*, 746–747. [CrossRef]

57. Plantan, I.; Selic, L.; Mesar, T.; Anderluh, P.S.; Oblak, M.; Prezelj, A.; Hesse, L.; Andrejasic, M.; Vilar, M.; Turk, D.; et al. 4-substituted trinems as broad spectrum beta-lactamase inhibitors: Structure-based design, synthesis, and biological activity. *J. Med. Chem.* **2007**, *50*, 4113–4121. [CrossRef]

58. O'Boyle, N.M.; Greene, L.M.; Keely, N.O.; Wang, S.; Cotter, T.S.; Zisterer, D.M.; Meegan, M.J. Synthesis and biochemical activities of antiproliferative amino acid and phosphate derivatives of microtubule-disrupting beta-lactam combretastatins. *Eur. J. Med. Chem.* **2013**, *62*, 705–721. [CrossRef]

59. Spek, A.L.; Vandersteen, F.H.; Jastrzebski, J.T.B.H.; Vankoten, G. Trans-3-amino-1-methyl-4-phenyl-2-azetidinone, C10H12N2O. *Acta Crystallogr. C* **1994**, *50*, 1933–1935. [CrossRef]

60. Kabak, M.; Senoz, H.; Elmali, A.; Adar, V.; Svoboda, I.; Dusek, M.; Fejfarova, K. Synthesis and x-ray crystal structure determination of n-p-methylphenyl-4-benzoyl-3,4-diphenyl-2-azetidinone. *Crystallogr. Rep.* **2010**, *55*, 1220–1222. [CrossRef]

61. Lara-Ochoa, F.; Espinosa-Perez, G. A new synthesis of combretastatins a-4 and ave-8062a. *Tetrahedron Lett.* **2007**, *48*, 7007–7010. [CrossRef]

62. Combes, S.; Barbier, P.; Douillard, S.; McLeer-Florin, A.; Bourgarel-Rey, V.; Pierson, J.T.; Fedorov, A.Y.; Finet, J.P.; Boutonnat, J.; Peyrot, V. Synthesis and biological evaluation of 4-arylcoumarin analogues of combretastatins. Part 2. *J. Med. Chem.* **2011**, *54*, 3153–3162. [CrossRef]

63. Messaoudi, S.; Treguier, B.; Hamze, A.; Provot, O.; Peyrat, J.F.; De Losada, J.R.; Liu, J.M.; Bignon, J.; Wdzieczak-Bakala, J.; Thoret, S.; et al. Isocombretastatins a versus combretastatins a: The forgotten isoca-4 isomer as a highly promising cytotoxic and antitubulin agent. *J. Med. Chem.* **2009**, *52*, 4538–4542. [CrossRef]

64. Cushman, M.; Nagarathnam, D.; Gopal, D.; He, H.M.; Lin, C.M.; Hamel, E. Synthesis and evaluation of analogues of (z)-1-(4-methoxyphenyl)-2-(3,4,5-trimethoxyphenyl)ethene as potential cytotoxic and antimitotic agents. *J. Med. Chem.* **1992**, *35*, 2293–2306. [CrossRef]

65. Flynn, B.L.; Flynn, G.P.; Hamel, E.; Jung, M.K. The synthesis and tubulin binding activity of thiophene-based analogues of combretastatin a-4. *Bioorg. Med. Chem. Lett.* **2001**, *11*, 2341–2343. [CrossRef]

66. Chaudhary, A.; Pandeya, S.N.; Kumar, P.; Sharma, P.P.; Gupta, S.; Soni, N.; Verma, K.K.; Bhardwaj, G. Combretastatin a-4 analogs as anticancer agents. *Mini Rev. Med. Chem.* **2007**, *7*, 1186–1205. [CrossRef]

67. Devkota, L.; Lin, C.M.; Strecker, T.E.; Wang, Y.; Tidmore, J.K.; Chen, Z.; Guddneppanavar, R.; Jelinek, C.J.; Lopez, R.; Liu, L.; et al. Design, synthesis, and biological evaluation of water-soluble amino acid prodrug conjugates derived from combretastatin, dihydronaphthalene, and benzosuberene-based parent vascular disrupting agents. *Bioorg. Med. Chem.* **2016**, *24*, 938–956. [CrossRef]

68. Mousset, C.; Giraud, A.; Provot, O.; Hamze, A.; Bignon, J.; Liu, J.M.; Thoret, S.; Dubois, J.; Brion, J.D.; Alami, M. Synthesis and antitumor activity of benzils related to combretastatin a-4. *Bioorg. Med. Chem. Lett.* **2008**, *18*, 3266–3271. [CrossRef]

69. Hughes, L.; Malone, C.; Chumsri, S.; Burger, A.M.; McDonnell, S. Characterisation of breast cancer cell lines and establishment of a novel isogenic subclone to study migration, invasion and tumourigenicity. *Clin. Exp. Metastasis* **2008**, *25*, 549–557. [CrossRef]

70. National Cancer Institute Division of Cancer Treatment and Diagnosis. Available online: https://dtp.Cancer.Gov (accessed on 25 February 2019).

71. *National Cancer Institute Biological Testing Branch*; National Cancer Institute: Bethesda, MD, USA. Available online: https://dtp.Nci.Nih.Gov/branches/btb/hfa.Html (accessed on 16 January 2019).

72. Vichai, V.; Kirtikara, K. Sulforhodamine b colorimetric assay for cytotoxicity screening. *Nat. Protoc.* **2006**, *1*, 1112–1116. [CrossRef]

73. Smith, S.M.; Wunder, M.B.; Norris, D.A.; Shellman, Y.G. A simple protocol for using a ldh-based cytotoxicity assay to assess the effects of death and growth inhibition at the same time. *PLoS ONE* **2011**, *6*, e26908. [CrossRef]

74. Furlong, E.E.; Keon, N.K.; Thornton, F.D.; Rein, T.; Martin, F. Expression of a 74-kda nuclear factor 1 (nf1) protein is induced in mouse mammary gland involution. Involution-enhanced occupation of a twin nf1 binding element in the testosterone-repressed prostate message-2/clusterin promoter. *J. Biol. Chem.* **1996**, *271*, 29688–29697. [CrossRef]

75. Murtagh, J.; McArdle, E.; Gilligan, E.; Thornton, L.; Furlong, F.; Martin, F. Organization of mammary epithelial cells into 3d acinar structures requires glucocorticoid and jnk signaling. *J. Cell Biol.* **2004**, *166*, 133–143. [CrossRef]

76. Shen, C.H.; Shee, J.J.; Wu, J.Y.; Lin, Y.W.; Wu, J.D.; Liu, Y.W. Combretastatin a-4 inhibits cell growth and metastasis in bladder cancer cells and retards tumour growth in a murine orthotopic bladder tumour model. *Br. J. Pharmcol.* **2010**, *160*, 2008–2027. [CrossRef]

77. Greene, L.M.; O'Boyle, N.M.; Nolan, D.P.; Meegan, M.J.; Zisterer, D.M. The vascular targeting agent combretastatin-a4 directly induces autophagy in adenocarcinoma-derived colon cancer cells. *Biochem. Pharmcol.* **2012**, *84*, 612–624. [CrossRef]

78. *Tubulin Polymerization Assay Kit Manual (CDS03 and BK006)*; Cytoskeleton: Denver, CO, USA, 2009; pp. 1–18.

79. Barbier, P.; Tsvetkov, P.O.; Breuzard, G.; Devred, F. Deciphering the molecular mechanisms of anti-tubulin plant derived drugs. *Phytochem. Rev.* **2014**, *13*, 157–169. [CrossRef]

80. Castedo, M.; Perfettini, J.-L.; Roumier, T.; Andreau, K.; Medema, R.; Kroemer, G. Cell death by mitotic catastrophe: A molecular definition. *Oncogene* **2004**, *23*, 2825–2837. [CrossRef]

81. Vitale, I.; Antoccia, A.; Cenciarelli, C.; Crateri, P.; Meschini, S.; Arancia, G.; Pisano, C.; Tanzarella, C. Combretastatin ca-4 and combretastatin derivative induce mitotic catastrophe dependent on spindle checkpoint and caspase-3 activation in non-small cell lung cancer cells. *Apoptosis* **2007**, *12*, 155–166. [CrossRef]

82. Cenciarelli, C.; Tanzarella, C.; Vitale, I.; Pisano, C.; Crateri, P.; Meschini, S.; Arancia, G.; Antoccia, A. The tubulin-depolymerising agent combretastatin-4 induces ectopic aster assembly and mitotic catastrophe in lung cancer cells h460. *Apoptosis* **2008**, *13*, 659–669. [CrossRef]

83. Simoni, D.; Romagnoli, R.; Baruchello, R.; Rondanin, R.; Rizzi, M.; Pavani, M.G.; Alloatti, D.; Giannini, G.; Marcellini, M.; Riccioni, T.; et al. Novel combretastatin analogues endowed with antitumor activity. *J. Med. Chem.* **2006**, *49*, 3143–3152. [CrossRef]

84. O'Boyle, N.M.; Carr, M.; Greene, L.M.; Knox, A.J.S.; Lloyd, D.G.; Zisterer, D.M.; Meegan, M.J. Synthesis, biochemical and molecular modelling studies of antiproliferative azetidinones causing microtubule disruption and mitotic catastrophe. *Eur. J. Med. Chem.* **2011**, *46*, 4595–4607. [CrossRef]

85. Fortin, S.; Lacroix, J.; Cote, M.F.; Moreau, E.; Petitclerc, E.; Gaudreault, R.C. Quick and simple detection technique to assess the binding of antimicrotubule agents to the colchicine-binding site. *Biol. Proced. Online* **2010**, *12*, 113–117. [CrossRef]

86. Canela, M.D.; Perez-Perez, M.J.; Noppen, S.; Saez-Calvo, G.; Diaz, J.F.; Camarasa, M.J.; Liekens, S.; Priego, E.M. Novel colchicine-site binders with a cyclohexanedione scaffold identified through a ligand-based virtual screening approach. *J. Med. Chem.* **2014**, *57*, 3924–3938. [CrossRef]

87. Carr, M.; Greene, L.M.; Knox, A.J.; Lloyd, D.G.; Zisterer, D.M.; Meegan, M.J. Lead identification of conformationally restricted beta-lactam type combretastatin analogues: Synthesis, antiproliferative activity and tubulin targeting effects. *Eur. J. Med. Chem.* **2010**, *45*, 5752–5766. [CrossRef]

88. Molecular Operating Environment (MOE); C.C.G.I.; (1010 Sherbooke St. West, Suite #910, Montreal, QC, Canada). Personal communications, 2016.

89. Elmeligie, S.; Taher, A.T.; Khalil, N.A.; El-Said, A.H. Synthesis and cytotoxic activity of certain trisubstituted azetidin-2-one derivatives as a cis-restricted combretastatin a-4 analogues. *Arch. Pharm. Res.* **2017**, *40*, 13–24. [CrossRef]

90. Georg, G.I.; He, P.; Kant, J.; Mudd, J. N-vinyl and n-unsubstituted beta-lactams from 1-substituted 2-aza-1,3-butadienes. *Tetrahedron Lett.* **1990**, *31*, 451–454. [CrossRef]

91. Arroyo, Y.; Sanz-Tejedor, M.A.; Alonso, I.; Garcia-Ruano, J.L. Synthesis of optically pure vic-sulfanyl amines mediated by a remote sulfinyl group. *Org. Lett.* **2011**, *13*, 4534–4537. [CrossRef]

92. Sandhar, R.K.; Sharma, J.R.; Manrao, M.R. Reaction of acetylacetone with benzal-4-fluoroanilines and antifungal potential of the products. *J. Indian Counc. Chem.* **2005**, *22*, 32–34.

93. Dehno Khalaji, A.; Fejfarova, K.; Dusek, M. N,N'-bis(3,4-dimethoxy-benzyl-idene)butane-1,4-diamine. *Acta Crystallogr. Sect. E Struct. Rep. Online* **2009**, *65*, o1773. [CrossRef]

94. Khalaji, A.D.; Weil, M.; Gotoh, K.; Ishida, H. 4-bromo-N-(3,4,5-trimethoxy-benzyl-idene)aniline. *Acta Crystallogr. Sect. E Struct. Rep. Online* **2009**, *65*, o436. [CrossRef]

95. Yang, Z. Synthesis and in vitro biological activity evaluation of the derivatives of combretastatin a-4. *Lett. Drug Des. Discov.* **2006** *3*, 544–546. [CrossRef]

96. Cushman, M.; He, H.M.; Lin, C.M.; Hamel, E. Synthesis and evaluation of a series of benzylaniline hydrochlorides as potential cytotoxic and antimitotic agents acting by inhibition of tubulin polymerization. *J. Med. Chem.* **1993**, *36*, 2817–2821. [CrossRef]

97. Gaidhane, M.K.; Ghatole, A.M.; Lanjewar, K.R. Novel synthesis and antimicrobial activity of novel schiff base derived quinoline and their beta-lactam derivatives. *Int. J. Pharm. Pharm. Sci.* **2013**, *5*, 421–426.

98. Malebari, A.M.; Greene, L.M.; Nathwani, S.M.; Fayne, D.; O'Boyle, N.M.; Wang, S.; Twamley, B.; Zisterer, D.M.; Meegan, M.J. Beta-lactam analogues of combretastatin a-4 prevent metabolic inactivation by glucuronidation in chemoresistant ht-29 colon cancer cells. *Eur. J. Med. Chem.* **2017**, *130*, 261–285. [CrossRef]

99. Meegan, M.J.; Zisterer, D.M.; Carr, M.; Greene, T.; O'Boyle, N.; Greene, L. Combretastatin Derivatives and Uses Therefor. European Patent WO 2011073211, 23 June 2011.

100. Wang, Y.L.; Liu, M.; Zhou, P.; Feng, K.; Ding, K.; Wang, X. Diaryl-B-Lactam Compound and Preparation Method and Pharmaceutical Use Thereof. Chinese Patent WO 2017167183, 5 October 2017.

101. Promega Corporation. *Cytotox 96® Non-Radioactive Cytotoxicity Assay*; Promega Cytotox 96 Nonradioactive Cytotoxicity Assay Protocol; Promega Corporation: Fitchburg, WI, USA, 2016.

102. *Bruker Apex2 v2012.12-0*; Bruker Axs Inc.: Madison, Wi, USA, 2012.

103. Sheldrick, G.M. A short history of shelx. *Acta Crystallogr. A* **2008**, *64*, 112–122. [CrossRef]

104. Sheldrick, G.M. Shelxt—Integrated space-group and crystal-structure determination. *Acta Crystallogr. A Found. Adv.* **2015**, *71*, 3–8. [CrossRef]

105. Sheldrick, G.M. Crystal structure refinement with shelxl. *Acta Crystallogr. C Struct. Chem.* **2015**, *71*, 3–8. [CrossRef]

106. Dolomanov, O.V.; Bourhis, L.J.; Gildea, R.J.; Howard, J.A.K.; Puschmann, H. Olex2: A complete structure solution, refinement and analysis program. *J. Appl. Crystallogr.* **2009**, *42*, 339–341. [CrossRef]

107. Sadabs; (Bruker Axs Inc., Madison, WI, USA); Sheldrick, G.M.; (University of Göttingen, Göttingen, Germany). Personal communications, 2014.

108. Crystalclear Rigaku Molecular Structure Corporation Inc.; (The Woodlands, TX, USA). Personal communications, 2000.

109. Pflugrath, J.W. The finer things in x-ray diffraction data collection. *Acta Crystallogr. D Biol. Crystallogr.* **1999**, *55*, 1718–1725. [CrossRef]

110. *Molecular Operating Environment (MOE) Version 2015.10*; Chemical Computing Group Inc.: Montreal, QC, Canada, 2016.

Can the Efficacy of [^{18}F]FDG-PET/CT in Clinical Oncology be Enhanced by Screening Biomolecular Profiles?

Hazel O'Neill [1],*, Vinod Malik [2], Ciaran Johnston [2], John V Reynolds [1] and Jacintha O'Sullivan [1]

[1]   Trinity Translational Medicine Institute, Department of Surgery, Trinity College Dublin,
     D08W9RT Dublin, Ireland; reynoldsjv@stjames.ie (J.V.R.); osullij4@tcd.ie (J.O.S.)
[2]   Department of Radiology, St. James's Hospital, D08 X4RX Dublin, Ireland; malikvi@tcd.ie (V.M.);
     cjohnston@stjames.ie (C.J.)
*   Correspondence: oneillhm@tcd.ie

Abstract: Positron Emission Tomography (PET) is a functional imaging modality widely used in clinical oncology. Over the years the sensitivity and specificity of PET has improved with the advent of specific radiotracers, increased technical accuracy of PET scanners and incremental experience of Radiologists. However, significant limitations exist—most notably false positives and false negatives. Additionally, the accuracy of PET varies between cancer types and in some cancers, is no longer considered a standard imaging modality. This review considers the relative influence of macroscopic tumour features such as size and morphology on 2-Deoxy-2-[^{18}F]fluoroglucose ([^{18}F]FDG) uptake by tumours which, though well described in the literature, lacks a comprehensive assessment of biomolecular features which may influence [^{18}F]FDG uptake. The review aims to discuss the potential influence of individual molecular markers of glucose transport, glycolysis, hypoxia and angiogenesis in addition to the relationships between these key cellular processes and their influence on [^{18}F]FDG uptake. Finally, the potential role for biomolecular profiling of individual tumours to predict positivity on PET imaging is discussed to enhance accuracy and clinical utility.

Keywords: [^{18}F]FDG PET/CT; biomarker profiling; cancer

1. Introduction

1.1. Positron Emission Tomography

Positron emission tomography (PET) is an imaging modality used in the diagnosis, staging, restaging and monitoring of cancer. It involves the administration of selected labelled molecules that localise in malignant tissues. These molecules integrate into metabolic pathways or act as receptor ligands in cancer cells, concentrating in tumours. Examples include non-specific tracers of metabolism and cell membrane synthesis such as [^{11}C]Choline, [^{11}C]Acetate and 2-Deoxy-2-[^{18}F]fluoroglucose ([^{18}F]FDG) and specific tracers such as tyrosine kinase inhibitors that localise exclusively to overexpressed epithelial growth factor receptors on cancer cells [1]. Clinically the most widely used tracer is glucose analogue [^{18}F]FDG, a marker of cellular metabolism. Detection of [^{18}F]FDG is the basis of functional cancer imaging and is the focus of this review.

1.2. 2-Deoxy-2-[^{18}F]fluoroglucose ([^{18}F]FDG)

[^{18}F]FDG undergoes cellular uptake via the same mechanisms as glucose and other hexoses: passive diffusion, sodium dependent transport mechanisms and via specific glucose uptake transporters (GLUTs). GLUTs are expressed on the membranes of most cells and facilitate transmembrane glucose transport [2]. Thirteen GLUT subtypes are described with GLUT-1 and GLUT-3 most commonly expressed on cancer cells [2]. Upon entering the cell, [^{18}F]FDG undergoes an initial phosphorylation reaction via hexokinase. Structural modifications produced by the hexose-[^{18}F]FDG bond prevent its catabolism or extracellular transport at a high rate via glucose-6-phosphatase, hence metabolically "trapping" [^{18}F]FDG [3].

The detection of [^{18}F]FDG uptake relies on the ability of the PET detector to detect the natural radioactive decay of fluorine-18 attached to this glucose analogue. This occurs by beta+ decay which involves the conversion of fluorine to oxygen, releasing a positron which travels approximately 1mm before colliding with an electron, becoming neutralised and undergoing an annihilation reaction, producing a pair of gamma rays emitted at $180°$ from each other. These are detected by the scanner which draws a line of response between the rays. The crossing point of several lines of response indicates the area of greatest [^{18}F]FDG uptake. Abnormal regions of [^{18}F]FDG uptake are detected by comparison with the low overall background activity [3]. Standard uptake value (SUV) is a measure of [^{18}F]FDG uptake by tissues and this is calculated by the division of the activity detected in the region of interest by the injected dose per unit body weight [3].

[^{18}F]FDG competes with glucose for uptake by metabolically active tissue. It localises in tissues with a greater metabolic rate such as tumours, brain, salivary glands, myocardium, gastrointestinal tract, bladder, thyroid and gonads. [^{18}F]FDG uptake has also been noted in brown adipose tissue in 2.3–4% of patients [3]. Thus, PET is not specific to cancerous tissues but those tissues with a greater than average metabolic rate offering functional information about the metabolic state of tissues. The advent of PET-CT has made it feasible to visualize the anatomical and metabolic properties of the tumour simultaneously.

1.3. Limitations: False Positives and Negatives

[^{18}F]FDG-PET scanning is not without limitations, in particular false positives and false negatives impacting on sensitivity and specificity. False positives occur in tissues more metabolically active than background tissue such as inflammatory foci, limiting the specificity of [^{18}F]FDG-PET. False positives can result in additional investigation, inappropriate treatment and altered clinical management with increased costs. Pancreatic cancer, commonly detected at a late stage, lacks an accurate method of detection often hindered by the difficulty in differentiating pancreatitis from pancreatic cancer and compounded by pancreatitis often accompanying cancer. Kubota et al. revealed that 24% of [^{18}F]FDG uptake in pancreatic cancer is consumed by local inflammatory cells, demonstrating the poor specificity of [^{18}F]FDG-PET in differentiating pancreatitis from cancer [4].

Thoracic diseases including tuberculomas, sarcoidosis, cryptococcosis and radiation fibrosis are a common source of false positive results, necessitating further invasive testing [3]. Immunosuppressed cancer patients or recipients of prior radiation are at increased risk of suffering from one of these conditions, effecting the efficacy of [^{18}F]FDG-PET in cancer follow up or diagnosis of lung metastases.

False negatives are another major limitation to [^{18}F]FDG-PET scanning where appropriate scanning fails to detect malignancy. Some of the underlying biology underpinning these false negative results will be outlined later in this review.

1.4. Clinical Importance

[^{18}F]FDG-PET has a significant role in the diagnosis, staging, restaging, prognosis and monitoring of response to therapy in cancer. The functional information on tissue metabolism allows for identification of tumours otherwise undetectable on standard imaging modalities. PET has also had an impact on the treatment planning of cancer patients. Identification of occult metastases by PET alters the clinical management of patients, by avoiding futile surgery in favour of palliative interventions. Despite its usefulness, there is scope to improve the accuracy of PET by addressing the limitations outlined above.

2. Factors Affecting the Clinical Efficacy of PET

2.1. Gross Features

2.1.1. Tumour Size

Small tumour size has been associated with decreased [18F]FDG uptake, accounting for false negative results in many studies [5–9]. This is most notable in the breast cancer setting where the persistent correlation between small tumour size and false negativity has meant that the National Comprehensive Cancer Network (NCCN) no longer endorses PET for evaluating stage I, II or operable stage III invasive disease [10]. A recent systematic review confirmed that [18F]FDG-PET does not have sufficient sensitivity to detect breast tumours <10 mm and is therefore not a recommended first line imaging modality for the initial assessment of primary breast tumours [5]. In bronchoalveolar lung cancer, a study with lung nodules <10 mm identified a negative PET scan in 20% of patients [8]. [18F]FDG uptake in cervical cancer is also influenced by size with a significant association between SUV and tumour size (r = 0.456, p = 0.025) [9]. In oral squamous cell carcinoma (SCC) higher T stage (3 and 4) have increased [18F]FDG uptake compared to lower T stages (1 and 2) [2]. Despite the evidence, small tumour size cannot exclusively cause false negatives. Higashi et al. identified a large 33 mm false negative tumour in their pancreatic study and highlighted that size alone does not influence decreased tumour [18F]FDG uptake [11].

2.1.2. Tumour Grade

Aggressive lesions are associated with higher metabolism and increased [18F]FDG uptake compared to slow growing, less invasive types [5]. Tumour grade has been strongly associated with increased [18F]FDG uptake in breast, musculoskeletal and brain tumours however no correlation exists with mucinous tumours of the GI tract and lung [12,13]. In cervical cancer, Yen et al. reported higher [18F]FDG uptake in poorly differentiated, aggressive tumours compared to lower grade tumours in their 2004 study [9].

2.1.3. Cellularity

The content of the tumour mass, in particular the cellular concentration has an association with [18F]FDG uptake. Poor [18F]FDG uptake by cystic mucinous, or signet ring tumours is attributed to fewer tumour cells forming the tumour mass [13]. Kim et al. and Higashi et al. have both reported a large difference in peak SUVs in mucinous bronchoalveolar carcinoma compared to cell-dense SCC or adenocarcinoma (AC) cancer types [14,15]. One large study by Higashi et al. revealed 57% of bronchoalveolar carcinoma patients as negative on PET while Berger et al. noted false negatives in 40% of patients with mucinous tumours [13,15]. Cellularity is also postulated to be linked to more rapid proliferation, increased likelihood of hypoxia and glycolysis, translating into increased [18F]FDG uptake [16].

2.2. Molecular Features

2.2.1. Heterogeneity

The heterogeneity of the tumour microenvironment dictates the varied intratumoral uptake of [18F]FDG resulting in both false negatives and underestimations of tumour size [17]. Establishing these microenvironmental characteristics that influence [18F]FDG uptake is therefore important in order to optimise the clinical reliability of PET.

Currently, intratumoral variations in [18F]FDG uptake are not clearly defined in clinical practice when staging or planning radiation treatment in cancer, potentially misdiagnosing more extensive disease. Knowledge of tumour micro-environmental factors could augment PET efficacy with accurate prediction of tumour volume and disease extent with biomolecular profiles having a potential role [17].

2.2.2. Metabolism

The preferential role for glycolysis over oxidative phosphorylation in cancer cells forms the basis of effective PET imaging. Glycolysis associated protein expression has been extensively studied with GLUT-1 and GLUT-3 overexpressed in a range of cancer types [18,19]. The evidence for correlating GLUT expression and [^{18}F]FDG uptake is strong. Kurokawa et al. showed a positive correlation between [^{18}F]FDG uptake and GLUT-1 expression [20]. Similarly Kunkel et al. associated high GLUT-1 to increased SUV in oral SCC [21] while Tian et al. confirmed this, no linear relationship between expression and [^{18}F]FDG uptake was noted rather only overexpression facilitates increased SUVs [2].

The increased expression of GLUT-1 and GLUT-3 compared with other GLUT subtypes in cancer cells is in theory due to their significance in facilitating basal glucose transport in cells. They are vital in maintaining glycolysis despite a relative deficiency of glucose in the poorly perfused tumour microenvironment. GLUT-1 and GLUT-3 are therefore largely responsible for facilitating the Warburg effect, that is the preferential use of aerobic glycolysis by tumours compared with oxidative phosphorylation- and satisfying the abnormal glucose requirements of cancer cells. This provides some explanation for increased [^{18}F]FDG uptake associated with these biomarkers of metabolism [2].

The metabolic profile of distant tumour metastasis differs from the primary tumour in some cases. Kurata et al. revealed elevated GLUT-3 and GLUT-5 in liver metastases compared to the primary lung cancer [22]. This differential expression of metabolic markers may present a limitation in biomolecular profiling for enhancing PET as some primary and secondary tumours appear to differ in their protein expression.

Despite several studies correlating high GLUT-1 and [^{18}F]FDG uptake, some studies have revealed discrepant results postulating involvement of other metabolic factors. In oesophageal squamous cell cancer (SCC) hexokinase (HK) II had a higher correlation with [^{18}F]FDG uptake than GLUT-1 expression [23]. Although not as prominent in influencing [^{18}F]FDG uptake as GLUT, HK have been noted to strengthen the statistical significance of GLUT correlation with increased [^{18}F]FDG uptake. Studies in oesophageal SCC and breast cancer could not demonstrate a significant correlation between tumour SUV and HK expression; on logistic regression however HK was identified as adding significance to the correlation between SUV and GLUT-1 expression [19]. This demonstrates the combined role of intracellular FDG transport via GLUTs with the commencement of glycolysis facilitated by HK.

The discordance in metabolic markers of [^{18}F]FDG uptake between studies may not be an artefact but a source of biological significance. Correlations have been documented between GLUT expression and tumour aggressiveness as well as inflammation of normal tissue. Experimental models have shown GLUT-1 and 3 to be overexpressed in both tumour and inflammation though GLUT-1 was higher in tumour tissue while GLUT-3 was higher in inflammatory lesions [24]. This differential expression of biomarkers between cancer and inflammation, both of which exhibit increased [^{18}F]FDG uptake on PET could potentially form some basis for differentiating benign from malignant lesions.

GLUT-1 appears to be the most prominently investigated GLUT in relation to [^{18}F]FDG uptake. Though the studies described above have identified that GLUT-1 overexpression relates to increased [^{18}F]FDG uptake, the correlation seems to vary between cancer types, something that may in part be attributable to the degree of tumour hypoxia (vide infra). Understanding and identifying cancers which exhibit the greatest correlation between GLUT-1 and [^{18}F]FDG uptake could help highlight these cancers by means of a viable biomarker.

2.2.3. Hypoxia

Hypoxia inducible factor 1-alpha (HIF-1α) is known to regulate glucose metabolism and consequently influence the regulation of [^{18}F]FDG uptake. In the absence of oxygen, HIF-1α binds hypoxia response elements (HREs) causing expression of hypoxia responding genes related to angiogenesis, glycolysis and oxygen delivery. The underlying reasoning behind this mechanism is the cell's attempt to prevent death; a mechanism manipulated by cancer in its expression of HIF-1α.

HIF-1α acts as an essential transcription factor involved in regulating metabolic functions by targeting a number of metabolism related proteins (Table 1) [25]. In addition, HIF-1α influences the relative contribution from metabolic function to overall energy production depending on the hypoxic state of the cell. Thus, the tumour hypoxic state affects the relative uptake of [^{18}F]FDG. Pugachev et al. showed a positive correlation between [^{18}F]FDG uptake and pimonidazole staining which identified hypoxic areas of tumour [17]. This supports the Dearling et al. study which revealed [^{18}F]FDG uptake 1.26 times higher in hypoxic tumour regions versus normoxic areas [26].

Tumour necrosis has also been positively associated with [^{18}F]FDG uptake in breast cancer [19]. This is probable due to the pre-necrotic hypoxic environment activating glycolysis and increasing [^{18}F]FDG uptake. This theory is supported by pre-necrotic changes in cancer demonstrating increased [^{18}F]FDG uptake.

Table 1. Targets of HIF-1α. Adapted from Denko et al. [25].

Target Genes	Metabolic Function
GLUT-1/GLUT-3	Cellular Glucose Entry
HKII	Phosphorylation
PGI, PFK1, Aldolase, TPI, GAPDH, PGK, PGM, enolase, PK, PFKFB1-4	Glycolysis
LDHA	Pyruvate>Lactate Conversion
MCT4	Cellular Lactate Removal
PDK1, MXI1	Decreased Mitochondrial Activity
COX4I2, Lon Protease	O$_2$ Consumption in Hypoxia

GLUT: Glucose uptake transporter; HK: Hexokinase; PGI: Glucose-6-phosphate isomerase; PFK: Phosphofructokinase; TPI: Triose phosphate isomerase; GAPDH: Glyceraldehyde 3-phosphate dehydrogenase; PGK: phosphoglycerate kinase; PGM: phosphoglucomutase; PK: pyruvate kinase; PFKFB: 6-phosphofructo-2-kinase/fructose-2,6-biphosphatase; LDHA: Lactate Dehydrogenase A; MCT: Monocarboxylate transporter; PDK: Pyruvate dehydrogenase kinase; MXI: MAX-interacting protein; COX: Cytochrome c oxidase.

2.2.4. Angiogenesis

Tumour blood vessel status including microvascular blood volume (measured on functional MRI) and microvessel density has also been associated with variations in [^{18}F]FDG uptake [19,27]. Though few studies exist regarding blood flow distribution in cancer, the evidence reveals that blood flow varies with the site, size, type of tumour and micro-vessel density [17]. Histologically identical tumours can also vary in their rates and distribution of blood flow [28]. The impact of angiogenesis on [^{18}F]FDG uptake has been established in few cancer types such as breast cancer and malignant glioma where micro-vessel density and microvascular blood volume have been associated with increased [^{18}F]FDG uptake [19,27].

The influence of angiogenesis on [^{18}F]FDG uptake has led to investigation of the potential role of [^{18}F]FDG PET in monitoring response to anti-angiogenic therapies such as bevacizumab. De Bruyne et al. demonstrated that low [^{18}F]FDG uptake following bevacizumab therapy was associated with improved progression free survival in metastatic colorectal cancer [29]. Additionally, Colavolpe et al. showed that low [^{18}F]FDG uptake on PET following bevacizumab treatment for glioma predicted longer progression-free survival, postulating reduced tumour angiogenesis, resulting in lower SUVs [30]. Similarly Goshen et al. concluded that pre and post bevacizumab [^{18}F]FDG PET was superior in predicting pathological response to bevacizumab compared to standard restaging CT for metastatic colorectal cancer [31].

2.3. Interplay of Biological Features

Identifying individual biological features that influence [^{18}F]FDG uptake is complicated by many of the biological processes being intricately linked. HIF-1α, expressed in hypoxia, regulates several key genes involved in angiogenesis and metabolism. Additionally, angiogenesis and metabolism influence each other and in turn have an impact of hypoxia.

For cellular [18F]FDG uptake to occur, it must reach the tumour site, making perfusion of the tumour facilitated by angiogenesis a key feature in controlling [18F]FDG metabolism [23]. Furthermore, metabolic demands in cancer influence hypoxia which induces vascular endothelial growth factor (VEGF) expression, facilitating blood vessel formation and tumour perfusion. Rapidly proliferating cells also require increased levels of glucose and differentiation has been correlated to [18F]FDG uptake [12,32,33]. When metabolic needs go unaddressed necrosis occurs causing inflammation with additional glucose demands and hypoxia. This intricate interplay between biological features highlights factors influencing [18F]FDG uptake are multifactorial and complex with interpretation of their combined effect on [18F]FDG uptake more important than any individual feature. Figure 1 illustrates this complex interplay of cellular processes.

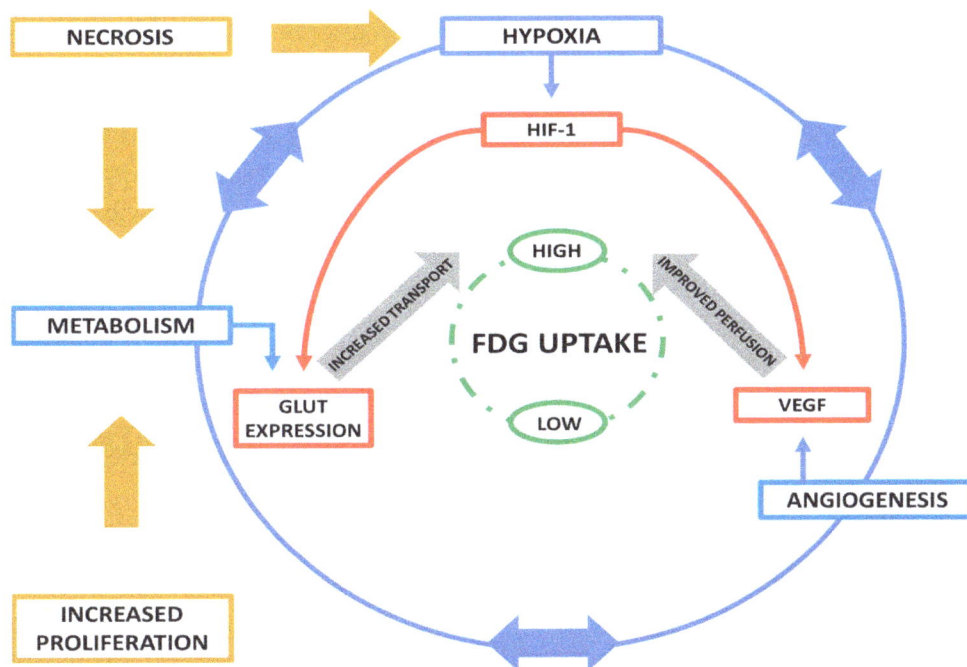

Figure 1. Biomolecular influences on [18F]FDG uptake. Metabolism, hypoxia and angiogenesis all play a role in glucose and therefore [18F]FDG uptake via their associated biomolecular proteins (GLUT, HIF-1α and VEGF respectively). Interrelationships exist between metabolism, hypoxia and angiogenesis such that they play a role in regulating each other. Proliferation and necrosis-induced inflammation increase overall tumoral energy requirements, also driving metabolism and contributing to this complex network.

2.4. Other Factors

2.4.1. P-glycoprotein

Elevated expression of P-glycoprotein has been associated with decreased [18F]FDG uptake [34]. In hepatocellular carcinoma (HCC), both in vivo and in vitro models showed decreased [18F]FDG uptake with increased P-glycoprotein expression [35]. This suggests that [18F]FDG was a substrate of this drug efflux pump, with high levels of expression leading to reduced [18F]FDG uptake. Decreased [18F]FDG uptake and associate high P-glycoprotein expression have been observed in lung cancer and cholangiocarcinoma patients [34].

2.4.2. Tumour Suppressor Genes

Tumour suppressor gene expression has been shown to influence SUVs. Vousden et al. demonstrated that p53 plays a significant role in cell metabolism and other essential cellular functions [36]. As p53 is mutated in up to 50% of tumours, and wild type p53 is anti-Warburg, promoting mitochondrial oxidative phosphorylation, the impact of p53 in promoting glycolysis is consequently potentially of great importance. Several studies have observed that variations in [^{18}F]FDG uptake have been associated with mutated p53 [37,38]. In breast cancer, tumours with p53 mutations exhibit higher SUVs than those expressing the wild type protein [37]. In lung cancer, a statistically significant difference in [^{18}F]FDG uptake was noted between cancers with no mutated tumour suppressors (Rb, P16, P27 and P53) and cancers with alterations which exhibited higher uptake values [38].

2.4.3. Patient Factors

Multiple patient related factors are known to cause variable [^{18}F]FDG uptake [39]. Patient size and body composition affects distribution of [^{18}F]FDG and this is important considering the increasing prevalence of obesity and obesity-associated cancers [39]. Furthermore, high plasma glucose levels reduce [^{18}F]FDG uptake [23]—an issue to account for in the diabetic and pre-diabetic setting. It is proposed that decreased [^{18}F]FDG uptake is a result of the high glucose levels competing with [^{18}F]FDG for cellular uptake [40]. The significance of glucose levels on FDG uptake remains controversial—while some studies report a significant effect of glucose levels on SUV, others dispute this [40–43]. The introduction of a 'glycaemia modified SUV' has been proposed, though there is no evidence of a linear relationship between glycaemia and SUV [11].

As blood glucose levels influence [^{18}F]FDG uptake, drugs that can alter these levels need to be considered. In diabetics, drugs such as insulin or metformin, their dosage and administration time from commencement of PET scan could affect the reliability of PET. Consequently, cancer patients with comorbidities and drugs used to treat them can play a role in influencing [^{18}F]FDG uptake. Corticosteroids may also affect [^{18}F]FDG uptake. Zhao et al. compared the effect of prednisolone therapy on [^{18}F]FDG uptake in granuloma and cancer xenograft rat models identifying that corticosteroids decreased [^{18}F]FDG uptake in the granuloma models but not the cancerous lesions [44]. The potential that corticosteroids could help differentiate between inflammatory and cancerous lesions needs to be further validated as it could enhance the accuracy of PET scanning.

3. Optimising PET with Biomolecular Profiling

3.1. Stratification

It is evident from the literature that PET is a clinically useful diagnostic and prognostic imaging modality in oncology. However, variations in [^{18}F]FDG uptake between patients highlight the apparent influence of tumour biology on PET accuracy and thus its efficacy. As stated herein, gross and molecular tumour features in addition to inherent patient characteristics play a role in influencing [^{18}F]FDG uptake. If the relative influence of each of these factors could be ascertained both clinically and molecularly, it could be employed to enhance the accuracy of PET. The addition of biomolecular testing to PET imaging could also improve the sensitivity in identifying certain tumours. In an era where multimodal therapy is becoming increasingly utilized, the improved information obtained on the tumour could facilitate development of diagnostic algorithms for stratification of patients into appropriate treatment regimens.

This theory has been trailed by Hoeben et al. who investigated the significance of biomolecular profiling in mouse xenograft models, aiming to determine if combining immunohistochemistry (IHC) and [^{18}F]FDG-PET parameters could reliably stratify Head and Neck cancers (HNC) into clusters [45]. By using [^{18}F]FDG-PET as a biomarker and adding an IHC criterion, this group aimed to enhance prognostic prediction and facilitate appropriate treatment selection. Using 14 HNC lines grafted into mice, they revealed a distinct selection of biomarkers related to metabolism, proliferation, hypoxia and perfusion that could match tumours consistently to the correct cell line with high reliability [45]. The potential of combining [^{18}F]FDG-PET with biomolecular profiling added value in terms of providing diagnostic and prognostic information.

3.2. Diagnosis and Predicting Prognosis

[^{18}F]FDG avidity on PET is in itself a 'biomarker,' with studies citing it as a predictor of prognosis at diagnosis and post treatment in head and neck cancer (HNC) and oesophageal cancer [46–48]. In HNC pre-treatment high [^{18}F]FDG uptake is associated with poor survival [49]. Conversely, HNC with an increased [^{18}F]FDG pre-treatment had a better response to radiotherapy [46].

In oesophageal cancer, increased [^{18}F]FDG uptake is also associated with poor prognosis compared to low [^{18}F]FDG uptake [47,48]. Studies have also revealed however that SUVmax is nota prognostic parameter [50,51].

[^{18}F]FDG uptake in oesophageal cancer is also identified as a predictor of lymph node disease, disease free survival (DFS) and recurrence [50,51]. A significant correlation between [^{18}F]FDG uptake and tumour recurrence has also been noted in other cancer types [23,52–54]. The prognostic potential of [^{18}F]FDG uptake in combination with biomarkers of tumour metabolism has also been evaluated. In oral SCC associations were found between increased [^{18}F]FDG uptake in combination with increased GLUT-1 expression and poorer survival while another study showed similar results with GLUT-3 [21,55].

As described above, FDG uptake has been proposed as a prognostic biomarker in some small HNC and oesophageal cancer studies. Whether increased SUVs in smaller tumours predict a worse prognosis compared to decreased SUVs in larger tumours is not clearly defined from this research. It appears that several factors are responsible for predicting outcomes in combination with [^{18}F]FDG uptake. By identifying molecular features that affect [^{18}F]FDG uptake for individual cancers, biomolecular profiling could advance the role of PET in stratifying tumours and increase its efficacy. Table 2 outlines biomarkers and their associated influence on [^{18}F]FDG uptake published to date.

4. Profiling Specific Cancer Types

The relationship between [^{18}F]FDG uptake and tumour biology is not clearly defined with conflicting results between cancer types and subtypes with no definite consensus on which biomarkers are relevant for specific cancer types.

Discordance between studies regarding PET biomarkers can be attributed to variations in study design. Higashi et al. demonstrated in their pancreatic study that the numerical value of SUVs varied between different studies and between PET machines [11]. They suggest that SUV should not be used as an absolute value in the evaluation of [^{18}F]FDG uptake rather broader categories of positive or negative uptake results are more important than absolute values [11].

Biological features and technical differences have both caused discordance in establishing the most appropriate and reliable biomarkers in relation to PET. However, there is evidence for specific biomarkers to predict levels of FDG uptake in some cancer types which are outlined below.

4.1. Oesophageal Cancer

PET's ability to identify metastases not detected by conventional workup have been highlighted in oesophageal cancer [52]. Prediction of prognosis based on tumour SUVs has been shown with pathologic response and DFS correlated with SUV changes following induction therapy [53,54]. Importantly, 10–20% of oesophageal cancers are [^{18}F]FDG negative on PET, demonstrating the need for biomolecular profiling to help identify this sub-group of tumours [56].

Potential biomarkers include size and GLUT-1 expression which positively correlate with SUV [23]. Taylor et al. could not identify a correlation between several prominent tumour markers and SUVmax, namely EGRF, P53, cyclin D1 and VEGF [57]. Although Schreurs et al. observed a significant relationship between HKII and SUVmax there were no significant relationships between GLUT-1, HK-1, HIF-Iα 1, VEGF-C, p53 and Ki-67 with SUV [58].

4.2. Breast Cancer

PET is not recommended for staging or follow-up in operable breast cancer as per the NCCN guidelines on account of the high rate of false negatives, largely attributed to small tumour size [10,59]. As a result, PET is not available to all breast cancer patients. Development of biomolecular profiles could help increase its accuracy by identifying tumours with likely poor [^{18}F]FDG uptake. Recommended markers which indicate increased [^{18}F]FDG uptake are GLUT-1 and HK-1 [19].

4.3. Non-Small Cell Lung Cancer (NSCLC)

The histological differences between NSCLC subtypes have revealed varied results in relation to PET accuracy. Several studies have suggested a high frequency of false negatives in bronchoalveolar carcinoma is due to decreased cellularity an assertion disproved by Yap et al. They showed sensitivity of [^{18}F]FDG PET in bronchoalveolar carcinoma to be high overall with the introduction of more precise classification guidelines by the World Health Organisation [60]. GLUT-1, GLUT-3 and Ki-67 are potential biomarkers which have been positively correlated with increased [^{18}F]FDG uptake in NSCLC [61].

4.4. Glioma

A SR on glioma revealed that [^{18}F]FDG-PET has a sensitivity of 0.77 (95% CI, 0.66–0.85) and specificity of 0.78 (95% CI, 0.54–0.91) [62]. The only biomarker identified influencing [^{18}F]FDG uptake is VEGF [63]. The practicality of using biomolecular profiling to increase sensitivity is made difficult by the inability to obtaining tumour samples as these tumours are often unresectable.

4.5. Head and Neck Cancer

Gronroos et al. revealed that an increased [^{18}F]FDG uptake is associated with a more aggressive phenotype and therefore high P53 and VEGF expression [64]. Detecting the presence or absence of these markers in HNC could enhance accuracy of PET. A recent study by Rasmussen et al. reported a positive correlation between SUVmax and β-tubulin-1 index and significant negative correlations between SUV max and Bcl-2 and P16 [65].

Table 2. Metabolic, hypoxic and angiogenic biomarkers affecting [^{18}F]FDG uptake in different cancer types. A positive association (+) indicates [^{18}F]FDG uptake increased with biomarker. A negative association (−) indicates [^{18}F]FDG uptake decreased with biomarker. A null association (0) indicates biomarker expression was unrelated to [^{18}F]FDG uptake.

Cancer Type	[^{18}F]FDG Uptake Association	Biomarker	Function	Reference
Oesophageal SCC	+	HK-I	Metabolism	[19]
	+	HK-II *	Metabolism	[19]
	−	HK-II	Metabolism	[58]
	+	VEGF	Angiogenesis	[66]
	0	VEGF	Angiogenesis	[57,66]
	0	KI67	Proliferation	[23]
Oesophageal AC	+	GLUT-1	Metabolism	[23,57]
	−	HK-II	Metabolism	[58]
	0	HIF-1α	Hypoxia	[58]
	0	VEGF	Angiogenesis	[23]
	0	P53	TSG	[58]
	0	Ki67	Proliferation	[58]

Table 2. *Cont.*

Cancer Type	[^{18}F]FDG Uptake Association	Biomarker	Function	Reference
Breast	+	GLUT-1	Metabolism	[19]
	+	HK-1	Metabolism	[19]
	0	HK-II **	Metabolism	[19]
	0	HK-III	Metabolism	[19]
	0	HIF-1α	Hypoxia	[19]
	0	VEGF	Angiogenesis	[19]
Head and Neck	−	GLUT-1	Metabolism	[2,21,64]
	+	GLUT-3	Metabolism	[2]
	+	VEGF	Angiogenesis	[64]
Oral SCC	+	GLUT-1 **	Metabolism	[2,21,67]
	+	GLUT-3 **	Metabolism	[2,21]
	+	HK-II	Metabolism	[67]
	+	HIF-1α	Hypoxia	[67]
Cervical	+	GLUT-1	Metabolism	[9,68]
	+	HK-II	Metabolism	[68]
Pancreatic	+	GLUT-1	Metabolism	[18]
Ovarian	+	GLUT-1	Metabolism	[20]
NSCLC	+	GLUT-1	Metabolism	[61,69]
	+	GLUT-3	Metabolism	[61]
	0	GLUT-3	Metabolism	[69]
	+	HIF-1α	Hypoxia	[69]
	0	Ki-67	Proliferation	[69]
Glioma	+	VEGF	Angiogenesis	[63]
Gastric	0	GLUT-1	Metabolism	[70]
	0	HKII	Metabolism	[70]
	+	HIF-1α	Hypoxia	[70]
	0	PCNA	Proliferation	[70]
Colorectal	+	HIF-1α	Hypoxia	[71]
	0	PCNA	Proliferation	[71]
Musculoskeletal	+	GLUT-1	Metabolism	[72]
	+	HK-II	Metabolism	[72]
Hodgkin's Lymphoma	+	GLUT-1	Metabolism	[73]
	0	GLUT-3	Metabolism	[73]
	0	HK-II	Metabolism	[73]
Thyroid	0	GLUT-1	Metabolism	[74]
	0	GLUT-3	Metabolism	[74]
	0	HK-II	Metabolism	[74]
	+	VEGF	Angiogenesis	[74]

* No significant correlation between these biomarkers and SUV though in logistic regression they added value to GLUT-1 correlation. ** These biomarkers were only found to correlate with increased SUV when overexpressed.

5. Conclusions and Future Directions

The influence of biomolecular markers on [^{18}F]FDG uptake has been established and is clearly linked with hypoxia, metabolism and angiogenesis. Despite this, a definite consensus is lacking on associations between biomarkers, [^{18}F]FDG uptake and cancer. Considerable variation and heterogeneity in study design including small sample size, variation in PET algorithms employed between centres; the diverse molecular markers examined and the lack of validation are clearly an issue limiting firm conclusions, and further research is clearly warranted. Biomolecular profiling can articulate the true significance of [^{18}F]FDG uptake while also addressing the limitations of PET in clinical oncology such as false negative results. There is a compelling case that the integration of biomolecular profiling and [^{18}F]FDG PET could enhance diagnosis, improve prognosis prediction and facilitate appropriate stratification of patients to treatment regimens based on a clear characterisation of the tumour, but this needs to be validated in rigorous scientific study.

Author Contributions: Conceptualization: J.V.R., J.O.S., C.J.; Methodology: V.M., H.O.N., J.O.S.; Software: N/A; Validation: N/A; Formal Analysis: N/A; Investigation: H.O.N., V.M., J.O.S.; Resources: J.O.S.; Data Curation: N/A; Writing—original draft preparation: H.O.N.; Writing—review and editing: C.J., J.V.R.; Visualization: H.O.N., J.O.S., V.M.; Supervision: J.V.R., J.O.S., C.J.; Project; Administration: J.O.S.; Funding Acquisition: N/A.

References

1. Slobbe, P.; Windhorst, A.D.; Stigter-van Walsum, M.; Schuit, R.C.; Smit, E.F.; Niessen, H.G.; Solca, F.; Stehle, G.; van Dongen, G.A.; Poot, A.J. Development of [^{18}f]afatinib as new tki-pet tracer for egfr positive tumours. *Nucl. Med. Boil.* **2014**, *41*, 749–757. [CrossRef]

2. Tian, M.; Zhang, H.; Nakasone, Y.; Mogi, K.; Endo, K. Expression of glut-1 and glut-3 in untreated oral squamous cell carcinoma compared with fdg accumulation in a pet study. *Eur. J. Nucl. Med. Mol. Imaging* **2004**, *31*, 5–12. [CrossRef] [PubMed]

3. Chang, J.M.; Lee, H.J.; Goo, J.M.; Lee, H.Y.; Lee, J.J.; Chung, J.K.; Im, J.G. False positive and false negative fdg-pet scans in various thoracic diseases. *Korean J. Radiol.* **2006**, *7*, 57–69. [CrossRef] [PubMed]

4. Kubota, R.; Kubota, K.; Yamada, S.; Tada, M.; Ido, T.; Tamahashi, N. Active and passive mechanisms of [fluorine-18] fluorodeoxyglucose uptake by proliferating and prenecrotic cancer cells in vivo: A microautoradiographic study. *J. Nucl. Med.* **1994**, *35*, 1067–1075. [PubMed]

5. Warning, K.; Hildebrandt, M.G.; Kristensen, B.; Ewertz, M. Utility of 18fdg-pet/ct in breast cancer diagnostics—A systematic review. *Dan. Med. Bull.* **2011**, *58*, A4289.

6. Purohit, B.S.; Ailianou, A.; Dulguerov, N.; Becker, C.D.; Ratib, O.; Becker, M. Fdg-pet/ct pitfalls in oncological head and neck imaging. *Insights Imaging* **2014**, *5*, 585–602. [CrossRef] [PubMed]

7. Jo, I.; Zeon, S.K.; Kim, S.H.; Kim, H.W.; Kang, S.H.; Kwon, S.Y.; Kim, S.J. Correlation of primary tumour fdg uptake with clinicopathologic prognostic factors in invasive ductal carcinoma of the breast. *Nucl. Med. Mol. Imaging* **2015**, *49*, 19–25. [CrossRef] [PubMed]

8. Balogova, S.; Huchet, V.; Kerrou, K.; Nataf, V.; Gutman, F.; Antoine, M.; Ruppert, A.M.; Prignon, A.; Lavolee, A.; Montravers, F.; et al. Detection of bronchioloalveolar cancer by means of pet/ct and 18f-fluorocholine and comparison with 18f-fluorodeoxyglucose. *Nucl. Med. Commun.* **2010**, *31*, 389–397. [CrossRef] [PubMed]

9. Yen, T.C.; See, L.C.; Lai, C.H.; Yah-Huei, C.W.; Ng, K.K.; Ma, S.Y.; Lin, W.J.; Chen, J.T.; Chen, W.J.; Lai, C.R.; et al. ^{18}f-fdg uptake in squamous cell carcinoma of the cervix is correlated with glucose transporter 1 expression. *J. Nucl. Med.* **2004**, *45*, 22–29.

10. Society of Nuclear Medicine and Molecular Imaging. NCCN Practice Guidelines: Narrative Summary of Indications for FDG Pet and PET/CT; 2016. Available online: http://snmmi.files.cms-plus.com/images/NCCN%20Narrative%20Summary%20Feb%202016.pdf (accessed on 22 January 2019).

11. Higashi, T.; Saga, T.; Nakamoto, Y.; Ishimori, T.; Fujimoto, K.; Doi, R.; Imamura, M.; Konishi, J. Diagnosis of pancreatic cancer using fluorine-18 fluorodeoxyglucose positron emission tomography (fdg pet)—Usefulness and limitations in "clinical reality". *Ann. Nucl. Med.* **2003**, *17*, 261–279. [CrossRef] [PubMed]

12. Adler, L.P.; Blair, H.F.; Makley, J.T.; Williams, R.P.; Joyce, M.J.; Leisure, G.; al-Kaisi, N.; Miraldi, F. Noninvasive grading of musculoskeletal tumours using pet. *J. Nucl. Med.* **1991**, *32*, 1508–1512.

13. Berger, K.L.; Nicholson, S.A.; Dehdashti, F.; Siegel, B.A. Fdg pet evaluation of mucinous neoplasms: Correlation of fdg uptake with histopathologic features. *Am. J. Roentgenol.* **2000**, *174*, 1005–1008. [CrossRef] [PubMed]

14. Kim, B.T.; Kim, Y.; Lee, K.S.; Yoon, S.B.; Cheon, E.M.; Kwon, O.J.; Rhee, C.H.; Han, J.; Shin, M.H. Localized form of bronchioloalveolar carcinoma: Fdg pet findings. *Am. J. Roentgenol.* **1998**, *170*, 935–939. [CrossRef] [PubMed]

15. Higashi, K.; Ueda, Y.; Seki, H.; Yuasa, K.; Oguchi, M.; Noguchi, T.; Taniguchi, M.; Tonami, H.; Okimura, T.; Yamamoto, I. Fluorine-18-fdg pet imaging is negative in bronchioloalveolar lung carcinoma. *J. Nucl. Med.* **1998**, *39*, 1016–1020. [PubMed]

16. Norikane, T.; Yamamoto, Y.; Maeda, Y.; Kudomi, N.; Matsunaga, T.; Haba, R.; Iwasaki, A.; Hoshikawa, H.; Nishiyama, Y. Correlation of (18)f-fluoromisonidazole pet findings with hif-1alpha and p53 expressions in head and neck cancer: Comparison with (18)f-fdg pet. *Nucl. Med. Commun.* **2014**, *35*, 30–35. [CrossRef] [PubMed]

17. Pugachev, A.; Ruan, S.; Carlin, S.; Larson, S.M.; Campa, J.; Ling, C.C.; Humm, J.L. Dependence of fdg uptake on tumor microenvironment. *Int. J. Radiat. Oncol. Biol. Phys.* **2005**, *62*, 545–553. [CrossRef] [PubMed]

18. Higashi, T.; Tamaki, N.; Honda, T.; Torizuka, T.; Kimura, T.; Inokuma, T.; Ohshio, G.; Hosotani, R.; Imamura, M.; Konishi, J. Expression of glucose transporters in human pancreatic tumors compared with increased fdg accumulation in pet study. *J. Nucl. Med.* **1997**, *38*, 1337–1344.

19. Bos, R.; van Der Hoeven, J.J.; van Der Wall, E.; van Der Groep, P.; van Diest, P.J.; Comans, E.F.; Joshi, U.; Semenza, G.L.; Hoekstra, O.S.; Lammertsma, A.A.; et al. Biologic correlates of (18)fluorodeoxyglucose uptake in human breast cancer measured by positron emission tomography. *J. Clin. Oncol.* **2002**, *20*, 379–387. [CrossRef]

20. Kurokawa, T.; Yoshida, Y.; Kawahara, K.; Tsuchida, T.; Okazawa, H.; Fujibayashi, Y.; Yonekura, Y.; Kotsuji, F. Expression of glut-1 glucose transfer, cellular proliferation activity and grade of tumor correlate with [f-18]-fluorodeoxyglucose uptake by positron emission tomography in epithelial tumors of the ovary. *Int. J. Cancer* **2004**, *109*, 926–932. [CrossRef]

21. Kunkel, M.; Reichert, T.E.; Benz, P.; Lehr, H.A.; Jeong, J.H.; Wieand, S.; Bartenstein, P.; Wagner, W.; Whiteside, T.L. Overexpression of glut-1 and increased glucose metabolism in tumors are associated with a poor prognosis in patients with oral squamous cell carcinoma. *Cancer* **2003**, *97*, 1015–1024. [CrossRef]

22. Kurata, T.; Oguri, T.; Isobe, T.; Ishioka, S.; Yamakido, M. Differential expression of facilitative glucose transporter (glut) genes in primary lung cancers and their liver metastases. *Jpn. J. Cancer Res. GANN* **1999**, *90*, 1238–1243. [CrossRef] [PubMed]

23. Westerterp, M.; Sloof, G.W.; Hoekstra, O.S.; Ten Kate, F.J.; Meijer, G.A.; Reitsma, J.B.; Boellaard, R.; van Lanschot, J.J.; Molthoff, C.F. 18fdg uptake in oesophageal adenocarcinoma: Linking biology and outcome. *J. Cancer Res. Clin. Oncol.* **2008**, *134*, 227–236. [CrossRef] [PubMed]

24. Mochizuki, T.; Tsukamoto, E.; Kuge, Y.; Kanegae, K.; Zhao, S.; Hikosaka, K.; Hosokawa, M.; Kohanawa, M.; Tamaki, N. Fdg uptake and glucose transporter subtype expressions in experimental tumor and inflammation models. *J. Nucl. Med.* **2001**, *42*, 1551–1555. [PubMed]

25. Denko, N.C. Hypoxia, hif1 and glucose metabolism in the solid tumour. *Nat. Rev. Cancer* **2008**, *8*, 705–713. [CrossRef]

26. Dearling, J.L.; Flynn, A.A.; Sutcliffe-Goulden, J.; Petrie, I.A.; Boden, R.; Green, A.J.; Boxer, G.M.; Begent, R.H.; Pedley, R.B. Analysis of the regional uptake of radiolabeled deoxyglucose analogs in human tumor xenografts. *J. Nucl. Med.* **2004**, *45*, 101–107. [PubMed]

27. Aronen, H.J.; Pardo, F.S.; Kennedy, D.N.; Belliveau, J.W.; Packard, S.D.; Hsu, D.W.; Hochberg, F.H.; Fischman, A.J.; Rosen, B.R. High microvascular blood volume is associated with high glucose uptake and tumor angiogenesis in human gliomas. *Clin. Cancer Res.* **2000**, *6*, 2189–2200. [PubMed]

28. Laking, G.; Price, P. Radionuclide imaging of perfusion and hypoxia. *Eur. J. Nucl. Med. Mol. Imaging* **2010**, *37* (Suppl. 1), S20–S29. [CrossRef] [PubMed]

29. De Bruyne, S.; Van Damme, N.; Smeets, P.; Ferdinande, L.; Ceelen, W.; Mertens, J.; Van de Wiele, C.; Troisi, R.; Libbrecht, L.; Laurent, S.; et al. Value of dce-mri and fdg-pet/ct in the prediction of response to preoperative chemotherapy with bevacizumab for colorectal liver metastases. *Br. J. Cancer* **2012**, *106*, 1926–1933. [CrossRef]

30. Colavolpe, C.; Chinot, O.; Metellus, P.; Mancini, J.; Barrie, M.; Bequet-Boucard, C.; Tabouret, E.; Mundler, O.; Figarella-Branger, D.; Guedj, E. Fdg-pet predicts survival in recurrent high-grade gliomas treated with bevacizumab and irinotecan. *Neuro Oncol.* **2012**, *14*, 649–657. [CrossRef]

31. Goshen, E.; Davidson, T.; Zwas, S.T.; Aderka, D. Pet/ct in the evaluation of response to treatment of liver metastases from colorectal cancer with bevacizumab and irinotecan. *Technol. Cancer Res. Treat.* **2006**, *5*, 37–43. [CrossRef]

32. Crippa, F.; Seregni, E.; Agresti, R.; Chiesa, C.; Pascali, C.; Bogni, A.; Decise, D.; De Sanctis, V.; Greco, M.; Daidone, M.G.; et al. Association between [^{18}f]fluorodeoxyglucose uptake and postoperative histopathology, hormone receptor status, thymidine labelling index and p53 in primary breast cancer: A preliminary observation. *Eur. J. Nucl. Med.* **1998**, *25*, 1429–1434. [CrossRef] [PubMed]

33. Schulte, M.; Brecht-Krauss, D.; Heymer, B.; Guhlmann, A.; Hartwig, E.; Sarkar, M.R.; Diederichs, C.G.; Schultheiss, M.; Kotzerke, J.; Reske, S.N. Fluorodeoxyglucose positron emission tomography of soft tissue tumours: Is a non-invasive determination of biological activity possible? *Eur. J. Nucl. Med.* **1999**, *26*, 599–605. [CrossRef]

34. Smith, T.A. Influence of chemoresistance and p53 status on fluoro-2-deoxy-d-glucose incorporation in cancer. *Nucl. Med. Biol.* **2010**, *37*, 51–55. [CrossRef]

35. Seo, S.; Hatano, E.; Higashi, T.; Nakajima, A.; Nakamoto, Y.; Tada, M.; Tamaki, N.; Iwaisako, K.; Kitamura, K.; Ikai, I.; et al. P-glycoprotein expression affects 18f-fluorodeoxyglucose accumulation in hepatocellular carcinoma in vivo and in vitro. *Int. J. Oncol.* **2009**, *34*, 1303–1312.

36. Berkers, C.R.; Maddocks, O.D.; Cheung, E.C.; Mor, I.; Vousden, K.H. Metabolic regulation by p53 family members. *Cell Metab.* **2013**, *18*, 617–633. [CrossRef]

37. Groheux, D.; Giacchetti, S.; Moretti, J.L.; Porcher, R.; Espie, M.; Lehmann-Che, J.; de Roquancourt, A.; Hamy, A.S.; Cuvier, C.; Vercellino, L.; et al. Correlation of high 18f-fdg uptake to clinical, pathological and biological prognostic factors in breast cancer. *Eur. J. Nucl. Med. Mol. Imaging* **2011**, *38*, 426–435. [CrossRef]

38. Sasaki, M.; Sugio, K.; Kuwabara, Y.; Koga, H.; Nakagawa, M.; Chen, T.; Kaneko, K.; Hayashi, K.; Shioyama, Y.; Sakai, S.; et al. Alterations of tumor suppressor genes (rb, p16, p27 and p53) and an increased fdg uptake in lung cancer. *Ann. Nucl. Med.* **2003**, *17*, 189–196. [CrossRef] [PubMed]

39. Adams, M.C.; Turkington, T.G.; Wilson, J.M.; Wong, T.Z. A systematic review of the factors affecting accuracy of suv measurements. *Am. J. Roentgenol.* **2010**, *195*, 310–320. [CrossRef] [PubMed]

40. Bares, R.; Klever, P.; Hauptmann, S.; Hellwig, D.; Fass, J.; Cremerius, U.; Schumpelick, V.; Mittermayer, C.; Bull, U. F-18 fluorodeoxyglucose pet in vivo evaluation of pancreatic glucose metabolism for detection of pancreatic cancer. *Radiology* **1994**, *192*, 79–86. [CrossRef]

41. Friess, H.; Langhans, J.; Ebert, M.; Beger, H.G.; Stollfuss, J.; Reske, S.N.; Buchler, M.W. Diagnosis of pancreatic cancer by 2[^{18}f]-fluoro-2-deoxy-d-glucose positron emission tomography. *Gut* **1995**, *36*, 771–777. [CrossRef]

42. Zimny, M.; Bares, R.; Fass, J.; Adam, G.; Cremerius, U.; Dohmen, B.; Klever, P.; Sabri, O.; Schumpelick, V.; Buell, U. Fluorine-18 fluorodeoxyglucose positron emission tomography in the differential diagnosis of pancreatic carcinoma: A report of 106 cases. *Eur. J. Nucl. Med.* **1997**, *24*, 678–682. [CrossRef] [PubMed]

43. Diederichs, C.G.; Staib, L.; Glatting, G.; Beger, H.G.; Reske, S.N. Fdg pet: Elevated plasma glucose reduces both uptake and detection rate of pancreatic malignancies. *J. Nucl. Med.* **1998**, *39*, 1030–1033.

44. Zhao, S.; Kuge, Y.; Nakada, K.; Mochizuki, T.; Takei, T.; Okada, F.; Tamaki, N. Effect of steroids on [^{18}f]fluorodeoxyglucose uptake in an experimental tumour model. *Nucl. Med. Commun.* **2004**, *25*, 727–730. [CrossRef] [PubMed]

45. Hoeben, B.A.; Starmans, M.H.; Leijenaar, R.T.; Dubois, L.J.; van der Kogel, A.J.; Kaanders, J.H.; Boutros, P.C.; Lambin, P.; Bussink, J. Systematic analysis of 18f-fdg pet and metabolism, proliferation and hypoxia markers for classification of head and neck tumors. *BMC Cancer* **2014**, *14*, 130. [CrossRef] [PubMed]

46. Rege, S.; Safa, A.A.; Chaiken, L.; Hoh, C.; Juillard, G.; Withers, H.R. Positron emission tomography: An independent indicator of radiocurability in head and neck carcinomas. *Am. J. Clin. Oncol.* **2000**, *23*, 164–169. [CrossRef]

47. Sepesi, B.; Raymond, D.P.; Polomsky, M.; Watson, T.J.; Litle, V.R.; Jones, C.E.; Hu, R.; Qiu, X.; Peters, J.H. Does the value of pet-ct extend beyond pretreatment staging? An analysis of survival in surgical patients with esophageal cancer. *J. Gastrointest. Surg.* **2009**, *13*, 2121–2127. [CrossRef]

48. Suzuki, A.; Xiao, L.; Hayashi, Y.; Macapinlac, H.A.; Welsh, J.; Lin, S.H.; Lee, J.H.; Bhutani, M.S.; Maru, D.M.; Hofstetter, W.L.; et al. Prognostic significance of baseline positron emission tomography and importance of clinical complete response in patients with esophageal or gastroesophageal junction cancer treated with definitive chemoradiotherapy. *Cancer* **2011**, *117*, 4823–4833. [CrossRef]

49. Minn, H.; Lapela, M.; Klemi, P.J.; Grenman, R.; Leskinen, S.; Lindholm, P.; Bergman, J.; Eronen, E.; Haaparanta, M.; Joensuu, H. Prediction of survival with fluorine-18-fluoro-deoxyglucose and pet in head and neck cancer. *J. Nucl. Med.* **1997**, *38*, 1907–1911.

50. Chatterton, B.E.; Ho Shon, I.; Baldey, A.; Lenzo, N.; Patrikeos, A.; Kelley, B.; Wong, D.; Ramshaw, J.E.; Scott, A.M. Positron emission tomography changes management and prognostic stratification in patients with oesophageal cancer: Results of a multicentre prospective study. *Eur. J. Nucl. Med. Mol. Imaging* **2009**, *36*, 354–361. [CrossRef]

51. Gillies, R.S.; Middleton, M.R.; Han, C.; Marshall, R.E.; Maynard, N.D.; Bradley, K.M.; Gleeson, F.V. Role of positron emission tomography-computed tomography in predicting survival after neoadjuvant chemotherapy and surgery for oesophageal adenocarcinoma. *Br. J. Surg.* **2012**, *99*, 239–245. [CrossRef]

52. Meyers, B.F.; Downey, R.J.; Decker, P.A.; Keenan, R.J.; Siegel, B.A.; Cerfolio, R.J.; Landreneau, R.J.; Reed, C.E.; Balfe, D.M.; Dehdashti, F.; et al. The utility of positron emission tomography in staging of potentially operable carcinoma of the thoracic esophagus: Results of the american college of surgeons oncology group z0060 trial. *J. Thorac. Cardiovasc. Surg.* **2007**, *133*, 738–745. [CrossRef] [PubMed]

53. Cerfolio, R.J.; Bryant, A.S. Maximum standardized uptake values on positron emission tomography of esophageal cancer predicts stage, tumor biology and survival. *Ann. Thorac. Surg.* **2006**, *82*, 391–394; discussion 394–395. [CrossRef] [PubMed]

54. Rizk, N.; Downey, R.J.; Akhurst, T.; Gonen, M.; Bains, M.S.; Larson, S.; Rusch, V. Preoperative ^{18}[f]-fluorodeoxyglucose positron emission tomography standardized uptake values predict survival after esophageal adenocarcinoma resection. *Ann. Thorac. Surg.* **2006**, *81*, 1076–1081. [CrossRef] [PubMed]

55. Baer, S.; Casaubon, L.; Schwartz, M.R.; Marcogliese, A.; Younes, M. Glut3 expression in biopsy specimens of laryngeal carcinoma is associated with poor survival. *Laryngoscope* **2002**, *112*, 393–396. [CrossRef]

56. Van Westreenen, H.L.; Heeren, P.A.; van Dullemen, H.M.; van der Jagt, E.J.; Jager, P.L.; Groen, H.; Plukker, J.T. Positron emission tomography with f-18-fluorodeoxyglucose in a combined staging strategy of esophageal cancer prevents unnecessary surgical explorations. *J. Gastrointest. Surg.* **2005**, *9*, 54–61. [CrossRef] [PubMed]

57. Taylor, M.D.; Smith, P.W.; Brix, W.K.; Wick, M.R.; Theodosakis, N.; Swenson, B.R.; Kozower, B.D.; Jones, D.R. Correlations between selected tumor markers and fluorodeoxyglucose maximal standardized uptake values in esophageal cancer. *Eur. J. Cardio-Thorac. Surg.* **2009**, *35*, 699–705. [CrossRef] [PubMed]

58. Schreurs, L.M.; Smit, J.K.; Pavlov, K.; Pultrum, B.B.; Pruim, J.; Groen, H.; Hollema, H.; Plukker, J.T. Prognostic impact of clinicopathological features and expression of biomarkers related to (18)f-fdg uptake in esophageal cancer. *Ann. Surg. Oncol.* **2014**, *21*, 3751–3757. [CrossRef] [PubMed]

59. Kumar, R.; Chauhan, A.; Zhuang, H.; Chandra, P.; Schnall, M.; Alavi, A. Clinicopathologic factors associated with false negative fdg-pet in primary breast cancer. *Breast Cancer Res. Treat.* **2006**, *98*, 267–274. [CrossRef]

60. Yap, C.S.; Schiepers, C.; Fishbein, M.C.; Phelps, M.E.; Czernin, J. Fdg-pet imaging in lung cancer: How sensitive is it for bronchioloalveolar carcinoma? *Eur. J. Nucl. Med. Mol. Imaging* **2002**, *29*, 1166–1173. [CrossRef] [PubMed]

61. Marom, E.M.; Aloia, T.A.; Moore, M.B.; Hara, M.; Herndon, J.E., 2nd; Harpole, D.H., Jr.; Goodman, P.C.; Patz, E.F., Jr. Correlation of fdg-pet imaging with glut-1 and glut-3 expression in early-stage non-small cell lung cancer. *Lung Cancer* **2001**, *33*, 99–107. [CrossRef]

62. Nihashi, T.; Dahabreh, I.J.; Terasawa, T. Diagnostic accuracy of pet for recurrent glioma diagnosis: A meta-analysis. *Am. J. Neuroradiol.* **2013**, *34*, 944–950, s941-911. [CrossRef] [PubMed]

63. Cher, L.M.; Murone, C.; Lawrentschuk, N.; Ramdave, S.; Papenfuss, A.; Hannah, A.; O'Keefe, G.J.; Sachinidis, J.I.; Berlangieri, S.U.; Fabinyi, G.; et al. Correlation of hypoxic cell fraction and angiogenesis with glucose metabolic rate in gliomas using 18f-fluoromisonidazole, 18f-fdg pet and immunohistochemical studies. *J. Nucl. Med.* **2006**, *47*, 410–418. [PubMed]

64. Grönroos, T.J.; Lehtiö, K.; Söderström, K.-O.; Kronqvist, P.; Laine, J.; Eskola, O.; Viljanen, T.; Grénman, R.; Solin, O.; Minn, H. Hypoxia, blood flow and metabolism in squamous-cell carcinoma of the head and neck: Correlations between multiple immunohistochemical parameters and pet. *BMC Cancer* **2014**, *14*, 876. [CrossRef] [PubMed]

65. Rasmussen, G.B.; Vogelius, I.R.; Rasmussen, J.H.; Schumaker, L.; Ioffe, O.; Cullen, K.; Fischer, B.M.; Therkildsen, M.H.; Specht, L.; Bentzen, S.M. Immunohistochemical biomarkers and fdg uptake on pet/ct in head and neck squamous cell carcinoma. *Acta Oncol.* **2015**, *54*, 1408–1415. [CrossRef] [PubMed]

66. Kobayashi, M.; Kaida, H.; Kawahara, A.; Hattori, S.; Kurata, S.; Hayakawa, M.; Hirose, Y.; Uchida, M.; Kage, M.; Fujita, H.; et al. The relationship between glut-1 and vascular endothelial growth factor expression and 18f-fdg uptake in esophageal squamous cell cancer patients. *Clin. Nucl. Med.* **2012**, *37*, 447–452. [CrossRef] [PubMed]

67. Yamada, T.; Uchida, M.; Kwang-Lee, K.; Kitamura, N.; Yoshimura, T.; Sasabe, E.; Yamamoto, T. Correlation of metabolism/hypoxia markers and fluorodeoxyglucose uptake in oral squamous cell carcinomas. *Oral Surg. Oral Med. Oral Pathol. Oral Radiol.* **2012**, *113*, 464–471. [CrossRef] [PubMed]

68. Tong, S.Y.; Lee, J.M.; Ki, K.D.; Choi, Y.J.; Seol, H.J.; Lee, S.K.; Huh, C.Y.; Kim, G.Y.; Lim, S.J. Correlation between fdg uptake by pet/ct and the expressions of glucose transporter type 1 and hexokinase ii in cervical cancer. *Int. J. Gynecol. Cancer* **2012**, *22*, 654–658. [CrossRef]

69. Van Baardwijk, A.; Dooms, C.; van Suylen, R.J.; Verbeken, E.; Hochstenbag, M.; Dehing-Oberije, C.; Rupa, D.; Pastorekova, S.; Stroobants, S.; Buell, U.; et al. The maximum uptake of (18)f-deoxyglucose on positron emission tomography scan correlates with survival, hypoxia inducible factor-1alpha and glut-1 in non-small cell lung cancer. *Eur. J. Cancer* **2007**, *43*, 1392–1398. [CrossRef]

70. Takebayashi, R.; Izuishi, K.; Yamamoto, Y.; Kameyama, R.; Mori, H.; Masaki, T.; Suzuki, Y. [^{18}f]fluorodeoxyglucose accumulation as a biological marker of hypoxic status but not glucose transport ability in gastric cancer. *J. Exp. Clin. Cancer Res.* **2013**, *32*, 34. [CrossRef]

71. Izuishi, K.; Yamamoto, Y.; Sano, T.; Takebayashi, R.; Nishiyama, Y.; Mori, H.; Masaki, T.; Morishita, A.; Suzuki, Y. Molecular mechanism underlying the detection of colorectal cancer by 18f-2-fluoro-2-deoxy-d-glucose positron emission tomography. *J. Gastrointest. Surg.* **2012**, *16*, 394–400. [CrossRef]

72. Hamada, K.; Tomita, Y.; Qiu, Y.; Zhang, B.; Ueda, T.; Myoui, A.; Higuchi, I.; Yoshikawa, H.; Aozasa, K.; Hatazawa, J. 18f-fdg-pet of musculoskeletal tumors: A correlation with the expression of glucose transporter 1 and hexokinase II. *Ann. Nucl. Med.* **2008**, *22*, 699–705. [CrossRef] [PubMed]

73. Shim, H.K.; Lee, W.W.; Park, S.Y.; Kim, H.; Kim, S.E. Relationship between fdg uptake and expressions of glucose transporter type 1, type 3 and hexokinase-ii in reed-sternberg cells of hodgkin lymphoma. *Oncol. Res.* **2009**, *17*, 331–337. [CrossRef] [PubMed]

74. Kim, B.H.; Kim, I.J.; Kim, S.S.; Kim, S.J.; Lee, C.H.; Kim, Y.K. Relationship between biological marker expression and fluorine-18 fluorodeoxyglucose uptake in incidentally detected thyroid cancer. *Cancer Biother. Radiopharm.* **2010**, *25*, 309–315. [CrossRef] [PubMed]

Cytotoxic Effects of Newly Synthesized Heterocyclic Candidates Containing Nicotinonitrile and Pyrazole Moieties on Hepatocellular and Cervical Carcinomas

Amira A. El-Sayed [1,*], **Abd El-Galil E. Amr** [2,3,*], **Ahmed K. EL-Ziaty** [1] **and Elsayed A. Elsayed** [4,5]

[1]   Laboratory of Synthetic Organic Chemistry, Chemistry Department, Faculty of Science, Ain Shams University, Abbassia, Cairo 11566, Egypt; ahm512@gmail.com

[2]   Pharmaceutical Chemistry Department, Drug Exploration & Development Chair (DEDC), College of Pharmacy, King Saud University, Riyadh 11451, Saudi Arabi

[3]   Applied Organic Chemistry Department, National Research Center, Cairo, Dokki 12622, Egypt

[4]   Zoology Department, Bioproducts Research Chair, Faculty of Science, King Saud University, Riyadh 11451, Saudi Arabiap; eaelsayed@ksu.edu.sa

[5]   Chemistry of Natural and Microbial Products Department, National Research Centre, Dokki 12622, Cairo, Egypt

*   Correspondence: aamr@ksu.edu.sa (A.E.-G.E.A.); amira_aa47@hotmail.com (A.A.E.-S.);

Academic Editor: Qiao-Hong Chen

Abstract: In this study, a series of newly synthesized substituted pyridine **9, 11–18**, naphthpyridine derivative **10** and substituted pyrazolopyridines **19–23** by using cycnopyridone **8** as a starting material. Some of the synthesized candidates are evaluated as anticancer agents against different cancer cell lines. In vitro cytotoxic activities against hepatocellular and cervical carcinoma cell lines were evaluated using standard MTT assay. Different synthesized compounds exhibited potential in vitro cytotoxic activities against both HepG2 and HeLa cell lines. Furthermore, compared to standard positive control drugs, compounds **13** and **19** showed the most potent cytotoxic effect with IC$_{50}$ values of 8.78 ± 0.7, 5.16 ± 0.4 µg/mL, and 15.32 ± 1.2 and 4.26 ± 0.3 µg/mL for HepG2 and HeLa cells, respectively.

Keywords: cyanopyridone; substituted pyridine; pyridotriazine; pyrazolopyridine; thioxotriazopyridine; anticancer activity; HepG2; HeLa

1. Introduction

Multicomponent reactions (MCR) "in which three or more starting materials react to form a product" play a significant role in the synthesis of heterocyclic compounds with pharmaceutical and chemical importance [1]. Several nicotinonitriles have been constructed via (MCR) and showed antitumor [2], antimicrobial [3], and antioxidant [4] activities. Also nicotinonitriles have been utilized as a scaffold for the synthesis of heterocyclic compounds containing a pyridine moiety with antimicrobial and antiviral activities [5]. A series of nicotinonitriles **1–3** (Figure 1) and have been synthesized and anti-proliferative [6], anti-Alzheimer's [7], and anti-inflammatory [8] activities.

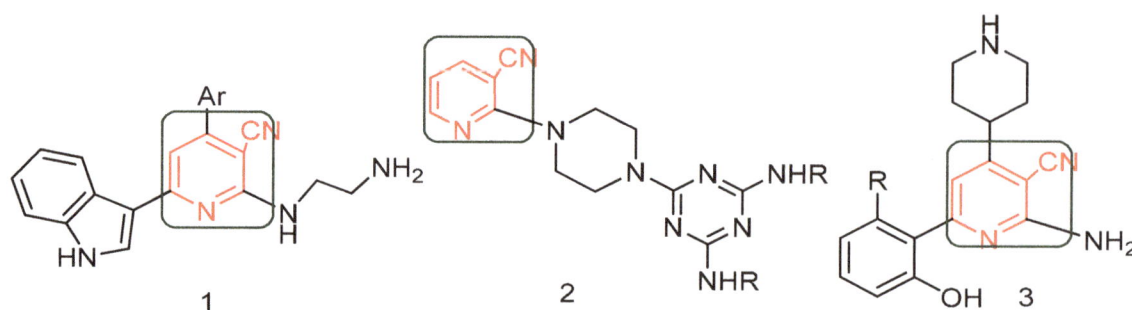

Figure 1. Nicotinonitriles with anti-proliferative, anti-Alzheimer's anti-inflammatory activities.

The pyrazole moiety is both pharmacologically and medicinally significant [9]. A series of pyrazoles **4–7** (Figure 2) has been reported as anti-inflammatory activity by Bekhit et al. [10], they observed that the synthesized pyrazoles showed more anti-inflammatory activity than the standard indomethacin [11]. Trisubstituted pyrazoles have been constructed by Christodoulou et al. (2010) [11] and evaluated as anti-angiogenic agents; these derivatives showed a potent anti-angiogenic efficacy and moreover inhibited the growth of Mammary gland breast cancer (MCF-7) and cervical carcinoma (Hela) [12]. Recently novel derivatives of pyrazoles **5,6** have been prepared as antimicrobial [13] and anticonvulsant [14] agents. The pyrazole **7** has been prepared by Bonesi et al. (2010) [15] and showed effective Angiotensin -1-Converting Enzyme (ACE) inhibitor activity [15].

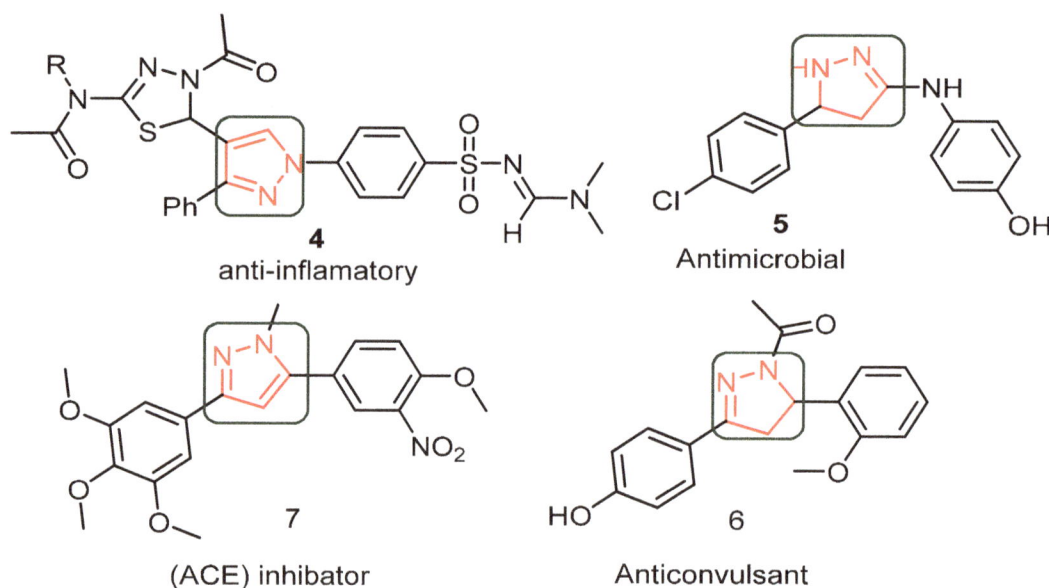

Figure 2. Pyrazoles as anti-inflammatory antimicrobial and anticonvulsant activities.

Based on the previous facts about the importance of pyrazoles and nicotinonitriles in medicinal chemistry, we have herein synthesized of some novel heterocyclic candidates containing nicotinonitrile and pyrazole moieties and tested their anticancer activity.

2. Results

2.1. Chemistry

The nicotinonitriles were obtained by two different ways, from the reaction of chalcone with ethylcyanoacetate, ammonium acetate and drops of piperidine as a base and from one pot four components reaction of methylketone, aldehyde, ethylcyanoacetate, ammonium acetate and drops of piperidine as a base [15]. In prolongation of our work in the synthesis of heterocyclic compounds and evaluation of their medicinal importance [16–27] and based on the literature survey about the pharmacological and medicinal importance of pyrazoles and nicotinonitriles, we have devoted our efforts to design and synthesize novel heterocyclic compounds containing pyrazol and nicotine-nitrile moieties, 4-(3-(4-fluorophenyl)-1-phenyl-1*H*-pyrazol-4-yl)-2-hydroxy-6-(naphthalen-1-yl)-nicotinenitrile **8** has been obtained by reacting of 1-acetylnaphthalene (**A**), 3-(4-fluorophenyl)-1-phenyl-1*H*-pyrazole-4-carbaldehyde (**B**), ethyl 2-cyanoacetate, ammonium acetate and piperidine (Scheme 1).

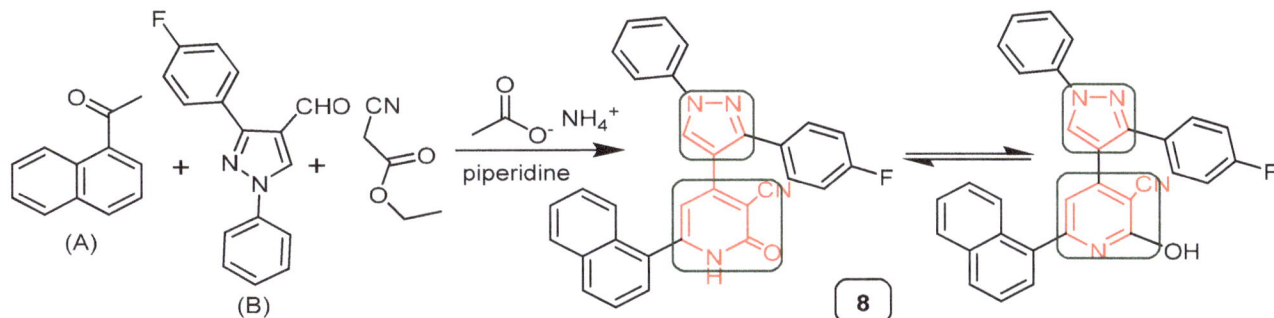

Scheme 1. Synthesis of compound **8** as starting material.

The structure of the nicotinonitrile **8** has been confirmed from its spectral data. IR spectrum showing absorption frequencies at ν 3159 cm^{-1}, 2220 cm^{-1} and ν 1647 cm^{-1} for OH, C≡N and C=N groups, respectively. Also, ^{1}H-NMR spectrum of the assigned compound displayed signals at δ 12.89 ppm (disappeared with D$_2$O) corresponding to acidic OH. A compelling evidence for the structure of **8** was provided by ^{13}C-NMR spectrum that showed a singlet signal at δ 149.8, 139.3 and 139.3 ppm for C-OH, C=N and C≡N groups respectively. Mass spectra of **8** showed [M$^+$] at *m/z* (%) 482 (22). Treatment of **8** with ethylchloroacetate afforded compound **9**, which was hydrazinolysis with NH$_2$NH$_2$ to give the corresponding cyclized product **10**.

Remediation of the nicotinonitrile derivative **8** with malononitrile in the presence of few drops of piperidine afforded 1,8-naphthyridine-3-carbonitrile derivative **11**. Chlorination of **8** by a mixture of (POCl$_3$/PCl$_5$) afforded 2-chloronicotinonitrile derivative **12**, which was reacted with malono nitrile as a carbon nucleophile gave the nicotinonitrile derivative **13**. Reaction of **12** with primary and secondary amines, namely, *o*-aminothiophenol, morpholine, 1-methylpiperazine and hydrazine hydrate gave novel nicotinonitriles **14**, **15a**, **b** and **16** (Scheme 2). The mechanism formation route of compound **11** has been shown in Figure 3.

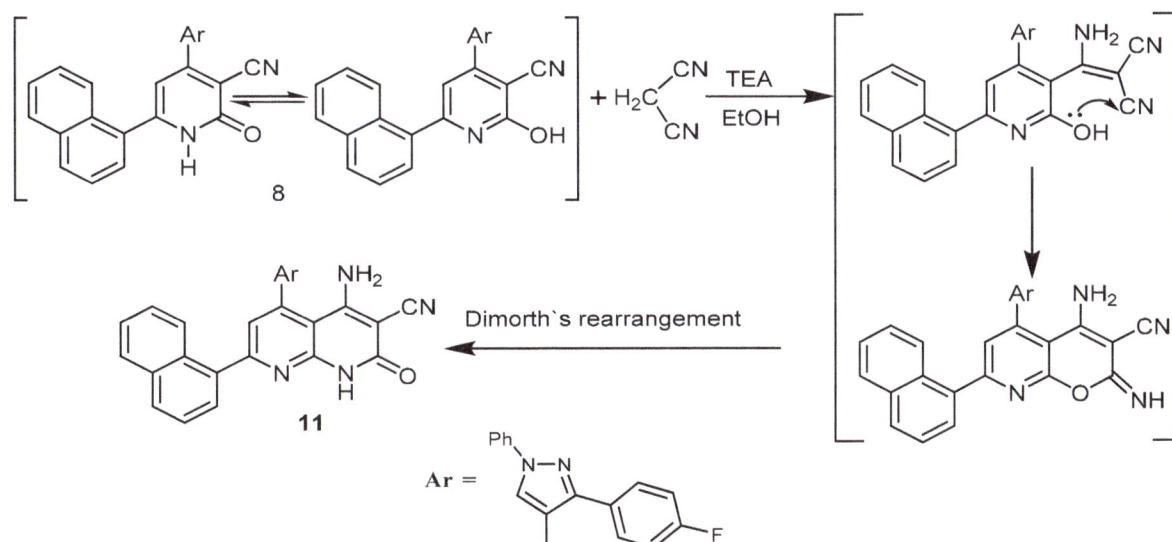

Figure 3. The mechanism formation route of compound **11**.

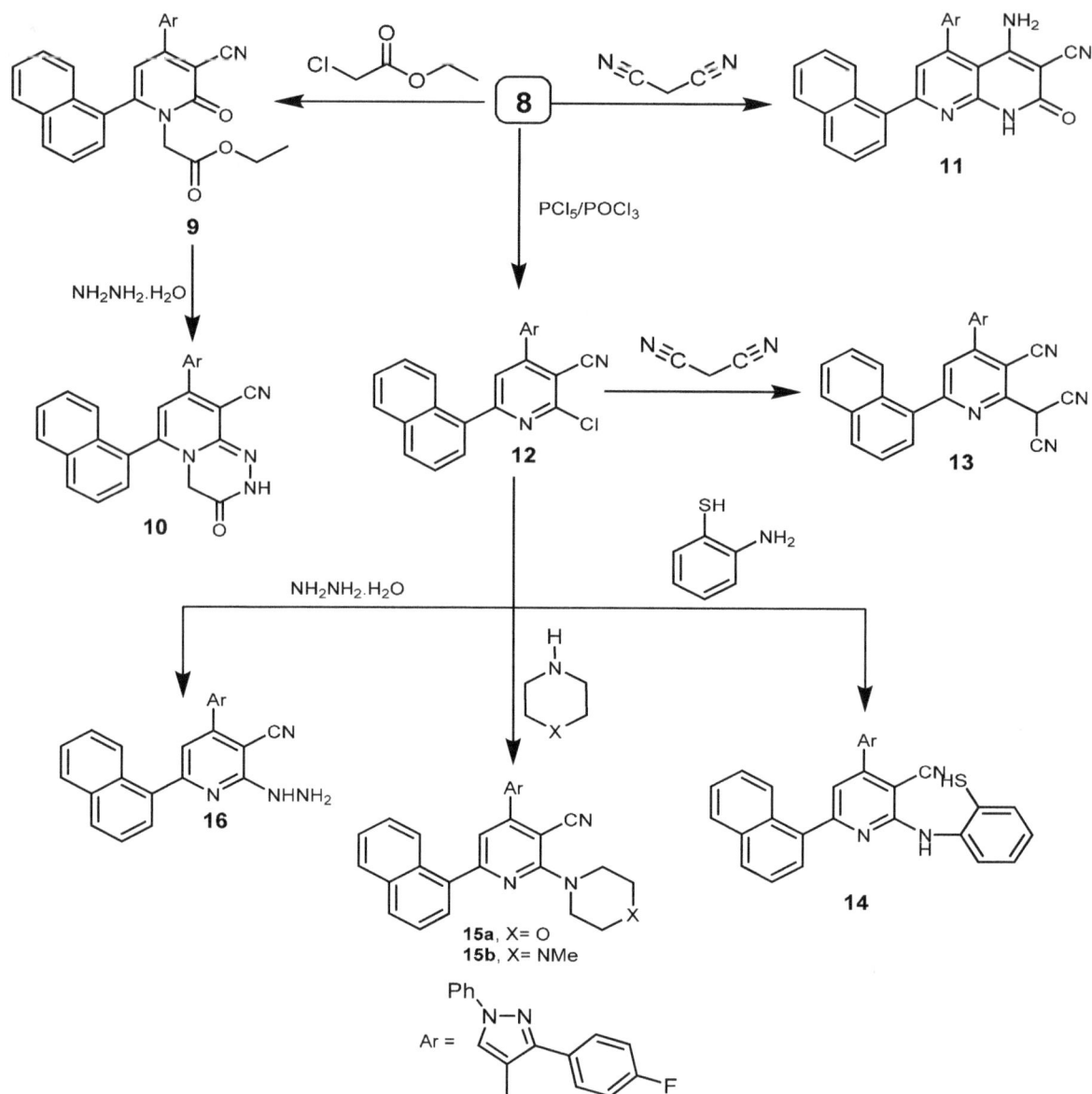

Scheme 2. Synthetic route for compounds 9–16.

Compound **16** was utilized as a building block for novel nicotinonitriles containing two pyrazole moieties. 2-Pyrazolyl nicotinonitrile derivatives **17** and **18** were prepared by treatment of **16** with acetyl acetone and 4,4,4,-trifluoro-1-(thiophen-2-yl)butane-1,3-dione, respectively. Treatment of **16** with acetic anhydride and acetic acid afforded pyrazolopyridine derivative **19**. The derivative **16** was treated with acetic anhydride to afford the *N*-acetyl pyrazolopyridine as a sole product **20**. The structure of compound **20** was confirmed chemically by acetylation of the amino pyrazopyridine **19** (Scheme 3).

Treatment of **16** with 4-chlorobenzaldehyde and/or tetrachlorophthalic anhydride in the presence of acetic acid afforded the cyclized **19** followed by condensation to give the Schiff's base **21** and tetra chloroisoindoline **22**, respectively. The structures of **21** and **22** were confirmed chemically by condensation of compound **19** with 4-chlorobenzaldehyde and/or tetrachlorophthalic anhydride to provide compounds **21** and **22**, respectively. Treatment of hydrazinyl derivative **16** with CS$_2$ in the presence of alcoholic KOH provided thioxotriazolo pyridine derivative **23** (Scheme 3).

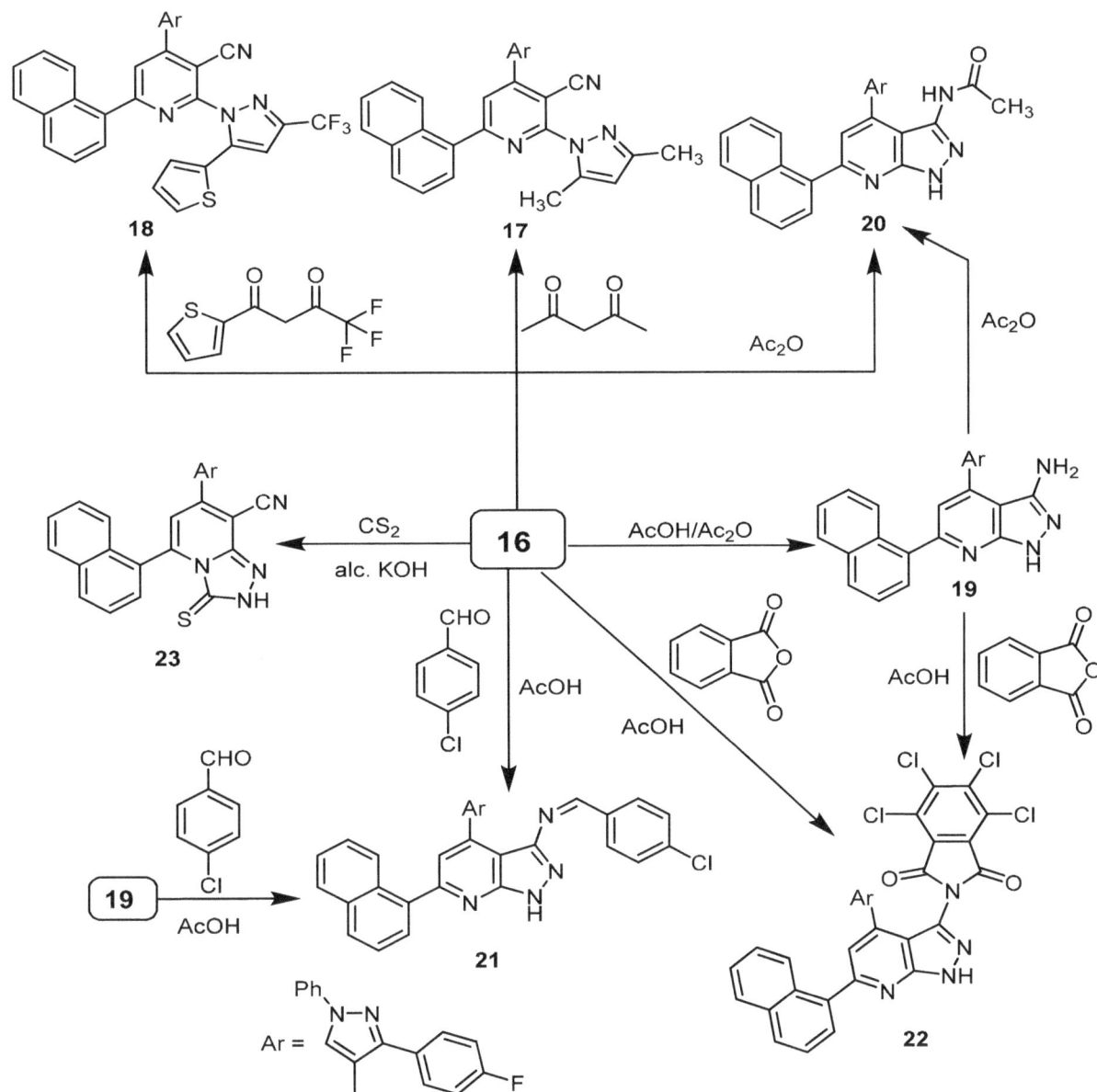

Scheme 3. Synthetic route for compounds **17–23**.

2.2. Cytotoxic Activity

The newly synthesized compounds were screened for their anticancer potentials against hepatocellular carcinoma HepG2 and cervical carcinoma HeLa. The cytotoxicity of the compounds was determined using MTT assay and DOX as a positive control [28–31].

The cytotoxic activities of the novel synthesized compounds **8–23** were estimated and the obtained results are presented in Figure 4. In general, it can be seen that all synthesized compounds exhibited cytotoxic activities against both tested cancer cell lines. Moreover, it can be seen that both cells reacted in a dose-dependent manner toward the applied concentrations. Additionally, both tested cell lines varied in their response toward different synthesized compounds. Furthermore, based on the IC_{50} values (Table 1) obtained for the tested compounds, it can be seen that cytotoxic activities ranged from very strong to non-cytotoxic. Compounds **13** and **19** exhibited the most potent cytotoxic effect (very strong activity) with IC_{50} 8.78 ± 0.7, 5.16 ± 0.4 µg/mL, and 15.32 ± 1.2 and 4.26 ± 0.3 µg/mL for HepG2 and HeLa cells, respectively. Furthermore, it can be noticed that **Cpd. 19** exhibited more or less stronger activity similar to DOX towards HepG2 cells, (IC_{50} 5.16 ± 0.4 and 4.50 ± 0.2 µg/mL, respectively). On the other hand, it was stronger by about 23.5% than DOX against HeLa cells (4.50 ±

0.2 and 5.57 ± 0.4 µg/mL, respectively). Additionally, **Cpd. 18** showed very strong activity towards HcLa cells with IC$_{50}$value of 7.67 ± 0.6 µg/mL, while it exhibited strong activity towards HepG2 cells (IC$_{50}$ 16.70 ± 1.3 µg/mL). Moreover, **Cpd. 14** showed strong cytotoxic activities towards both tested cell lines (IC$_{50}$values 12.20 ± 1.0 and 19.44 ± 1.4 µg/mL for HepG2 and HeLa cells, respectively). Meanwhile, **Cpds. 16** and **22** showed moderate and strong activities towards both cell lines. **Cpd. 16** showed IC$_{50}$value of 33.45 ± 2.3 and 10.37 ± 0.9 µg/mL against HepG2 and HeLa cells, respectively. Also, **Cpd. 22** showed IC$_{50}$ of 26.64 ± 1.9 and 9.33 ± 0.8 µg/mL for HepG2 and HeLa cells, respectively. On the other hand, **Cpd. 17** showed strong activity towards HepG2 cells (IC$_{50}$ 20.00 ± 1.7 µg/mL) and moderate activity towards HeLa cells (IC$_{50}$ 35.58 ± 2.6 µg/mL). Finally, **Cpds. 9**, **10**, **11**, **12**, **15a**, **b**, **17**, **20**, **21** and **23** showed activities ranging from moderate to non-cytotoxic, with IC$_{50}$ values ranging from 24.83 ± 1.8 to >100 µg/mL.

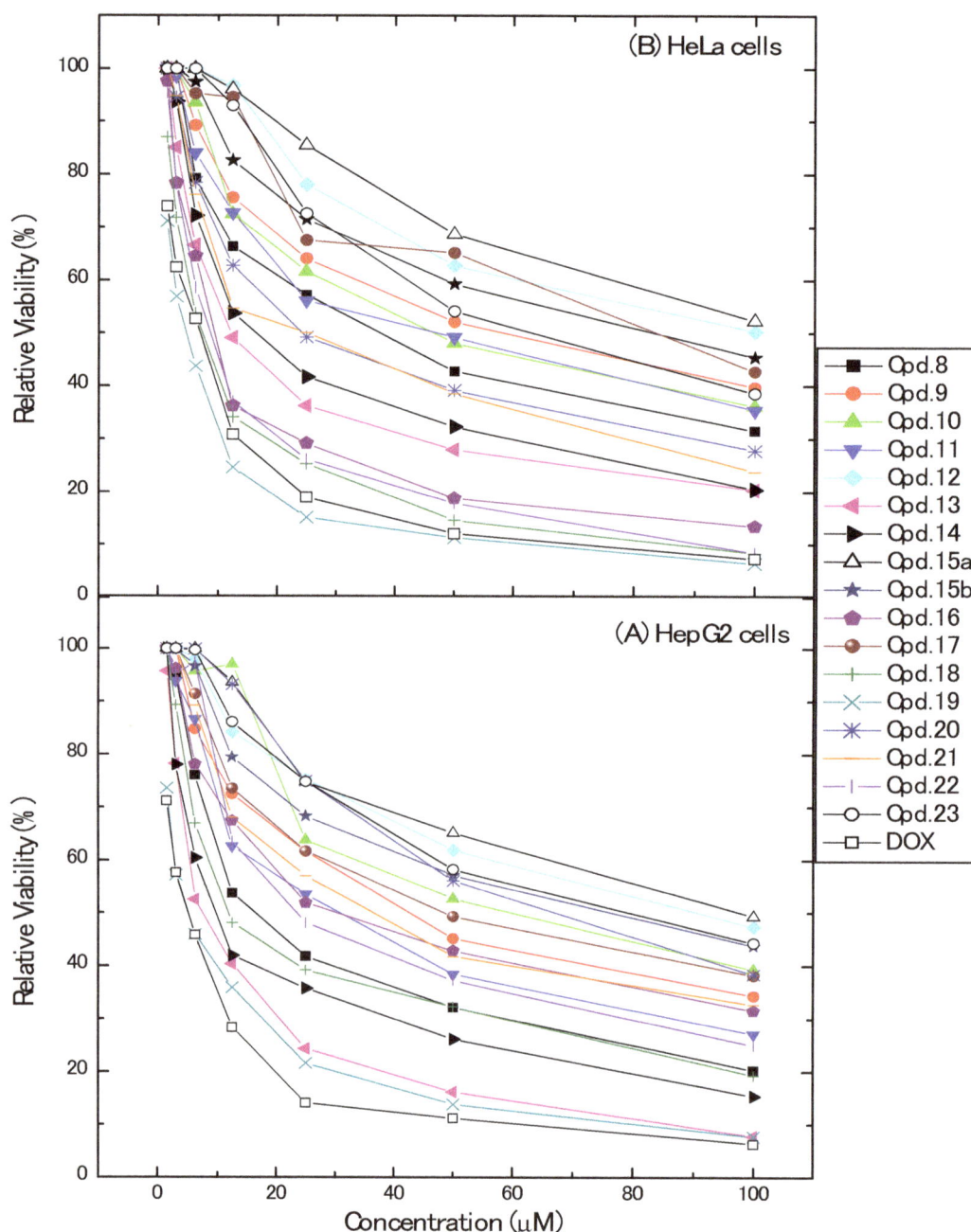

Figure 4. Relative viabilities of HepG2 and HeLa cells as affected by different synthesized compounds.

Table 1. IC_{50} values obtained for the tested compounds against both HepG2 and HeLa cell lines.

Compound	IC_{50} (µM) *	
	HepG2	HeLa
8	20.00 ± 1.7	35.58 ± 2.6
9	42.95 ± 3.2	55.00 ± 3.7
10	56.57 ± 3.4	47.02 ± 3.4
11	30.22 ± 2.1	43.64 ± 3.3
12	83.82 ± 4.5	89.72 ± 4.7
13	8.87 ± 0.70	15.32 ± 1.2
14	12.20 ± 1.0	19.44 ± 1.4
15a	90.05 ± 5.1	>100
15b	68.19 ± 3.7	75.05 ± 4.5
16	33.45 ± 2.3	10.37 ± 0.9
17	49.66 ± 3.2	65.91 ± 4.1
18	16.70 ± 1.3	7.67 ± 0.60
19	5.16 ± 0.40	4.26 ± 0.30
20	64.39 ± 3.6	28.15 ± 2.2
21	37.42 ± 2.5	24.83 ± 1.8
22	26.64 ± 1.9	9.33 ± 0.80
23	73.48 ± 4.0	62.07 ± 3.9
Doxorubicin	4.50 ± 0.20	5.57 ± 0.40

* IC_{50}: 1–10 is (very strong), 11–20 is (strong), 21–50 is (moderate), 51–100 is (weak) and above is 100 (non-cytotoxic).

3. Discussion

During current work, multi-component reaction strategy was used to synthesize of compound **8**, which was used as a building block for preparing **16** new derivatives. The cytotoxic potential of the new prepared compounds has been evaluated against HepG2 and HeLa cells. Results obtained showed potential cytotoxic activities against both cell lines. Compounds **13** and **19** showed the most cytotoxic effects (IC_{50} 8.78 ± 0.7 and 5.16 ± 0.4 µg/mL, for HepG2 cells, and 15.32 ± 1.2 and 4.26 ± 0.3 µg/mL for HeLa cells, respectively). Also, results showed that both tested cell lines varied in their response toward different synthesized compounds. This can be attributed to the inherent differences in both cell lines in terms of membrane structure and organization, hence different cell lines react differently towards different compounds [32–35].

Different activities of the prepared compounds may be attributed to the structure–activity relationship of these compounds. It can be seen that conversion of **Cpd. 12** to **13**, **14** and **16**, **18**, **19** and **22** altered the cytotoxicity from weak to moderate and strong activity towards two cell lines. This explained due to the introduction of two more nitrile groups, which significantly increased the activity. Compound **14** exhibited very strong activity due to the entity of the SH and NH groups, which may be added to any unsaturated group in DNA (thia or aza Michael addition) or the formation of hydrogen bonds with either one of the nucleo-bases of the DNA, thus causing DNA damage. Furthermore, the cytotoxicity of **Cpd. 16** may be due to the intermolecular hydrogen bonding of NH and NH_2 groups with DNA moieties. Additionally, conversion of **Cpd. 16** to **18**, **19** and **22** increased their cytotoxic activities against both cell lines. Introducing thiophene ring increases the cytotoxic effect of **Cpd. 18** beside the effect of the pyrazole ring and the trifluoromethyl group. Additionally, introducing pyrazole ring bearing NH_2 group to **Cpd. 16** increases the cytotoxic effect of **Cpd. 19** to very strong effect against both cell lines. The introduction of chloroiso- indoline-1,3-dione increases the cytotoxic effects of **Cpd. 22**. The chloro- group, with more electron withdrawing properties, may be the crucial for tumor cell inhibition beside the effect of the isoindoline-1,3-dioneas moderate cytokine inhibitor in cancer cells.

4. Materials and Methods

4.1. Chemistry

"Melting points reported are inaccurate. IR spectra were registered on Shimadzu FT-IR 8300 E (Shimadzu Corporation, Kyoto, Japan) spectrophotometer using the (KBr) disk technique. ^{1}H-NMR spectra were determined on a Varian Spectrophotometer at 400 MHz using (TMS) as an internal reference and DMSO-d_6 as solvent using (TMS) as internal standard. All chemical shifts (δ) are uttered in ppm. The mass spectra were determined using (MP) model MS-5988 and Shimadzu single focusing mass spectrophotometer (70 eV). Elemental analysis was investigated by Elemental analyzer Vario EL III".

4.1.1. Synthesis of 4-(3-(4-fluorophenyl)-1-phenyl-1H-pyrazol-4-yl)-2-hydroxy-6-(naphthalen-1-yl)-nicotinenitrile (8)

A mixture of 1-acetyl naphthalene (**A**) (1.7 g, 0.01 mol), ethyl cyanoacetate (1.3 g, 0.01 mol), aldehyde (**B**) (3.6 g, 0.01 mol), ammonium acetate (5.40 g, 0.07 mol) and three drops of piperidine in ethanol (20 mL) was heated under reflux for 3 h. The obtained precipitate was filtered off, washed with cold water, dried and crystallized from ethanol/dioxane to give compound 8. Yield 75%, yellow powder, m.p. > 300 °C; IR (KBr): ν (cm^{-1}) 3159 (OH), 2220 (C≡N), 1647 (C=N); ^{1}H-NMR (DMSO-d_6): δ (ppm) 12.89 (s, 1H, OH, disappeared by D$_2$O), 9.80 (s, 1H, pyrazole-H), 8.39–7.78 (m, 7H, Ar-H for naphthalene), 7.75–7.37 (m, 10H, Ar-H). ^{13}C NMR (DMSO-d_6): δ (ppm) 149.8 (C-OH), 139.3 (C=N), 119.3 (C≡N), 139.4, 134.3, 133.8, 133.5, 131.6, 131.2, 131.0, 130.9, 130.4, 130.3, 130.2, 129.9, 129.4, 129.3, 129.2, 129.1, 128.9, 128.2, 127.8, 127.6, 127.0, 125.6, 125.1, 117.4, 114.8 (Ar-CH), 40.6, 39.9 (aliph-C); MS m/z (ESI): 482 [M$^+$] (22), 465 (21), 440 (12), 237 (100), 204; Anal. Calcd. for C$_{31}$H$_{19}$FN$_4$O (482.50): C, 77.17; H, 3.97; N, 11.61. Found C, 76.98; H, 3.78; N, 11.52%.

4.1.2. Synthesis of ethyl 2-(3-cyano-4-(3-(4-fluorophenyl)-1-phenyl-1H-pyrazol-4-yl)-6-(naphthalene-1-yl)-2-oxopyridin-1(2H)-yl)acetate (9)

A mixture of 8 (4.84 g, 0.01 mol), ethylchloroacetate (1.22 g, 0.01 mol) and K$_2$CO$_3$ (2.2 g, 0.015 mol) in (CH$_3$)$_2$O (40 mL) was heated under reflux for 24 h, concentrated and poured on water; the obtained precipitate was collected by filteration off, dried and crystallized from EtOH/dioxane to give 9. Yield 74%, m.p. 158–160 °C; IR (KBr): ν (cm^{-1}) 2204 (C≡N), 1751 (C=O ester), 1651 (C=O pyridine); ^{1}H-NMR (DMSO-d_6): δ (ppm) 9.15 (s, 1H, pyrazole-5H), 8.10–7.49 (m, 7H, Ar-H for naphthalene), 7.48–7.33 (m, 10H, Ar-H), 4.16 (q, 2H, -CH$_2$ ester), 3.40 (s, 2H, -CH$_2$), 1.20 (t, 3H, -CH$_3$, ester); MS m/z (ESI): 568 [M$^+$] (2.5), 495 (65), 237 (80), 127 (100); Anal. Calcd. for C$_{35}$H$_{25}$FN$_4$O$_3$ (568.60): C, 73.93; H, 4.43, N, 9.85. Found C, 73.80; H, 4.21; N, 9.64%.

4.1.3. Synthesis of 8-(3-(4-fluorophenyl)-1-phenyl-1H-pyrazol-4-yl)-6-(naphthalen-1-yl)-3-oxo-3,4-dihydro-2H-pyrido[2,1-c][1,2,4]triazine-9-carbonitrile (10)

A mixture of 9 (5.7 g, 0.01 mol), NH$_2$NH$_2$ηH$_2$O (2 mL, 0.04 mol) and EtOH (20 mL) was heated under reflux for 3 h. The outward appearance solid was filtered off, dried and crystallized from EtOH/dioxane to give 10. Yield 71%, yellow powder, m.p. > 300 °C; IR (KBr): ν (cm^{-1}) 3209 (NH), 2218 (C≡N), 1647 (C=O); ^{1}H-NMR (DMSO-d_6): δ (ppm) 12.38 (s, 1H, NH, disappeared in D$_2$O), 9.13 (s, 1H, pyrazole-5H), 8.87–7.65 (m, 7H, Ar-H for naphthalene), 7.63–6.85 (m, 10H, Ar-H), 6.10 (s, 2H, CH$_2$). ^{13}C-NMR (DMSO-d_6): δ (ppm) 165.8 (C=O), 139.7 (C=N), 136.1 (C=N), 133.8, 133.4, 131.7, 130.9, 130.8, 130.7, 130.6, 130.3, 130.2, 130.1, 129.9, 129.7, 129.2, 129.1, 128.8, 128.5, 128.1, 127.3, 126.8, 125.8, 125.6, 119.2, 119.1, 118.9, 118.5, 117.6 (Ar-CH), 119.3 (C≡N), 40.5, 39.9 (2CH), 17.6 (CH$_2$); MS m/z (ESI): 519 [M$^+$ − OH] (82), 393 (64), 284 (100), 237 (68), 127 (56); Anal. Calcd. for C$_{33}$H$_{21}$FN$_6$O (536.50): C, 73.87; H, 3.94; N, 15.66. Found C, 73.68; H, 3.24; N, 15.06%.

4.1.4. Synthesis of 5-(3-(4-fluorophenyl)-1-phenyl-1H-pyrazol-4-yl)-7-(naphthalen-1-yl)-2-oxo-1,2-dihydro-1,8-naphthyridine-3-carbonitrile (11)

Refluxing of compound 8 (4.84 g, 0.01 mol) with malononitrile (0.015 mol) in ethanol (20 mL) in the presence of drops of TEA for 5 h, then cooled, poured on ice/water, neutralized with drops of conc. HCl. The obtained solid was collected by filtration, crystallized from EtOH/dioxane to afford 11. Yield 71%, pale brown powder, m.p. > 300 °C; IR (KBr): ν (cm^{-1}) 3386, 3273 (NH$_2$), 3158 (NH), 2218 (C≡N), 1646 (C=O), ^{1}H-NMR (DMSO-d$_6$): δ (ppm) 12.89 (s, 1H, NH, disappeared by D$_2$O), 9.08 (s, 1H, pyrazole-5H), 8.07–7.61 (m, 7H, Ar-H for naphthalene), 7.60–7.37 (m, 10H, Ar-H), 6.22 (s, 2H, NH$_2$, disappeared in D$_2$O). ^{13}C-NMR (DMSO-d$_6$): δ (ppm) 149.9 (C=O), 139.3 (C=N), 133.8, 133.5, 131.2, 131.1, 131.00 (2), 130.9, 130.4, 130.3 (2), 130.2, 129.9 (2), 129.4, 129.1, 128.9 (2), 128.2, 127.8(2), 127.6, 127.1 (2), 125.6, 125.2 (2), 117.4, 116.8, 110.0 (Ar-CH), 119.3 (C≡N), 40.6, 39.9 (2CH); MS m/z (ESI): 532 [M$^+$ − NH$_3$] (82), 516 (76), 440 (28), 310 (20), 237 (100); Anal. Calcd. for C$_{34}$H$_{21}$FN$_6$O (548.50): C, 74.44; H, 3.89; N, 15.32. Found C, 74.24; H, 3.25; N, 14.98%.

4.1.5. Synthesis of 2-chloro-4-(3-(4-fluorophenyl)-1-phenyl-1H-pyrazol-4-yl)-6-(naphthalen-1-yl)-nicotinenitrile (12)

A mixture of 8 (4.82 g, 0.01 mol), PCl$_5$ (3 g, 0.03 mol) and POCl$_3$ (5 mL, 0.03 mol) was heated under reflux for 8 h, then it was poured on crushed ice. The formed solid was filtered off, dried and crystallized from EtOH/dioxane to give 12. Yield 61%, yellow powder, m.p. 164–166 °C; IR (KBr): ν (cm^{-1}) 2227 (C≡N), 1628 (C=N); ^{1}H-NMR (DMSO-d$_6$): δ (ppm) 9.16 (s, 1H, pyrazole-5H), 8.35–7.63 (m, 7H, Ar-H for naphthalene), 7.61–7.39 (m, 10H, Ar-H). ^{13}C-NMR (DMSO-d$_6$): δ (ppm) 152.7, 150.0, 148.4, 139.2 (C=N), 135.3(C=N), 133.8, 131.5, 131.0, 130.4, 130.3, 130.2, 129.8, 129.5, 129.2 (2), 129.1, 127.9, 127.6, 126.9, 125.8 (2), 125.4, 125.1, 119.3 (C≡N), 116.6, 115.5, 107.8 (Ar-CH), 40.6, 39.9 (2CH); MS m/z (ESI): 503 [M$^+$ + 2] (6), 501 [M$^+$] (50), 465 (100), 237 (82); Anal. Calcd. for C$_{31}$H$_{18}$ClFN$_4$ (500.90): C, 74.32; H, 3.62; N, 11.84. Found C, 74.12; H, 3.26; N, 11.42%.

4.1.6. Synthesis of 2-[4-(3-(4-fluorophenyl)-1-phenyl-1H-pyrazol-4-yl)-6-(naphthalen-1-yl)-3-cyano-pyridinyl]malononitrile (13)

To a solution of 12 (5.0 g, 0.01 mol) in EtOH (20 mL), malononitrile (0.01 mol) and TEA (1 mL) were added. The reaction mixture was heated under for 3 h. After cooling, it was poured on water and neutralized with diluted HCl. The obtained solid was separated by filtration, washed with water, dried and crystallized from EtOH/dioxane to yield 13. Yield 76%, pale brown powder, m.p. 194–196 °C; IR (KBr): ν (cm^{-1}) 2203 (C≡N), ^{1}H-NMR (DMSO-d$_6$): δ (ppm) 9.15 (s, 1H, pyrazole-5H), 8.11–7.66 (m, 7H, Ar-H for naphthalene), 7.65–7.36 (m, 10H, Ar-H), 7.07 (s, 1H, CH of CH(CN)$_2$), MS m/z (ESI): 530 [M$^+$] (12), 440 (100), 237 (76), 204 (31); Anal. Calcd. for C$_{34}$H$_{19}$FN$_6$ (530.50): C, 76.97; H, 3.61; N, 15.84. Found C, 76.78; H, 3.42; N, 15.24%.

4.1.7. Synthesis of 14 and 15a,b

A mixture of 2-chloronicotinonitrile 12 (5.0 g, 0.01 mol) and the appropriate amine, namely, o-aminothiophenol, morpholine or 2-methylpiperidine (0.01 mol) in EtOH (20 mL) was heated under reflux for 3 h, then it was poured on cold water, filtered off and crystallized from EtOH/dioxane to afford 14 and 15a,b, respectively.

4-(3-(4-Fluorophenyl)-1-phenyl-1H-pyrazol-4-yl)-2-(2-mercaptophenylamino)-6-(naphthalen-1-yl) nicotinonitrile (14). Yield 74%, brown powder, m.p. 108–110 °C; IR (KBr): ν (cm^{-1}) 3330 (NH), 2208 (C≡N), ^{1}H-NMR (DMSO-d$_6$): δ (ppm) 9.29 (s, 1H, pyrazole-5H), 9.06–8.54 (m, 4H, Ar-H, thionyl-H), 8.26–7.66 (m, 7H, Ar-H for naphthalene), 7.60–6.66 (m, 10H, Ar-H), 3.34 (s, 1H, NH, disappeared in D2O), 1.20 (s, 1H, SH, disappeared in D$_2$O). MS m/z (ESI): 589 [M$^+$] (32), 465 (82), 441 (62), 237 (100), 127(12), 124 (20); Anal. Calcd. for C$_{37}$H$_{24}$FN$_5$O (589.60): C, 75.36, H, 4.10; N, 11.88. Found C, 75.18; H, 4.05; N, 11.73%.

4-(3-(4-Fluorophenyl)-1-phenyl-1H-pyrazol-4-yl)-2-morpholino-6-(naphthalen-1-yl)nicotino-nitrile (**15a**). Yield 65%, pale brown powder, m.p. 130–133 °C; IR (KBr): ν (cm^{-1}) 2226 (C≡N), ^{1}H-NMR (DMSO-d$_6$): δ (ppm) 9.16 (s, 1H, pyrazole-5H), 8.71–7.56 (m, 7H, Ar-H for naphthalene), 7.55–7.15 (m, 10H, Ar-H), 3.76 (t, 4H, J = 8.8 Hz), 3.05 (t, 4H, J = 8.8 Hz), MS m/z (ESI): 552 [M$^+$] (52), 465 (28), 237 (100), 230 (7), 127 (12), 87 (22); Anal. Calcd. for C$_{35}$H$_{26}$FN$_5$O (551.60): C, 76.21; H, 4.75; N, 12.70. Found C, 75.98; H, 4.26; N, 12.31%.

4-(3-(4-Fluorophenyl)-1-phenyl-1H-pyrazol-4-yl)-2-(4-methylpiperazin-1-yl)-6-(naphthalen-1-yl) nicotinonitrile (**15b**). Yield 61%, brown powder, m.p. 156–158 °C; IR (KBr): ν (cm^{-1}) 2918 (aliph-H), 2227 (C≡N), ^{1}H-NMR (DMSO-d$_6$): δ (ppm) 9.18 (s, 1H, pyrazole-5H), 8.71–7.65 (m, 7H, Ar-H for naphthalene), 7.64–7.12 (m, 10H, Ar-H), 3.30–3.25 (m, 4H, 2CH$_2$), 2.43–2.23 (m, 4H, 2CH$_2$), 2.24 (s, 3H, CH$_3$), MS m/z (ESI): 564 [M$^+$] (27), 538 (25), 439 (12), 237 (100), 100 (23); Anal. Calcd. for C$_{35}$H$_{29}$FN$_6$ (564.60): C, 76.58, H, 5.18; N, 14.88. Found C, 75.98; H, 4.92; N, 14.72%.

4.1.8. Synthesis of 4-(3-(4-Fluorophenyl)-1-phenyl-1H-pyrazol-4-yl)-2-hydrazinyl-6-(naphthalen-1-yl) nicotinonitrile (16)

A mixture of the 2-chloronicotinonitrile **12** (5.0 g, 0.01 mol) and NH$_2$NH$_2$·H$_2$O (0.04 mol) in EtOH (20 mL) was heated under reflux for 4h. The obtained solid was collected by filtration, dried and crystallized from EtOH/dioxane to yield **16**. Yield 86%, yellow powder, m.p. 164–168 °C; IR (KBr): ν (cm^{-1}) 3417, 3310 (NH$_2$), 3199 (NH), 2206 (C≡N), ^{1}H-NMR (DMSO-d$_6$): δ (ppm) 9.16 (s, 1H, pyrazole-5H), 8.35–7.97 (m, 7H, Ar-H for naphthalene), 7.96–6.88 (m, 10H, Ar-H), 4.82 (s, 1H, NH, disappeared in D$_2$O), 3.43 (s, 2H, NH$_2$, disappeared in D$_2$O). ^{13}C-NMR (DMSO-d$_6$): δ (ppm) 149.3 (C-NHNH$_2$), 148.3, 139.7 (C≡N), 139.2, 138.5, 136.1 (C=N), 135.3, 134.0, 133.8, 131.7, 131.5, 131.0, 130.9, 130.4, 130.2, 130.1, 129.5, 129.1, 128.1, 127.9, 127.6, 127.3, 126.9, 126.7, 126.4, 125.8, 125.4, 119.3 (C≡N), 118.2 (Ar-CH), 40.6, 40.0 (2CH); MS m/z (ESI): 496 [M$^+$] (12), 465 (81), 440 (100), 237 (20), 204 (76); Anal. Calcd. for C$_{31}$H$_{21}$FN$_6$ (496.55): C, 74.99; H, 4.26; N, 16.93. Found C, 74.86; H, 4.12; N, 16.78%.

4.1.9. Synthesis of 17 and 18

A mixture of **16** (4.9 g, 0.01 mol), acetylacetone or 4,4,4-trifluoro-1-(thiophen-2-yl)butane-1,3-dione (0.01 mol) in EtOH (10 mL) and AcOH (4 mL) was heated reflux for 3 h. After cooling, the solid obtained was filtered off, dried and crystallized from EtOH/dioxane to afford **17** and **18**, respectively.

2-(3,5-Dimethyl-1H-pyrazol-1-yl)-4-(3-(4-fluorophenyl)-1-phenyl-1H-pyrazol-4-yl)-6-(naphthalen-1-yl)nicotinonitrile (**17**). Yield 85%, pale orange powder, m.p. 270–272 °C; IR (KBr): ν (cm^{-1}) 2209 (C≡N), 1620 (C=N), ^{1}H-NMR (DMSO-d$_6$): δ (ppm) 9.24 (s, 1H, pyrazole-5H), 8.17–7.96 (m, 7H, Ar-H for naphthalene), 7.66–7.35 (m, 10H, Ar-H), 7.25 (s, 1H, pyrazole-4H), 2.48 (s, 6H, 2 CH$_3$); MS m/z (ESI): 560 [M$^+$] (13), 533 (26), 438 (62), 237 (15), 95 (100); Anal. Calcd. for C$_{36}$H$_{25}$FN$_6$ (560.60): C, 77.13; H, 4.49; N, 14.99. Found C, 76.92; H, 4.32; N, 14.81%.

4-(3-(4-Fluorophenyl)-1-phenyl-1H-pyrazol-4-yl)-6-(naphthalen-1-yl)-2-(5-(thiophen-2-yl)-3-(tri-fluoromethyl)-1H-pyrazol-1-yl)nicotinonitrile (**18**). Yield 82%, dark yellow powder, m.p. 117–119 °C; IR (KBr): ν (cm^{-1}) 2209 (C≡N), ^{1}H-NMR (DMSO-d$_6$): δ (ppm) 8.92 (s, 1H, pyrazole-5H), 8.03–7.89 (m, 7H, Ar-H for naphthalene), 7.59–7.54 (m, 3H, thionyl-H), 7.53–7.33 (m, 10H, Ar-H), 6.88 (s, 1H, pyrazole-4H); MS m/z (ESI): 583 [M$^+$] (10), 465 (72), 237 (100), 299 (8), 217 (5); Anal. Calcd. for C$_{39}$H$_{22}$F$_4$N$_6$S (682.60): C, 68.61; H, 3.25; N, 12.31. Found C, 68.02; H, 3.12; N, 12.03%.

4.1.10. Synthesis of 19 and 20

A solution of **16** (4.9 g, 0.01 mol) in a mixture of AcOH/Ac$_2$O (10 mL) or in glacial AcOH (10 mL) was refluxed for 2 h, poured on ice/water, filtered off and crystallized from EtOH/dioxane to give **19** and **20**, respectively. Also, refluxing of **19** (0.5 g, 0.01 mol) in acetic anhydride (7 mL) afforded compound **20**.

4-(3-(4-Flurophenyl)-1-phenyl-1H-pyrazol-4-yl)-6-(naphthalen-1-yl)-1H-pyrazolo[3,4-b]pyridin-3-amine (**19**). Yield 84%, pale yellow powder, m.p. 140–143 °C; IR (KBr): ν (cm^{-1}) 3425–3354 (NH$_2$),

3198 (NH), ^{1}H-NMR (DMSO-d$_6$): δ (ppm) 8.92 (s, 1H, pyrazole-5H), 8.22–7.90 (m, 7H, Ar-H for naphthalene), 7.66–7.34 (m, 10H, Ar–H), 5.02 (s, 2H, NH2, disappeared in D$_2$O), 4.63 (s, 1H, NH, disappeared in D$_2$O); MS m/z (ESI): 496 [M$^+$] (28), 479 (76), 244 (50), 237 (100); Anal. Calcd. for C$_{31}$H$_{21}$FN$_6$ (496.52): C, 74.99; H, 4.26; N, 16.93. Found C, 74.76; H, 4.15; N, 16.82%.

N-(4-(3-(4-Flurophenyl)-1-phenyl-1H-pyrazol-4-yl)-6-(naphthalen-1-yl)-1H-pyrazolo-[3,4-b] pyridin-3-yl)acetamide (**20**). Yield 78%, yellow powder, m.p. 138–140 °C; IR (KBr): ν (cm^{-1}) 3196 (NH), 1690 (C=O), ^{1}H-NMR (DMSO-d$_6$): δ (ppm) 12.37 & 10.31 (s, NH, OH), 8.88 (s, 1H, pyrazole- 5H), 7.98–7.59 (m, 7H, Ar-H for naphthalene), 7.57–6.88 (m, 10H, Ar-H), 4.82 (s, 1H, NH, disappeared in D$_2$O), 2.73 (s, 3H, acetyl); MS m/z (ESI): 538 [M$^+$] (20), 479 (36), 244 (20), 237 (100); Anal. Calcd. for C$_{33}$H$_{23}$FN$_6$O (538.59): C, 73.59; H, 4.30; N, 15.60. Found C, 73.28; H, 4.19; N, 15.32%.

4.1.11. Synthesis of N-(4-chlorobenzylidene)-4-(3-(4-fluorophenyl)-1-phenyl-1H-pyrazol-4-yl)-6-(naphthalen-1-yl)-1H-pyrazolo[3,4-b]pyridine-3-amine (**21**)

A solution of **16** or **19** (0.01 mol) in AcOH (10 mL) in the presence of 4-chlorobenzaldehyde (0.01 mol) was heated under reflux for 2 h, left to precipitate, filtered and crystallized from EtOH/ dioxane to afford **21**. Yield 58%, yellow powder, m.p. 158–160 °C; IR (KBr): ν (cm^{-1}) 3192 (NH), ^{1}H-NMR (DMSO-d$_6$): δ (ppm) 9.89 (s, 1H, pyrazole-5H), 9.06 (s, 1H, N=C-H), 8.87–7.56 (m, 7H, Ar-H for naphthalene), 7.52–6.88 (m, 14H, Ar-H), 4.82 (s, 1H, NH, disappeared in D$_2$O); MS m/z (ESI): 621 [M$^+$] (15), 619 (48), 479 (20), 237 (80), 139 (35), 137 (100); Anal. Calcd. for C$_{38}$H$_{24}$ClFN$_6$ (619.10): C, 73.72; H, 3.91; N, 13.57. Found C, 73.25; H, 3.82; N, 13.27%.

4.1.12. Synthesis of 2-(4-(3-(4-fluorophenyl)-1-phenyl-1H-pyrazol-4-yl)-6-(naphthalen-1-yl)-1H-pyrazolo[3,4-b]-pyridin-3-yl)isoindoline-1,3-dione (**22**)

A mixture of **16** or **19** (0.01 mol) and tetrachlorophthalic anhydride (0.01 mol) in glacial acetic acid (10 mL) was refluxed for 1 h, poured on ice water, filtered off and crystallized from EtOH/dioxane to yield **22**. Yield 94%, yellow powder, m.p. 115–117 °C; IR (KBr): ν (cm^{-1}) 3196 (NH), 1785, 1731 (C=O); ^{1}H-NMR (DMSO-d$_6$): δ (ppm) 8.87 (s, 1H, pyrazole-5H), 8.04–7.56 (m, 7H, Ar-H for naphthalene), 7.55–7.33 (m, 10H, Ar-H), 4.28 (s, 1H, NH, disappeared in D$_2$O); Anal. Calcd. for C$_{39}$H$_{19}$Cl$_4$FN$_6$O$_2$ (764.42): C, 61.28; H, 2.51; N, 10.99. Found C, 61.00; H, 2.42; N, 10.89%.

4.1.13. Synthesis of 7-(3-(4-fluorophenyl)-1-phenyl-1H-pyrazol-4-yl)-5-(naphthalen-1-yl)-3-thioxo-2,3-dihydro[1,2,4]triazolo[4,3-a]pyridine-8-carbonitrile (**23**)

Solution of hydrazinyl derivative **16** (4.9 g, 0.01 mol) in alcoholic KOH (10%, 20 mL) and CS$_2$ (0.01 mol) was refluxed for 2 h, lift overnight, then poured on ice water, filtered off the solid obtained and crystallized from EtOH/dioxane to afford **23**. Yield 47% yellow powder, m.p. 288–290 °C; IR (KBr): ν (cm^{-1}) 3192 (NH), 2218 (C≡N), 1240 (C=S); ^{1}H-NMR (DMSO-d$_6$): δ (ppm) 8.73 (s, 1H, pyrazole-5H), 7.97–7.63 (m, 7H, Ar-H for naphthalene), 7.53–6.77 (m, 10H, Ar-H), 3.76 (s, 1H, NH, disappeared in D$_2$O). ^{13}C-NMR (DMSO-d$_6$): δ (ppm) 148.1 (C=S), 142.3, 138.7 (C=N), 133.8 (2), 133.4 (C=N), 131.7 (2), 131.2, 130.6 (2), 130.1, 129.9 (2), 129.4, 129.2 (2), 128.9, 128.4 (2), 126.9, 126.4 (2), 126.3 (2), 125.9 (2), 119.1 (C≡N), 110.0 (Ar-CH), 40.5, 39.9 (2CH); MS m/z (ESI): 538 [M$^+$] (45), 494 (18), 479 (10), 453 (50), 237 (100); Anal. Calcd. for C$_{32}$H$_{19}$FN$_6$S (538.60): C, 71.36; H, 3.56; N, 15.60. Found C, 71.31; H, 3.52; N, 15.58%.

4.2. Cytotoxicity Assay

4.2.1. Materials and Cell Lines

Hepatocellular carcinoma (HepG2) and cervical Carcinoma (HeLa) cell lines, ATCC, VA, USA, were used throughout the work. All used chemicals and reagents were of high purity-cell culture grade.

4.2.2. MTT Assay

Cytotoxic assay depends on the formation of purple formazan crystals by the action of dehydrogenase in living cells. Cells were cultured in RPMI-1640 medium supplemented with 10% fetal bovine serum, antibiotic solution (100 units/mL penicillin, 100 µg/mL streptomycin) at 37 °C in a 5% CO2 incubator. Cells were seeded in a 96-well plate (10^4 cells/well), and the plates were incubated for 48 h. Afterwards, cells were exposed to variable concentrations of prepared derivatives and incubation proceeded for further 24 h. After treatment, 20 µL of MTT solution (5 mg/mL) was added and incubated for 4 h. DMSO (100 µL/well) is added and the developed color density was measured at 570 nm using a plate reader (ELx 800, BioTek, Winuski, VT, USA). Relative cell viability was calculated as (Atreated/Auntreated) ×100 [36,37]. Results were compared with doxorubicin as a positive control.

5. Conclusions

During the current investigation, we synthesized a new building block; namely 4-(3-(4-fluorophenyl)-1-phenyl-1H-pyrazol-4-yl)-2-hydroxy-6-(naphthalen-1-yl)nicotinonitril, with the help of multicomponent reaction systems. From that compound, a series of **16** different nicotinonitril derivatives were synthesized, and their structural and spectral data were elucidated. Furthermore, in vitro cytotoxic activities against hepatocellular and cervical carcinoma cell lines were investigated. Obtained results revealed that different synthesized compounds showed promising in vitro cytotoxic activities against both HepG2 and HeLa cell lines. Compounds **13** and **19** showed the most potent cytotoxic effect (IC$_{50}$: 8.78 ± 0.7, 5.16 ± 0.4 µg/mL, and 15.32 ± 1.2 and 4.26 ± 0.3 µg/mL for HepG2 and HeLa cells, respectively.

Author Contributions: The listed authors contributed to this work as described in the following: A.A.E.-S. and A.K.E.-Z. synthesis, and interpreted the spectroscopic identification of the synthesized compounds, A.E.-G.E.A. and E.A.E. are interpreted the results, the experimental part and E.A.E. performed the revision before submission. All authors read and approved the final manuscript.

Acknowledgments: The authors are appreciative to Faculty of Science, Ain Shams University where the experimental part carried out in its laboratories and Faculty of Pharmaceutical, El-Masoura University to carry the anticancer activity in it.

References

1. Rajeswari, M.; Saluja, P.; Khurana, J.M. A facile and green approach for the synthesis of spiro[naphthalene-2,50-pyrimidine]-4-carbonitrile via a one-pot three-component condensation reaction using DBU as a catalyst. *Rsc. Adv.* **2016**, *6*, 1307–1312. [CrossRef]
2. El-Sayed, H.A.; Moustafa, A.H.; Haikal, A.Z.; Abu-El-Halawa, R.; El Ashry, E.H. Synthesis, antitumor and antimicrobial activities of 4-(4-chlorophenyl)-3-cyano-2-(b-o-glycosyloxy)-6-(thien-2-yl)nicotine- nitrile. *Eur. J. Med. Chem.* **2011**, *46*, 2948–2954. [CrossRef]
3. Kotb, E.R.; El-Hashash, M.A.; Salama, M.A.; Kalf, H.S.; Abdel Wahed, N.A.M. Synthesis and reactions of some novel nicotinonitrile derivatives for anticancer and antimicrobial evaluation. *Acta Chim. Slov.* **2009**, *56*, 908–919.
4. Hamdy, N.A.; Anwar, M.M.; Abu-Zied, K.M.; Awad, H.M. Synthesis, tumor inhibitory and antioxidant activity of new polyfunctionally 2-substituted 5,6,7,8-tetrahydronaphthalene derivatives containing pyridine, thioxopyridine and pyrazolopyridine moieties. *Acta Polo. Pharm. Drug Res.* **2013**, *70*, 987–1001.
5. Salem, M.S.; Sakr, S.I.; El-Senousy, W.M.; Madkour, H.M.F.; El-Senousy, W.M. Synthesis, Antibacterial, and Antiviral Evaluation of New Heterocycles Containing the Pyridine Moiety. *Arch. der Pharm.* **2013**, *346*, 766–773. [CrossRef]

6. El-Sayed, N.S.; Shirazi, A.N.; El-Meligy, M.G.; El-Ziaty, A.K.; Rowley, D.; Sun, J.; Nagib, Z.A.; Parang, K. Synthesis of 4-aryl-6-indolylpyridine-3-carbonitriles and evaluation of their anti-proliferative activity. *Tetra. Lett.* **2014**, *55*, 1154–1158. [CrossRef]

7. Ruiz, J.F.M.; Kedziora, K.; Keogh, B.; Maguire, J.; Reilly, M.; Windle, H.; Kelleher, D.P.; Gilmer, J.F. A double prodrug system for colon targeting of benzenesulfonamide COX-2 inhibitors. *Bioorganic Med. Chem. Lett.* **2011**, *21*, 6636–6640. [CrossRef]

8. Balsamo, A.; Coletta, I.; Guglielmotti, A.; Landolfi, C.; Mancini, F.; Martinelli, A.; Milanese, C.; Minutolo, F.; Nencetti, S.; Orlandini, E.; et al. Synthesis of heteroaromatic analogues of (2-aryl-1-cyclopentenyl-1-alkylidene)-(arylmethyloxy)amine COX-2 inhibitors: effects on the inhibitory activity of the replacement of the cyclopentene central core with pyrazole, thiophene or isoxazole ring. *Eur. J. Med. Chem.* **2003**, *38*, 157–168. [CrossRef]

9. Karrouchi, K.; Radi, S.; Ramli, Y.; Taoufik, J.; Mabkhot, Y.N.; Al-Aizari, F.A.; Al-Aizari, F.; Ansar, M.; A Al-Aizari, F.; Ansar, M. Synthesis and Pharmacological Activities of Pyrazole Derivatives: A Review. *Molecules* **2018**, *23*, 134. [CrossRef]

10. Bekhit, A.A.; Ashour, H.M.; Ghany, Y.S.A.; Bekhit, A.E.-D.A.; Baraka, A. Synthesis and biological evaluation of some thiazolyl and thiadiazolyl derivatives of 1H-pyrazole as anti-inflammatory antimicrobial agents. *Eur. J. Med. Chem.* **2008**, *43*, 456–463. [CrossRef]

11. Christodoulou, M.S.; Liekens, S.; Kasiotis, K.M.; Haroutounian, S.A. Novel pyrazole derivatives: Synthesis and evaluation of anti-angiogenic activity. *Bioorganic Med. Chem.* **2010**, *18*, 4338–4350. [CrossRef]

12. Bondock, S.; Fadaly, W.; Metwally, M.A. Synthesis and antimicrobial activity of some new thiazole, thiophene and pyrazole derivatives containing benzothiazole moiety. *Eur. J. Med. Chem.* **2010**, *45*, 3692–3701. [CrossRef] [PubMed]

13. Chimenti, F.; Bolasco, A.; Manna, F.; Secci, D.; Chimenti, P.; Befani, O.; Turini, P.; Giovannini, V.; Mondovi, B.; Cirilli, R.; et al. Synthesis and Selective Inhibitory Activity of 1-Acetyl-3,5-diphenyl-4,5-dihydro-(1H)-pyrazole Derivatives against Monoamine Oxidase. *J. Med. Chem.* **2004**, *47*, 2071–2074. [CrossRef]

14. Rashad, A.E.; Hegab, M.I.; Abdel-Megeid, R.E.; Micky, J.A.; Abdel-Megeid, F.M. Synthesis and antiviral evaluation of some new pyrazole and fused pyrazolopyrimidine derivatives. *Bioorganic Med. Chem.* **2008**, *16*, 7102–7106. [CrossRef]

15. Bonesi, M.; Loizzo, M.R.; Statti, G.A.; Michel, S.; Tillequin, F.; Menichini, F. The synthesis and Angiotensin Converting Enzyme (ACE) inhibitory activity of chalcones and their pyrazole derivatives. *Bioorganic Med. Chem. Lett.* **2010**, *20*, 1990–1993. [CrossRef]

16. Mahmoud, M.R.; El-Ziaty, A.K.; Abu El-Azm, F.S.M.; Ismail, M.F.; Shiba, S.A. Utility of Cyano-N-(2-oxo-1,2-dihydroindol-3-ylidene)acetohydrazide in the Synthesis of Novel Heterocycles. *J. Chem.* **2013**, *37*, 80–85. [CrossRef]

17. El-Sayed, N.S.; Shirazi, A.N.; El-Meligy, M.G.; El-Ziaty, A.K.; Nagieb, Z.A.; Parang, K.; Tiwari, R.K. Design, synthesis, and evaluation of chitosan conjugated GGRGDSK peptides as a cancer cell-targeting molecular transporter. *Int. J. Boil. Macromol.* **2016**, *87*, 611–622. [CrossRef]

18. El-Ziaty, A.K.; Shiba, S.A. Antibacterial activities of new (E) 2-cyano-3-(3,4-dimethoxyphenyl) -2-propenoylamide derivatives. *Synth. Commun.* **2007**, *37*, 4043–4057. [CrossRef]

19. Mahmoud, M.R.; Shiba, S.A.; El-Ziaty, A.K.; Abu El-Azm, F.S.M.; Ismail, M.F. Synthesis and reactions of novel 2,5-disubistituted 1,3,4-thiadiazoles. *Synth. Commun.* **2014**, *44*, 1094–1102. [CrossRef]

20. El-Shahawi, M.M.; El-Ziaty, A.K. Enaminonitrile as Building Block in Heterocyclic Synthesis: Synthesis of Novel 4H -Furo[2,3-d][1,3]oxazin-4-one and Furo[2,3- d]pyrimidin-4 (3H) -one Derivatives. *J. Chem.* **2017**, *2017*, 1–6. [CrossRef]

21. Mahmoud, M.R.; El-Ziaty, A.K.; Hussein, A.M. Synthesis and Spectral Characterization of Novel Thiazolopyridine and Pyrimidine Derivatives. *Synth. Commun.* **2013**, *43*, 961–978. [CrossRef]

22. Ismail, M.F.; El-Sayed, A.A. Synthesis and in-vitro antioxidant and antitumor evaluation of novel pyrazole-based heterocycles. *Iran. Chem. Soc.* **2019**, *16*, 921–937. [CrossRef]

23. Fahmy, A.F.M.; Rizk, S.A.; Hemdan, M.M.; El-Sayed, A.A.; Hassaballah, A.I. Efficient Green Synthesis and Computational Chemical Study of Some Interesting Heterocyclic Derivatives as Insecticidal Agents. *J. Chem.* **2018**, *55*, 2545–2555. [CrossRef]

24. Rizk, S.A.; El-Sayed, A.A.; Mounier, M.M.; El-Sayed, A.A. Synthesis of Novel Pyrazole Derivatives as Antineoplastic Agent. *J. Chem.* **2017**, *54*, 3358–3371. [CrossRef]

25. Fahmy, A.F.M.; El-Sayed, A.A.; Hemdan, M.M. Multicomponent synthesis of 4-arylidene-2-phenyl-5(4H)-oxazolones (azlactones) using a mechanochemical approach. *Chem. Central J.* **2016**, *10*, 59. [CrossRef]

26. Hemdan, M.M.; El-Sayed, A.A. Use of phthalimidoacetylisothiocyanate as a scaffold in synthesis of target heterocyclic systems with their antimicrobial assessment. *Chem. Pharm. Bull.* **2016**, *64*, 483–489. [CrossRef]

27. Hemdan, M.M.; El-Sayed, A.A. Synthesis of some new heterocycles derived from novel 2-(1,3-dioxisoindolin-2-yl)benzoyl isothiocyanate. *J. Heterocycl. Chem.* **2016**, *53*, 487–492. [CrossRef]

28. Metwally, M.; Gouda, M.; Harmal, A.N.; Khalil, A. Synthesis, antitumor, cytotoxic and antioxidant evaluation of some new pyrazolotriazines attached to antipyrine moiety. *Eur. J. Med. Chem.* **2012**, *56*, 254–262. [CrossRef] [PubMed]

29. Hossan, A.; Abu-Melha, H. Synthesis, mass spectroscopic studies, cytotoxicity evaluation and quantitative structure activity relationship of novel isoindolin-1,3-dione derivatives. *Chem. Process Eng. Res.* **2014**, *21*, 60–71.

30. Eissa, I.H.; El-Naggar, A.M.; El-Hashash, M.A. Design, synthesis, molecular modeling and biological evaluation of novel 1H-pyrazolo[3,4-b]pyridine derivatives as potential anticancer agents. *Bioorganic Chem.* **2016**, *67*, 43–56. [CrossRef]

31. Shaaban, S.; Negm, A.; Sobh, M.A.; Wessjohann, L.A. Organoselenocyanates and symmetrical diselenides redox modulators: Design, synthesis and biological evaluation. *Eur. J. Med. Chem.* **2015**, *97*, 190–201. [CrossRef]

32. Elsayed, E.A.; Farooq, M.; Dailin, D.; El-Enshasy, H.A.; Othman, N.Z.; Malek, R.; Danial, E.; Wadaan, M. In vitro and in vivo biological screening of kefiran polysaccharide produced by Lactobacillus kefiranofaciens. *Biomed. Res.* **2017**, *28*, 594–600.

33. Amr, A.E.-G.E.; El-Naggar, M.; Al-Omar, M.A.; Elsayed, E.A.; Abdalla, M.M. In Vitro and In Vivo Anti-Breast Cancer Activities of Some Synthesized Pyrazolinyl-estran-17-one Candidates. *Molecules* **2018**, *23*, 1572. [CrossRef]

34. Amr, A.E.-G.E.; Abo-Ghalia, M.H.; Moustafa, G.O.; Al-Omar, M.A.; Nossier, E.S.; Elsayed, E.A. Design, Synthesis and Docking Studies of Novel Macrocyclic Pentapeptides as Anticancer Multi-Targeted Kinase Inhibitors. *Molecules* **2018**, *23*, 2416. [CrossRef]

35. Dailin, D.J.; Elsayed, E.A.; Othman, N.Z.; Malek, R.; Phin, H.S.; Aziz, R.; Wadaan, M.; El Enshasy, H.A. Bioprocess development for kefiran production by *Lactobacillus kefiranofaciens* in semi industrial scale bioreactor. *Saudi J. Biol. Sci.* **2016**, *23*, 495–502. [CrossRef]

36. Mosmann, T. Rapid colorimetric assay for cellular growth and survival: Application to proliferation and cytotoxicity assays. *J. Immunol. Methods* **1983**, *65*, 55–63. [CrossRef]

37. Denizot, F.; Lang, R. Rapid colorimetric assay for cell growth and survival. Modifications to the tetrazolium dye procedure giving improved sensitivity and reliability. *J. Immunol. Methods* **1986**, *89*, 271–277. [CrossRef]

8

Role of Photoactive Phytocompounds in Photodynamic Therapy of Cancer

Kasipandi Muniyandi [1,2], **Blassan George** [1], **Thangaraj Parimelazhagan** [2] and **Heidi Abrahamse** [1,*]

[1] Laser Research Centre, Faculty of Health Sciences, University of Johannesburg, 17011, Doornfontein 2028, South Africa; kasim@uj.ac.za (K.M.); blassang@uj.ac.za (B.G.)

[2] Bioprospecting Laboratory, Department of Botany, School of Life Sciences, Bharathiar University, Coimbatore, Tamil Nadu 641046, India; drparimel@buc.edu.in

* Correspondence: habrahamse@uj.ac.za

Academic Editor: José Antonio Lupiáñez

Abstract: Cancer is one of the greatest life-threatening diseases conventionally treated using chemo- and radio-therapy. Photodynamic therapy (PDT) is a promising approach to eradicate different types of cancers. PDT requires the administration of photosensitisers (PSs) and photoactivation using a specific wavelength of light in the presence of molecular oxygen. This photoactivation exerts an anticancer effect via apoptosis, necrosis, and autophagy of cancer cells. Recently, various natural compounds that exhibit photosensitising potentials have been identified. Photoactive substances derived from medicinal plants have been found to be safe in comparison with synthetic compounds. Many articles have focused on PDT mechanisms and types of PSs, but limited attention has been paid to the phototoxic activities of phytocompounds. The reduced toxicity and side effects of natural compounds inspire the researchers to identify and use plant extracts or phytocompounds as a potent natural PS candidate for PDT. This review focusses on the importance of common photoactive groups (furanocoumarins, polyacetylenes, thiophenes, curcumins, alkaloids, and anthraquinones), their phototoxic effects, anticancer activity and use as a potent PS for an effective PDT outcome in the treatment of various cancers.

Keywords: photodynamic therapy; cancer; photosensitiser; natural compounds

1. Introduction

Cancer is one of the deadliest diseases reported in developed as well as developing countries [1]. It is mainly characterised by the uncontrolled cell growth and development of normal cells due to genetic alterations or exposure to the carcinogenic substances. The mutation of normal cells leads to abnormal cellular proliferation and develops into tumour [2]; this can be either benign, premalignant (non-cancerous) or malignant (cancerous) [3,4]. Presently surgery, radiotherapy, and chemotherapy either as monotherapy or as combined treatments are used in the treatment of cancer. However, these treatments frequently stimulate redundant side effects [2]. Many of the current chemotherapeutic drugs are of low molecular weight with high pharmacokinetic profiles [4]. Hence, in order to achieve the bioavailability and cytotoxicity induction, the drugs are administrated in high concentrations. In photodynamic therapy (PDT), photoactive drugs are generally administered systemically, but because of the precise application of light from the laser source, the cytotoxicity is attained in the tumour location. Due to the lesser drug specificity and toxicity to healthy cells, the chemotherapeutic drugs used in cancer treatments need to be improved.

Photodynamic therapy (PDT) is a promising minimally invasive therapy for the treatment of cancer. This involves the administration of photosensitiser (PS) and subsequent excitation of PS by light irradiation at a specific wavelength. The excited PS then reacts with cellular oxygen and produces reactive oxygen species (ROS). This reaction results in oxidising the cellular macromolecules surrounding tumour cells [5]. This remedial method has been developed over the last few years [6,7], and has not only been utilised in cancer treatment, but also in dermatological [8] and ophthalmic [9] conditions, including psoriasis and age-related diseases [10–12]. The use of photodynamic therapy to treat cancers has gained attention around the world [13,14]. The mechanism of PDT is based on various photocatalytic reactions that induce the destruction of cancer cells, and it has been clinically used for the treatment of cancer for over a decade [5]. In the first clinical PDT study reported by Granelli et al. [15], hematoporphyrin was used as a potent photosensitiser (PS) against glioma cancer cells. PDT destroys cancer cells through three fundamentally different pathways, namely, by damaging cancer cells over time, damaging vascular tissues that supply oxygen to cells, and finally by activating host immune response systems [13,16]. Combining PDT with chemotherapy, radiotherapy, and herbal therapy could be an emerging future methodology in cancer treatment. The combination therapy has more of a tendency to reduce the side effects when compared to monotherapy regimes and can significantly lower cancer cell proliferation by improving the drug uptake [17].

Since ancient times, herbal medicine from natural products has been utilised for treating various human ailments [18]. Most current medicines are derived from various medicinal plants, and it is evident that herbal extracts and their compounds should be examined as possible active lead components in cancer drug discoveries [19,20]. Nature is a valuable reserve for medicinal plants, and many of the pharmaceutically active compounds isolated from medicinal plants have not been tested for photoactive properties. There have been few studies attempting to identify new chemical compounds with photoactivity from plant extracts that can be used as potent natural PSs [21–25]. Hypericin (isolated from *Hypericum perforatum*) is a recognised plant-based PS used in PDT. The in vitro and in vivo studies reported that hypericin PS activated at 594 nm could destroy cancer cell proliferation effectively. The researchers already demonstrated that the effect of herbal extracts combined with illumination could significantly reduce cancer development by prohibiting metabolic viability and proliferation cancer cells [26–29].

Due to the low or no adverse side effects, herbal products have been used for the treatment of many more ailments than synthetic drugs. Studies have shown that plant-based compounds could be used in the treatment of various cancers [30]. Many phototoxic substances were subsequently reported in various plant species that are equally efficient as of conventional PSs [31]. These studies recommend that natural compounds with photosensitising abilities can be isolated from plants and used as alternatives for conventional PSs used in PDT. In this review, the underlying principles of PDT, PSs and plant-based photoactive compounds were addressed. This review mainly focused on the anticancer activity of furanocoumarins, polyacetylenes, thiophenes, curcumins, alkaloids and anthraquinones in relation to the light-absorbing properties.

2. Basic Principles of Photodynamic Therapy

Photodynamic therapy involves coordination with three individual factors, namely, the photosensitiser, oxygen, and light [7]. These components are not toxic to cells individually, but when irradiated, these can initiate a photochemical reaction that generates highly reactive singlet oxygen ($^1O_2$) and cause significant toxicity, leading to cell death. PDT is normally described in two stages, the first is administration of the PS and the second stage is the irradiation. Generally, the effect of PDT is affected by the PS type, dosage, light fluence, as well as exposure time. PDT can be used either before or after chemotherapy, radiotherapy, or surgery without compromise. The clinically approved PS should not accumulate in the body and does not develop resistant cancer cells. Pain during administration and continuous photosensitisation are the major drawbacks of PDT treatment. There are three types of lights ranges from 600 to 800 nm that are commonly used in PDT, namely, blue, red, and infrared lights. Among them, blue light penetrates the tissue the least when compared to red and infrared lights. The wavelengths below 800 nm are mostly used in PDT than higher wavelengths (above 800 nm) due to their lack of photodynamic reactions. The choice of light source is commonly based on PS nature, absorption spectra of PS, location, and size and characteristics of the infected tissue [7,32].

More than 300 chemical compounds have already been identified as potential candidates to be used as PSs. Amongst these, a few were authorised for clinical application in PDT, and others were medically evaluated, whereas some are still under examination [33,34]. We have tabulated some PSs which are used in various cancer treatments in Table 1. Photosensitisers are naturally or chemically produced compound conjugated with a visible light-absorbing chromophore group with a strong chemical absorbance. Choosing the correct PS is the most important phase in PDT for a successful outcome [33,34]. The purity and the presence of a tetrapyrrole structure with good storage stability are the preferable properties of most PSs used in PDT. The potent and effective PS should have the ability to initiate a photodynamic reaction after irradiation with 600–800 nm lights and should not cause any toxicity under dark conditions. It should be easily distinguishable from the body with no or minimum phototoxic side effects [35]. The better diffusion of PS through the cells after long administration might contribute to the effectiveness of PDT [36]. The production of a significant amount of ROS after irradiation that induces apoptosis with less inflammation is most likely to be a suitable PS for PDT application [37,38].

When a PS is subjected to a particular wavelength light, the electron of the outermost orbital will be shifted from the ground state (S0) to the first excited state (S1). Subsequently, the electromagnetic propulsion switches the molecule to an excited triplet state (T1) with a longer life span (Figure 1). In each of these excited states, PSs are quite unstable and lose their energy in the form of fluorescence, phosphorescence, and internal heat conversion. PSs in the T1 state may react photochemically in any of the two pathways. In the type 1 pathway, the excited PS reacts through an electron transfer process with the surrounding oxygen, which ultimately leads to generation of reactive oxygen species (ROS). Such free radicals communicate readily with the biomolecules (lipids, peptides, proteins, and nucleic acids) and destroy them [39,40]. In contrast, in the type 2 pathway, the energy is directly transferred from the T1 state of the PS to the S0-state oxygen. This results in the ground-state PS transformation and excited-state singlet reactive oxygen. The disruption caused by PDT is local because both singlet oxygen as well as free radicals have a short half-life between 10–300 nanoseconds and a small diffusion distance of 10–55 nm [41].

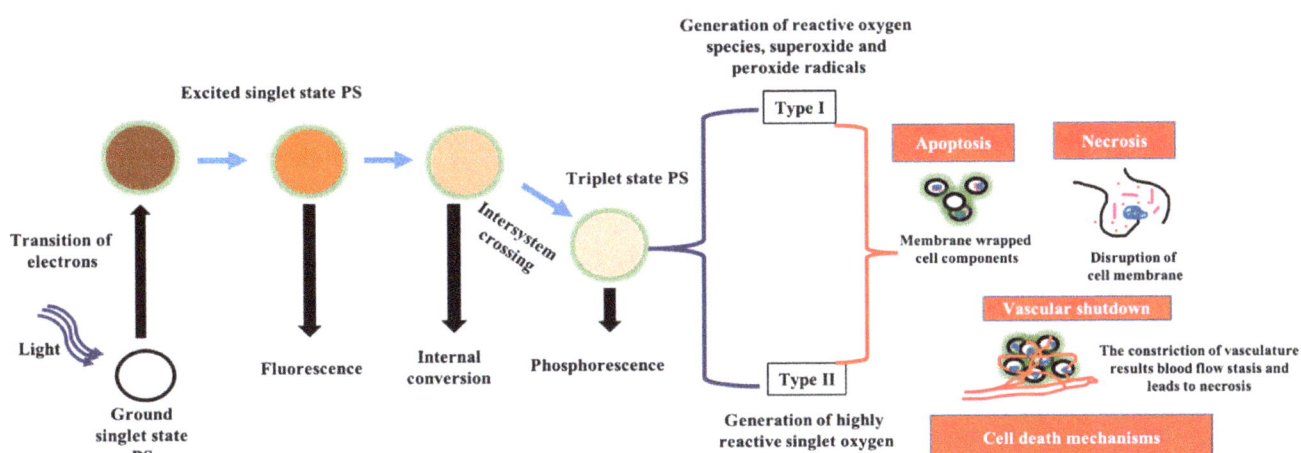

Figure 1. The general mechanism of photodynamic therapy.

Table 1. List of photosensitisers used in photodynamic therapy of various cancers.

Photosensitiser	Commercial Name	λ max (nm)	Structure	Type of Cancer	Reference
First-Generation Photosensitiser					
Hematoporphyrin derivatives	Photofrin Photoheme	630		Lung, bladder, skin, cervical, breast cancer.	[17,42]
Second-Generation Photosensitisers					
5-Aminolevulinic acid	Levulan Alasens	635		Bladder, skin, lung, ovary and gastrointestinal cancer.	[43–45]
Meta-tetra(hydroxyphenyl) chlorin	Foscan	652		Approved drug for the treatment of bronchial and oesophageal cancers.	[46–48]
Chlorin e6	MACEDACEPhotoditazine	664		Gynaecological diseases, prostate cancer, fibrosarcoma, Liver, brain, lung, and oral cancers.	[49–51]

Table 1. Cont.

Photosensitiser	Commercial Name	λ max (nm)	Structure	Type of Cancer	Reference
Benzoporphyrin	Visudyne	690		Prostate and skin cancer.	[52,53]
Texaphyrins	Lutrin, Antrin, Optrin, Xcytrin	720–760		Hepatocellular cancer, leukaemia, nasopharyngeal carcinoma, colon, prostate, bronchial and oesophageal cancers.	[54–58]
Phthalocyanines	Photosense	640–690		Breast, cervical, skin, lung, liver, colon and gastrointestinal cancers.	[17,59–61]
Purpurins	Purlytin	660		Breast cancer, prostate cancer and Kaposi's sarcoma.	[62–64]

3. PDT's Cancer Cell Death Mechanism

PDT's cancer cell death mechanism starts after the activation of administrated PS by a specific wavelength of light. The PS's hydrophilic, hydrophobic, and ionic charge-related interaction nature plays an important role in the targeting of particular cancer cell receptor (globulins and Low-Density Lipoprotein (LDL) receptors) [34]. After the activation of PSs, the cancer cell death mechanism might occur in three main pathways (Figure 1), namely, apoptosis, necrosis, and autophagy [33,65,66]. However, the level of cell death induced by PDT may be affected by various aspects, including subcellular localisation, bioavailability, the physicochemical nature of the PS, the cellular oxygen concentration, as well as the applied light intensity and wavelength [67]. In general, the light-absorbed PS interacts with cellular oxygen and highly produce ROS (hydroperoxides, superoxide, or hydroxyl radicals) as well as singlet oxygen ($^1O_2$). These produced ROS can induce cancerous cell death via the above-mentioned mechanisms. Both type 1 and 2 reactions may occur separately or in combination, but type 1 (generation of ROS followed by the apoptotic cell death mechanism) is commonly exhibited by most approved PSs [67].

4. PS from Natural Resources

The effectiveness of PDT is mainly based on the PS; it should possess all the properties of the PS as previously explained. The PS can be divided into first- and second-generation types. Hematoporphyrin and its derivative Photofrin®® were classified as first-generation PSs. After extensive studies, new and improved second-generation PSs, such as Levulan®®, Alasens®®, and Foscan have been introduced for PDT application (Table 1). Although these are widely used for various cancer treatments, their clinical usage is limited by various drawbacks such as lack of chemical purity, a longer half-life, accumulation in tissues and poor ability in relation to depth of tissue penetration [31–39].

Subsequently, there are some research reports on PSs with potent pharmaceutical properties to overcome the shortcomings of first- (Porphyrin based sensitisers) and second-generation (non-porphyrin derivatives) PSs [35–37]. These drawbacks of current PSs specifically imply the need for new PSs as anticancer agents from natural resources. The discovery of new PS compounds with anticipated pharmacological properties and clinical application is an inspiring task. Recently, a greater number of plant-based compounds have been reported for their anticancer activity, and these compounds are pharmaceutically very important for the development of potent drugs. The use of light to activate the bioactivities of natural products is generally called photopharmacology (a combination of photophysics and photochemistry). The absorption of lights ($\lambda < 350$ nm) by a molecule mainly depends on the chromophore compound attached (Figure 2) [36,37]. This review presents an overview of natural photoactive compounds as potent third-generation photosensitisers in the improvement of PSs in relation to their prospective application in cancer treatments.

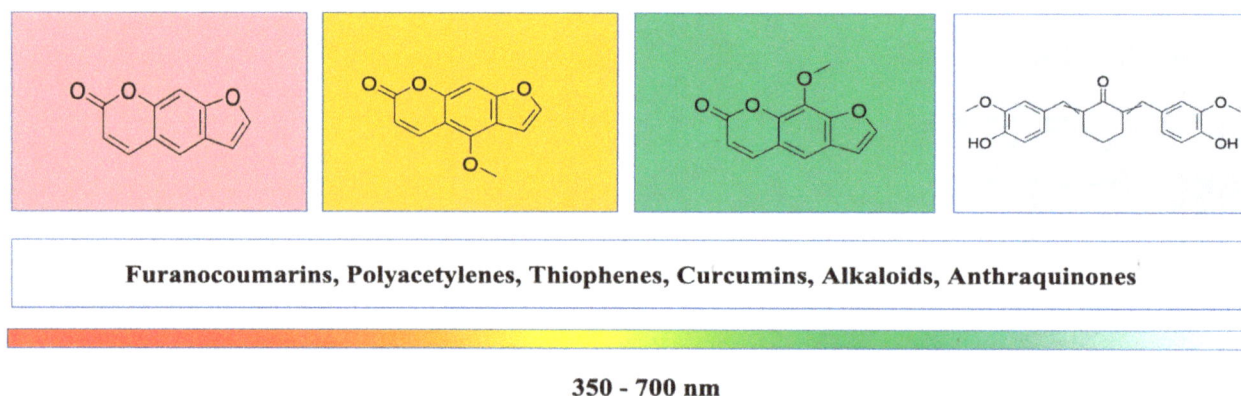

Furanocoumarins, Polyacetylenes, Thiophenes, Curcumins, Alkaloids, Anthraquinones

350 - 700 nm

Figure 2. Phototherapeutic window of natural compounds.

5. Natural Photoactive Compounds from Plants

The search for the natural compounds as efficient PSs has been progressively moving forward because of the side effects caused by current synthetic drugs. The advanced isolation, identification and characterisation techniques improved the extraction of desirable compounds from plants. Recently, using these advanced techniques, the isolation of natural photoactive compounds has become easy. Although there have been few studies attempting to identify new chemical compounds with photoactivity from plant extracts, this review discusses the photoactivity as well as the anticancer activity of some plant-based compounds such as furanocoumarins, polyacetylenes, thiophenes, curcumins, alkaloids and anthraquinones (Table 2).

Table 2. List of plant-based natural photoactive compounds with known photoactivity.

Name	Absorption Maxima	Chemical Property and Groups	Natural Sources	Possible Mode of Action	Reference
Furanocoumarins	333 nm	Aromatic compounds possessing a furan ring.	Angelicae dahuricae, Tetradium daniellii, Glehnia littoralis, Heracleum persicum, Syzygium Sps, Ruta graveolens, Ficus sps.	DNA intercalation under dark type 2 PDT reaction. Crosslinking and adduct formation with DNA and RNA. Cell membrane damage.	[68–70]
Polyacetylenes and Thiophenes	488 nm	Furanoacetylenes thiarubrines, thiophenes, polyacetylene (aliphatic compounds with more than three conjugated triple bonds), thiophenes (aromatic acetylenes; e.g., phenylheptatriyne).	Asteraceae spp, Heliopsisa, Rudbeckia spp, Arnica, Centaurea scabiosa, Tagetes erecta, Porophyllum obscurum, Echinops, Bidens, Ambrosia chamissonis, T. minuta, E. latifolius, E. sgrijissi, Rhaponticum uniflorum.	Membrane damage or erythrocyte leakage; type 1 and type 2 PDT reaction, as well as type 1 and 2 PDT mixed reaction.	[71–75]
Curcumins	420–480 nm	Dicinnamoylmethane, curcumin, curcuminoids, demethoxycurcumin, bisdemethoxycurcumin.	Curcuma longa.	Cell membrane is the primary target of curcuminoids. Induction of caspase-mediated cell death.	[76–78]
Alkaloids	360 nm	Chinolin alkaloids, pterins, benzylisoquinolines, beta-carbolines, harmine.	Guatteria blepharophylla, Berberis vulgaris, Sanguinaria Canadensis, Mahonia aquifolium Peganum harmala, Indigofera tinctoria.	Photo-oxidises histidine and tryptophan, resulting in DNA crosslinking. Photooxidation, type 1 PDT mechanism and targets mitochondria.	[79–87]
Anthraquinones	437 nm	Hydroxyanthraquinones, rhein, physcion, emodin, rubiadin, damnacanthol, soranjidiol, alizarin, purpurin, rubiadin, aloe-emodin, 1,5-dihydroxy przewalsquinone B, ziganein, uredinorubellins, caeruleoramularin, hypericin, cercosporin, elsinochromes A-C pleichrome, hypocrellin.	Polygonum cuspidatum, Heterophyllaea pustulata, H. lycioides Aloe vera, Rheum palmatum, Rumex crispus Polyathia suberosa, Dactylopius coccus, Xanthoria parietina, Drechslera avenae, Ramularia collo-cygni. H. perforatum, Fagopyrum esculentum.	Type 1 and 2 PDT action.	[88–91]

5.1. Furanocoumarins

The secondary metabolites, furanocoumarins (FC; Figure 3), are mostly present in higher plants. The photoactive furanocoumarins were mainly composed of a linear core, and the biological distribution, photochemistry and phototoxicity mechanisms of FC after PUVA (psoralen and long-wave ultraviolet radiation) irradiation were reported in previous study [92]. In terms of phototherapy, psoralen is activated in the wavelength range of 300–400 nm ultraviolet radiation to treat psoriasis, dermatitis, eczema, and other skin problems [92]. Over a few years, many researchers reported anticancer activity of FCs against various types of cancer such as breast, skin, and leukaemia. FCs modulate several pathways inducing cancer cell death by inhibiting signal transducer and activator of transcription 3 (STAT3), nuclear factor-κB (NF-κB), phosphatidylinositol-3-kinase and AKT protein expression (Figure 4). These pathways play a key role in tumour development through regular activation of several inflammatory genes. Studies show that FC displayed potent activity against breast cancer development by inhibiting STAT3 protein expression [93]. Panno et al. [92,93], demonstrated inhibition of breast cancer cell growth in a dose-dependent manner through activation of p53 and Bax, leading to the cleavage of caspase 9. In contrast, in leukaemia cells, FC inactivated the JAK (Janus-activated kinase), protein c-Src, and STAT3, and downregulated Bcl-xl and Bcl-2 proteins which are responsible for apoptosis [93–96]. The enhanced activity against the malignant melanoma cell line (A375) after UV irradiation of plant extracts containing FC also supported the possible photoactive nature of FCs [93–96]. The linear forms of furanocoumarins like psoralen and its derivatives 5-methoxypsoralen (5-MOP) and 8-methoxypsoralen (8-MOP) are reported to increase the cytotoxicity after irradiation by ultraviolet light in the 320–400 nm wavelength range against cutaneous T-cell lymphoma [97,98], and photoactivated psoralens induce apoptosis by forming adducts with DNA. This leads to the activation of p21waf/Cip and p53 and subsequently leads to cell death by the release of mitochondrial cytochrome c. The photoactivation of psoralen can also cause cell death by blocking oncogenic receptor tyrosine kinase signalling and the PI3K pathway by interfering with efficient recruitment of effector Akt kinase to the activated plasma membrane [92–104]. PUVA treatment was found effectively against B16F10 murine melanoma cells by cell cycle arrest in G2/M phases [93–96].

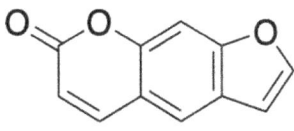

Psoralen

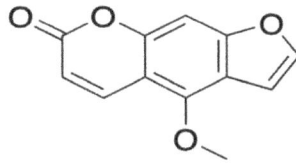

5-Methoxypsoralen

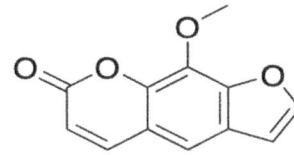

8-Methoxypsoralen

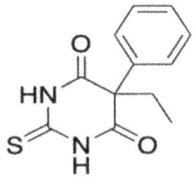

Thioxopyrimidine

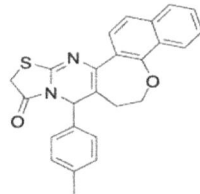

Thiazolopyrimidine

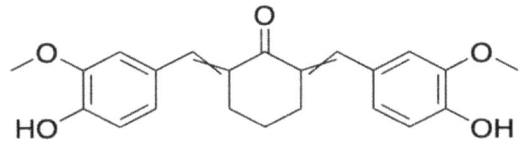

Curcuminoids

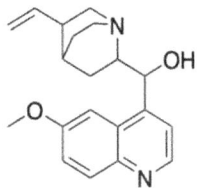

Quinine

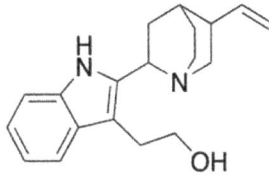

Cinchonamine

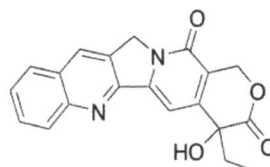

Camptothecin

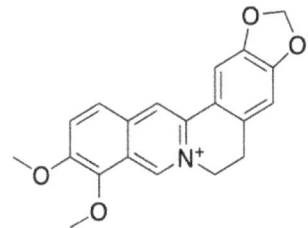

Berberine

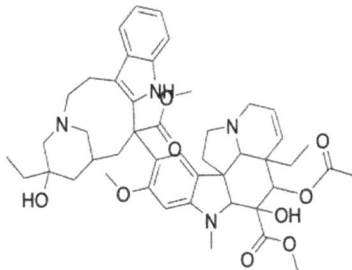

Vinblastine

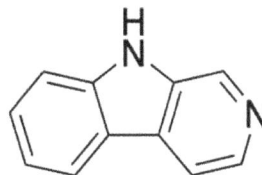

Beta-carboline

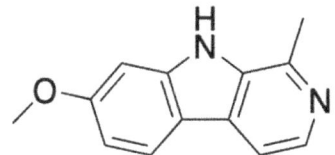

Harmine

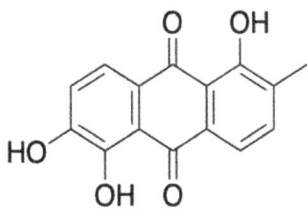

Morindone

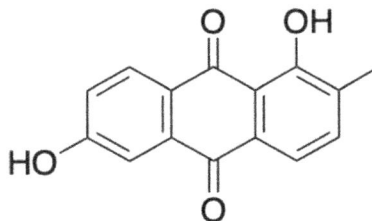

Soranjidiol

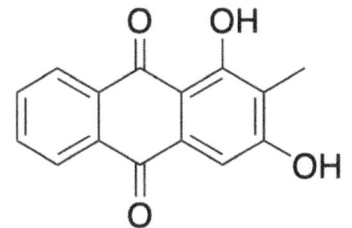

Rubiadin

Figure 3. Natural photoactive compounds presented in this review.

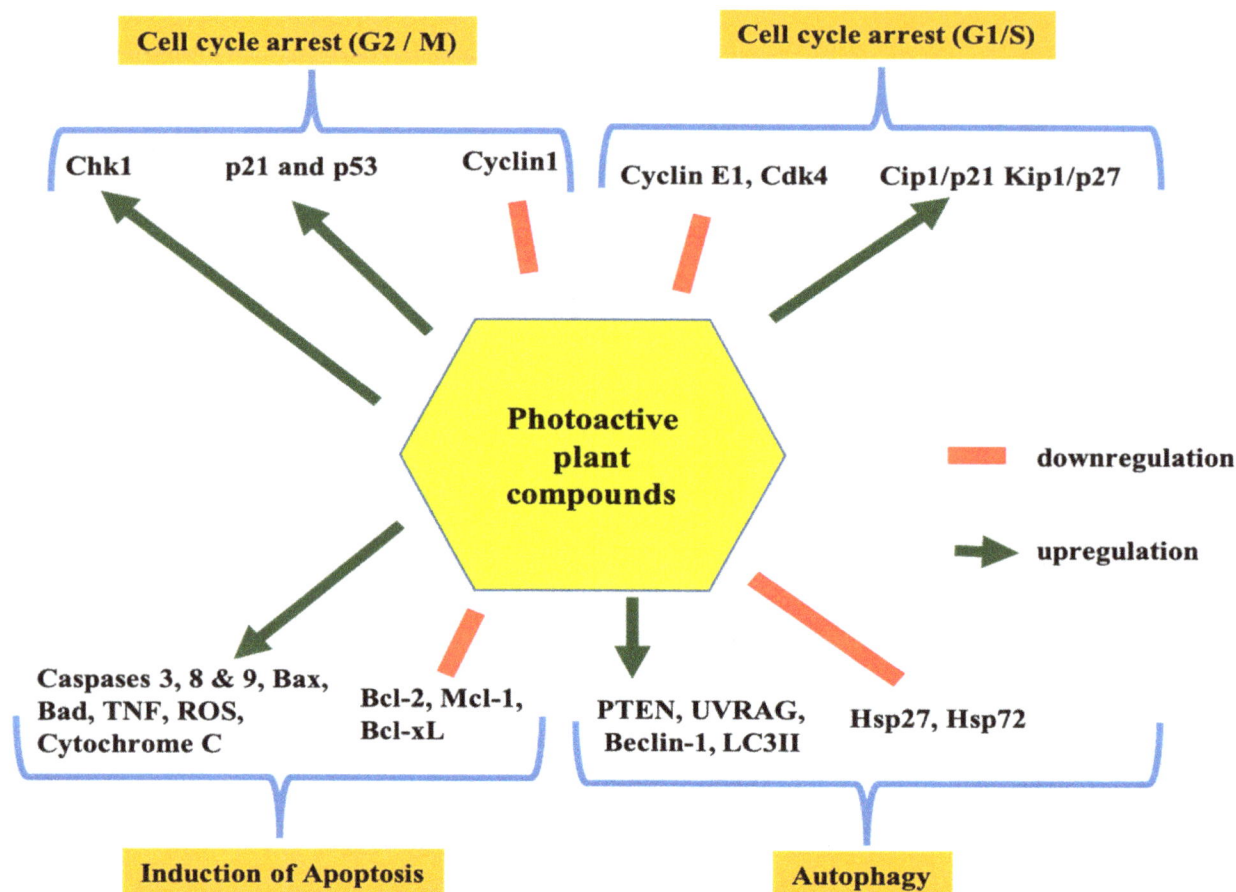

Figure 4. Common molecular targets of major photoactive compounds.

5.2. Polyacetylene and Thiophenes

These group compounds are characterised by a triple bond carbon–carbon molecule [75] and thiophenes compounds. Generally, the aliphatic compounds conjugated with three or more acetylenic bonds are considered phototoxic in nature. Among these, polyacetylenes compounds can produce $^1O_2$ under irradiation and thiophenes can provide high photo yield, leading to type 2 PDT reaction yields [105]. The polyacetylene and thiophenes compounds were reported to be activated or excited at a wavelength range of 314–350 nm absorbance maximum for the relevant photobiological effects [75]. The derivatives of these compounds were reported with a variety of potent biological activities, including analgesic, anti-inflammatory, antitumour, and antimicrobial activities. Some of the derivatives substituted by pyrimidines show antimicrobial, anti-inflammatory, and antitumour activities. A few numbers of thiophenes were reported for their cytotoxic effects against human cancer cell lines. *Echinops grijisii* root-derived thiophenes exhibited cytotoxicity against HL-60, K562 and MCF-7 cells [106]. Notably, derivatives such as thioxopyrimidine and thiazolopyrimidine were reported to possess anticancer activities against MCF-7 (breast adenocarcinoma), NCI-H460 (non-small cell lung cancer), and SF-268 (CNS cancer) cells. These acetylenic compounds and derivatives when combined with PDT might improve the efficacy of various cancer treatments [107–112]. The UV irradiation of some thiophenes also showed increased cytotoxic activities [113]; this might be due to their instable nature under UV radiation. Hence, the UV irradiation of polyacetylene and thiophene compounds can form free radicals that would induce cell death. Due to the ability to produce ROS after irradiation, these compounds can be used as an alternative PS from natural sources.

5.3. Curcumins

Curcumin (CU) is a plant-based therapeutic compound isolated from rhizome of *Curcuma longa* of the Zingiberaceae family. Curcuminoid is one of the most extensively studied plant-derived bioactive compounds [114]. Since the 1980s, the photobiological potential of CU was of great interest [115,116], and studies described CU as a desirable, highly promising photosensitiser [115,117–121]. The foremost property of CU is that it is biologically safe even at higher doses, and it can be easily produced on a large scale [117,122]. The photobleaching analysis reported the degradation profile of curcumin derivatives and its ability to produce singlet oxygen species [123]. CU was characterised by an absorption spectrum of 300–500 nm with a high extinction coefficient. This suggests that CU can induce a strong phototoxic reaction even at lower concentrations [124–126]. Curcumin is considered as a potential anticancer agent and inhibits cancer cell proliferation in breast, lung, colon, kidney, ovary, and liver cancers [114]. The in vitro and in vivo anticancer activity of curcumin has been proved by inhibition of various transcription factors such as NF-κB, AP-1, VEGF, iNOS, COX-2, 5-LOX, MMP-2, MMP-9 and IL-8, which are mainly responsible for angiogenesis and tumour growth [127,128]. The administration of curcumin significantly reduced the expression of the CDK4/cylin D1 complex by inhibiting p53 expression and causing the apoptotic process by inducing ROS generation. Furthermore, the enhanced antitumour activity was noted after UVB irradiation of curcumin by caspase activation on HaCaT (human keratinocyte cell) cells. It was also efficient against MCF-7 breast cancer cells at 30 J/cm^2 [77,78]. These data suggested that curcumin may act as a potent anticancer agent by preventing cancer progression, migration and invasion [129–131]. Dovigo et al. [132] found the light absorption ability of CU in the range of 300 and 500 nm with a maximum absorption at 430 nm, which might support its usage as a PS. The ROS-inducing and anticancer ability of CU makes it a potent candidate as a natural PS [133]. Nevertheless, Chan and Wu [134] observed that the photoactive nature of CU on human epidermal A431 carcinoma cells and the higher amount of CU also affect the irradiation penetration [132,134,135]. The irradiation of CU under a 290–320 nm UVB light source with the fluence of 100 mJ/cm^2 induced apoptosis in HaCaT keratinocyte cells [78]. Based on the above reports, CU can be used as a natural PS, and it can achieve high efficacy at a low concentration when combined with PDT. The existing PDT and photoactive reports on CU suggest that CU can be used as a potential and promising natural PS in PDT. In conclusion, CU can be a potent photosensitiser in the treatment of cancer and skin infections. Therefore, investigating the photodynamic potential of CU derivatives in terms of higher absorption and extinction coefficient will contribute to the increased efficacy of photodynamic toxicity.

5.4. Alkaloids

Alkaloids, a diverse secondary metabolites group from higher plants, contain a heterocyclic structure with a nitrogen atom in the ring [136]. Nitrogen-containing alkaloids are normally photoactive in nature, e.g., quinine and cinchonamine. The alkaloids were reported for many significant properties, such as analgesic and anticancer activity [136–139]. The alkaloids camptothecin and vinblastine are few alkaloids were successfully utilised as chemotherapeutic drugs [138,140]. The anticancer activity of alkaloids was proved by different studies by means of disturbing tumour progression by induction of cell cycle arrest at the G1 or G2/M phases, regulating cyclin-dependent kinase (CDK) and promoting apoptosis as well as autophagy in tumour cells. Furthermore, these compounds induce apoptosis by regulating Bax, Bcl-2, Bcl-xL, NF-κB and various caspase proteins [140–143]. In addition, the combination of alkaloids with chemotherapeutic drugs and irradiation also enhanced the biological activities [144,145]. Furthermore, alkaloids induce the formation of intracellular ROS in cancer cells, which leads to the destruction of cancer cell metabolism [140–143]. The photochemically best-known alkaloid is berberine; Luiza Andreazza et al. [146], Bhattacharyya et al. [147] and Inbaraj et al. [81] reported the antitumour activity of berberine upon UV and blue light irradiation. The irradiation of berberine at 410 nm proved to be effective in controlling brain cancer cell growth [146]. Beta-carboline and harmine are also a noticeable alkaloid with a photoactive nature and are reported to produce a significant amount of ROS after irradiation [148], which is considered an important feature of potent PSs. The photoactivity of harmine was proved by the UVA (long-wave ultraviolet radiation) irradiation against tumour cell lines [148]. Berberine was extensively investigated as a potential photosensitising agent for PDT [149–151]. The fluorescent active nature of berberine is indicated for its efficiency in PDT [149]; thus, berberine and its associated alkaloids can be used as a new candidate for photodynamic therapy [150]. Different studies have proved the photosensitising as well as ROS generation ability of alkaloids in the presence of a light source [151]. Therefore, berberine can be studied as a natural photosensitiser in PDT applications with minimal side effects.

5.5. Anthraquinones (AQ)

Anthraquinone are the largest group among natural quinones from higher plants, which, including naphthoquinones and benzoquinones, includes over 700 compounds, including emodin, physcion, catenarin and rhein [152,153]. The hydroxylation pattern, however, dictates the possibility of AQs' photopharmacological properties. Notably, AQs' aminoanthraquinone derivatives were studied extensively for their photoactive properties among the plant compounds due to their UV/vis absorption and photosensitising nature [154,155]. The AQs were reported as kinase and tyrosinase inhibitors as well as cytotoxicity agents. The *M. elliptica* AQs such as morindone, soranjidiol and rubiadin were also reported for their antitumour activity against lymphocytic leukaemia (P-388) cells [156]. The anthraquinones isolated from *H. pustulata* leaves and stem exhibited photosensitising properties by generation of singlet oxygen and/or superoxide anion radicals [157]. Comini et al. [158] reported that irradiation of AQs (soranjidiol and rubiadin) under visible radiation of 380–480 nm can promote the anti-proliferative effect on MCF-7 breast cancer cells. In addition, Montoya et al. [157] and Vittar et al. [159] also reported photosensitisation effects of AQs in Balb/c mice and their leukocyte-inhibiting ability in a dose-dependent manner by inducing apoptosis, necrosis, or autophagy. These study results show the photoactive nature of AQs to inhibit the proliferation of cancerous cells. Based on the previous studies and the above data, molecular targets responsible for the anticancer activity of AQs and major phytocompounds are summarised in Figure 4.

6. Theorical Studies for Assessing the Photoactivity of Natural Compounds

The development of various antitumor compounds with different molecular targets initiated an exciting field of investigation with recently developed theoretical studies. The theoretical studies including density functional theory (DFT) and time-dependent density functional theory (TD-DFT) were used to assess a series of photophysical properties, including absorption spectra, excitation energies (singlet and triplet) and spin–orbit matrix elements. All the reported compounds are potential UVA chemotherapeutic agents which require the lowest triplet-state energy for producing highly cytotoxic ROS [160,161].

7. Advantages and Scope of Natural PSs

The anticancer property of many plant extracts and bioactive compounds have been analysed, but not so much in terms of as sources of photosensitisers. Selecting proper PSs is the first step in PDT, and, to date, only a few PSs are clinically approved, such as Photofrin, Foscan and Levulan. The present study explored the common photoactive nature of various phytocompounds. Many of the natural photoactive compounds were reported for their non-toxicity against normal cells and toxicity towards cancer cells. The important property of a PS is the nontoxic nature during the absence of light. The increasing activity of extracts or phytocompounds after irradiation by light makes them good photosensitising candidates for PDT. Another important feature that makes photoactive plant compounds suitable photosensitisers is their absorption maxima at 400–700 nm, which is biologically compatible. The selective nature of these compounds is important in clinical PDT to overcome side effects. Future studies are warranted to isolate and evaluate these specific photoactive compounds from plants to be used as a potent PSs for PDT for cancer and related disorders [162,163].

8. Conclusions and Future Perspectives

As discussed in this review, plant-based photoactive compounds can be used as a natural PSs in PDT application. There are wide range of unknown natural compounds with different photoactive and phototoxic properties. This review summarises and encourages researchers to identify and elucidate natural photoactive plant-based compounds and to use them as alternatives for the synthesis PSs for a better PDT outcome. Furthermore, discovering natural phototoxic agents as PSs will be helpful to reduce toxicity and side effects and improve selectivity. In conclusion, use the plant-based PSs in PDT typically causes less and minimal adverse effects than other treatments that are commonly used in cancer therapies.

Author Contributions: Conceptualisation and writing, K.M.; review and editing, K.M., B.G., T.P. and H.A.; supervision, B.G., T.P. and H.A. The final version of the submitted manuscript was read and agreed by all the authors. All authors have read and agreed to the published version of the manuscript.

Acknowledgments: The authors sincerely thank the Science and Engineering Research Board (SERB), Department of Science and Technology (DST), Government of India and the Laser research centre, University of Johannesburg, South Africa for their support.

References

1. El-Hussein, A.; Harith, M.; Abrahamse, H. Assessment of DNA Damage after Photodynamic Therapy Using a Metallophthalocyanine Photosensitizer. *Int. J. Photoenergy* **2012**, *2012*, 1–10. [CrossRef]

2. Klug, W.S.; Cummings, M.R.; Spencer, C.A. *Concepts of Genetics*, 8th ed.; Pearson Education International: Upper Saddle River, NJ, USA, 2006.

3. Matés, J.M.; Segura, J.A.; Alonso, F.J.; Márquez, J.D. Intracellular redox status and oxidative stress: Implications for cell proliferation, apoptosis, and carcinogenesis. *Arch. Toxicol.* **2008**, *82*, 273–299. [CrossRef] [PubMed]

4. Santiago-Montero, R.; Sossa-Azuela, H.; Gutiérrez-Hernández, D.; Zamudio, V.; Hernández-Bautista, I.; Valadez-Godínez, S. Novel Mathematical Model of Breast Cancer Diagnostics Using an Associative Pattern Classification. *Diagnostics* **2020**, *10*, 136. [CrossRef] [PubMed]

5. Zhou, Z.; Song, J.; Nie, L.; Chen, X.S. Reactive oxygen species generating systems meeting challenges of photodynamic cancer therapy. *Chem. Soc. Rev.* **2016**, *45*, 6597–6626. [CrossRef] [PubMed]

6. Baskaran, R.; Lee, J.; Yang, S.-G. Clinical development of photodynamic agents and therapeutic applications. *Biomater. Res.* **2018**, *22*, 25. [CrossRef] [PubMed]

7. De Almeida, D.R.Q.; Terra, L.F.; Labriola, L.; Dos Santos, A.F.; Baptista, M.S. Photodynamic therapy in cancer treatment—An update review. *J. Cancer Metastasis Treat.* **2019**, *2019*, 10–20517. [CrossRef]

8. Nguyen, K.; Khachemoune, A. An update on topical photodynamic therapy for clinical dermatologists. *J. Dermatol. Treat.* **2019**, *30*, 732–744. [CrossRef]

9. Blasi, M.A.; Pagliara, M.M.; Lanza, A.; Sammarco, M.G.; Caputo, C.G.; Grimaldi, G.; Scupola, A. Photodynamic Therapy in Ocular Oncology. *Biomedicines* **2018**, *6*, 17. [CrossRef]

10. Choi, Y.M.; Adelzadeh, L.; Wu, J.J. Photodynamic therapy for psoriasis. *J. Dermatol. Treat.* **2014**, *26*, 202–207. [CrossRef]

11. Silva, A.M.; Siopa, J.R.; Martins-Gomes, C.; Teixeira, M.D.C.; Santos, D.J.; Pires, M.D.A.; Andreani, T. New strategies for the treatment of autoimmune diseases using nanotechnologies. *Emerg. Nanotechnol. Immunol.* **2018**, 135–163. [CrossRef]

12. Hatz, K.; Schneider, U.; Henrich, P.B.; Braun, B.; Sacu, S. Ranibizumab plus Verteporfin Photodynamic Therapy in Neovascular Age-Related Macular Degeneration: 12 Months of Retreatment and Vision Outcomes from a Randomized Study. *Ophthalmologia* **2014**, *233*, 66–73. [CrossRef] [PubMed]

13. Oniszczuk, A.; Wojtunik-Kulesza, K.A.; Oniszczuk, T.; Kasprzak, K. The potential of photodynamic therapy (PDT)—Experimental investigations and clinical use. *Biomed. Pharmacother.* **2016**, *83*, 912–929. [CrossRef] [PubMed]

14. Zhang, J.; Jiang, C.; Longo, J.P.F.; Azevedo, R.B.; Zhang, H.; Muehlmann, L.A. An updated overview on the development of new photosensitizers for anticancer photodynamic therapy. *Acta Pharm. Sin. B* **2017**, *8*, 137–146. [CrossRef] [PubMed]

15. Granelli, S.G.; Diamond, I.; McDonagh, A.F.; Wilson, C.B.; Nielsen, S.L. Photochemotherapy of glioma cells by visible light and hematoporphyrin. *Cancer Res.* **1975**, *35*, 2567–2570.

16. Abrahamse, H.; Hamblin, M.R. *Photomedicine and Stem Cells: The Janus Face of Photodynamic Therapy (PDT) to Kill Cancer Stem Cells, and Photobiomodulation (PBM) to Stimulate Normal Stem Cells*; Morgan & Claypool Publishers: Bristol, UK, 2017.

17. Moreira, L.M.; Dos Santos, F.V.; Lyon, J.P.; Maftoum-Costa, M.; Soares, C.P.; Da Silva, N.S. Photodynamic Therapy: Porphyrins and Phthalocyanines as Photosensitizers. *Aust. J. Chem.* **2008**, *61*, 741–754. [CrossRef]

18. Mohammadi, A.; Mansoori, B.; Baradaran, B. Regulation of miRNAs by herbal medicine: An emerging field in cancer therapies. *Biomed. Pharmacother.* **2017**, *86*, 262–270. [CrossRef]

19. Mohammadi, A.; Mansoori, B.; Aghapour, M.; Baradaran, B. Urtica dioica dichloromethane extract induce apoptosis from intrinsic pathway on human prostate cancer cells (PC3). *Cell. Mol. Boil.* **2016**, *62*, 78–83.

20. Mohammadi, A.; Mansoori, B.; Goldar, S.; Shanehbandi, D.; Khaze, V.; Mohammadnejad, L.; Baghbani, E.; Baradaran, B. Effects of Urtica dioica dichloromethane extract on cell apoptosis and related gene expression in human breast cancer cell line (MDA-MB-468). *Cell. Mol. Boil.* **2016**, *62*, 62–67.

21. Alali, F.Q.; Tawaha, K. Dereplication of bioactive constituents of the genus hypericum using LC-(+,−)-ESI-MS and LC-PDA techniques: Hypericum triquterifolium as a case study. *Saudi Pharm. J.* **2009**, *17*, 269–274. [CrossRef]

22. Bailly, C. Ready for a comeback of natural products in oncology. *Biochem. Pharmacol.* **2009**, *77*, 1447–1457. [CrossRef]

23. Mishra, B.B.; Tiwari, V.K. Natural products: An evolving role in future drug discovery. *Eur. J. Med. Chem.* **2011**, *46*, 4769–4807. [CrossRef] [PubMed]

24. Rodrigues, M.C. Photodynamic Therapy Based on Arrabidaea chica (Crajiru) Extract Nanoemulsion: In vitro Activity against Monolayers and Spheroids of Human Mammary Adenocarcinoma MCF-7 Cells. *J. Nanomed. Nanotechnol.* **2015**, *6*, 1–6. [CrossRef]

25. Tan, P.J.; Appleton, D.R.; Mustafa, M.R.; Lee, H.B. Rapid Identification of Cyclic Tetrapyrrolic Photosensitisers for Photodynamic Therapy Using On-line Hyphenated LC-PDA-MS Coupled with Photo-cytotoxicity Assay. *Phytochem. Anal.* **2011**, *23*, 52–59. [CrossRef]

26. Skalkos, D.; Gioti, E.; Stalikas, C.; Meyer, H.; Papazoglou, T.; Filippidis, G.; Papazoglou, T.G. Photophysical properties of Hypericum perforatum L. extracts—Novel photosensitizers for PDT. *J. Photochem. Photobiol. B Boil.* **2006**, *82*, 146–151. [CrossRef] [PubMed]

27. Zeisser-Labouèbe, M.; Lange, N.; Gurny, R.; Delie, F. Hypericin-loaded nanoparticles for the photodynamic treatment of ovarian cancer. *Int. J. Pharm.* **2006**, *326*, 174–181. [CrossRef] [PubMed]

28. Mirmalek, S.A.; Azizi, M.A.; Jangholi, E.; Yadollah-Damavandi, S.; Javidi, M.A.; Parsa, Y.; Parsa, T.; Salimi-Tabatabaee, S.A.; Kolagar, H.G.; Alizadeh-Navaei, R. Cytotoxic and apoptogenic effect of hypericin, the bioactive component of Hypericum perforatum on the MCF-7 human breast cancer cell line. *Cancer Cell Int.* **2016**, *16*, 3. [CrossRef]

29. Yonar, D.; Süloğlu, A.K.; Selmanoğlu, G.; Sünnetçioğlu, M.M. An Electron paramagnetic resonance (EPR) spin labeling study in HT-29 Colon adenocarcinoma cells after Hypericin-mediated photodynamic therapy. *BMC Mol. Cell Boil.* **2019**, *20*, 16. [CrossRef]

30. Aggarwal, B.B.; Ichikawa, H.; Garodia, P.; Weerasinghe, P.; Sethi, G.; Bhatt, I.D.; Pandey, M.K.; Shishodia, S.; Nair, M.G. From traditional Ayurvedic medicine to modern medicine: Identification of therapeutic targets for suppression of inflammation and cancer. *Expert Opin. Ther. Targets* **2006**, *10*, 87–118. [CrossRef]

31. Chaturvedi, D.; Singh, K.; Singh, V.K. Therapeutic and pharmacological aspects of photodynamic product chlorophyllin. *Eur. J. Biol. Res.* **2019**, *9*, 64–76.

32. Juzeniene, A.; Nielsen, K.P.; Moan, J. Biophysical Aspects of Photodynamic Therapy. *J. Environ. Pathol. Toxicol. Oncol.* **2006**, *25*, 7–28. [CrossRef]

33. George, B.P.; Abrahamse, H. A Review on Novel Breast Cancer Therapies: Photodynamic Therapy and Plant Derived Agent Induced Cell Death Mechanisms. *Anti-Cancer Agents Med. Chem.* **2016**, *15*, 1. [CrossRef]

34. Aniogo, E.C.; George, B.P.; Abrahamse, H. The role of photodynamic therapy on multidrug resistant breast cancer. *Cancer Cell Int.* **2019**, *19*, 91. [CrossRef] [PubMed]

35. Allison, R.R.; Sibata, C.H. Oncologic photodynamic therapy photosensitizers: A clinical review. *Photodiagn. Photodyn. Ther.* **2010**, *7*, 61–75. [CrossRef] [PubMed]

36. Chen, B.; Roskams, T.; De Witte, P.A.M. Antivascular tumor eradication by hypericin-mediated photodynamic therapy. *Photochem. Photobiol.* **2002**, *76*, 509. [CrossRef]

37. Ascencio, M.; Collinet, P.; Farine, M.; Mordon, S. Protoporphyrin IX fluorescence photobleaching is a useful tool to predict the response of rat ovarian cancer following hexaminolevulinate photodynamic therapy. *Lasers Surg. Med.* **2008**, *40*, 332–341. [CrossRef]

38. Garg, A.D.; Nowis, D.; Golab, J.; Vandenabeele, P.; Krysko, D.V.; Agostinis, P. Immunogenic cell death, DAMPs and anticancer therapeutics: An emerging amalgamation. *Biochim. Biophys. Acta (BBA) Rev. Cancer* **2010**, *1805*, 53–71. [CrossRef]

39. Castano, A.P.; Demidova, T.N.; Hamblin, M.R. Mechanisms in photodynamic therapy: Part three-Photosensitizer pharmacokinetics, biodistribution, tumor localization and modes of tumor destruction. *Photodiagn. Photodyn. Ther.* **2005**, *2*, 91–106. [CrossRef]

40. Ogilby, P.R. Singlet oxygen: There is indeed something new under the sun. *Chem. Soc. Rev.* **2010**, *39*, 3181. [CrossRef]

41. Oseroff, A.R.; Blumenson, L.R.; Wilson, B.D.; Mang, T.S.; Bellnier, D.A.; Parsons, J.C.; Frawley, N.; Cooper, M.; Zeitouni, N.; Dougherty, T.J. A dose ranging study of photodynamic therapy with porfimer sodium (Photofrin®) for treatment of basal cell carcinoma. *Lasers Surg. Med.* **2006**, *38*, 417–426. [CrossRef]

42. Juzeniene, A.; Juzenas, P.; Ma, L.-W.; Iani, V.; Moan, J. Effectiveness of different light sources for 5-aminolevulinic acid photodynamic therapy. *Lasers Med. Sci.* **2004**, *19*, 139–149. [CrossRef]

43. Lang, P. Methyl aminolaevulinate–photodynamic therapy: A review of clinical trials in the treatment of actinic keratoses and nonmelanoma skin cancer. *Yearb. Dermatol. Dermatol. Surg.* **2008**, *2008*, 322–323. [CrossRef]

44. Jeffes, E.W.; McCullough, J.L.; Weinstein, G.D.; Kaplan, R.; Glazer, S.D.; Taylor, J. Photodynamic therapy of actinic keratoses with topical aminolevulinic acid hydrochloride and fluorescent blue light. *J. Am. Acad. Dermatol.* **2001**, *45*, 96–104. [CrossRef] [PubMed]

45. Lu, K.; He, C.; Lin, W. A Chlorin-Based Nanoscale Metal–Organic Framework for Photodynamic Therapy of Colon Cancers. *J. Am. Chem. Soc.* **2015**, *137*, 7600–7603. [CrossRef] [PubMed]

46. Moore, C.M.; Nathan, T.; Lees, W.; Mosse, C.; Freeman, A.; Emberton, M.; Bown, S. Photodynamic therapy using meso tetra hydroxy phenyl chlorin (mTHPC) in early prostate cancer. *Lasers Surg. Med.* **2006**, *38*, 356–363. [CrossRef]

47. Grosjean, P.; Savary, J.-F.; Wagnières, G.; Mizeret, J.; Woodtli, A.; Theumann, J.-F.; Fontolliet, C.; Bergh, H.V.D.; Monnier, P. Tetra(m-hydroxyphenyl)chlorin clinical photodynamic therapy of early bronchial and oesophageal cancers. *Lasers Med. Sci.* **1996**, *11*, 227–235. [CrossRef]

48. Kessel, D. Pharmacokinetics of N-aspartyl chlorin e6 in cancer patients. *J. Photochem. Photobiol. B Boil.* **1997**, *39*, 81–83. [CrossRef]

49. Taber, S.W.; Fingar, V.H.; Coots, C.T.; Wieman, T.J. Photodynamic therapy using mono-L-aspartyl chlorin e6 (Npe6) for the treatment of cutaneous disease: A Phase I clinical study. *Clin. Cancer Res.* **1998**, *4*, 2741–2746.

50. Lagudaev, D.M. Sorokatyĭ Photodynamic therapy of prostatic adenoma. *Urologiia* **2007**, *4*, 34–37.

51. Momma, T.; Hamblin, M.R.; Wu, H.C.; Hasan, T. Photodynamic therapy of orthotopic prostate cancer with benzoporphyrin derivative: Local control and distant metastasis. *Cancer Res.* **1998**, *58*, 5425–5431.

52. Levy, J.G.; Waterfield, E.; Richter, A.M.; Smits, C.; Lui, H.; Hruza, L.; Anderson, R.R.; Salvatori, V. Photodynamic therapy of malignancies with benzoporphyrin derivative monoacid ring A. *Europto Biomedical Optics '93* **1994**, *2078*, 91–101. [CrossRef]

53. Young, S.W.; Woodburn, K.W.; Wright, M.; Mody, T.D.; Fan, Q.; Sessler, J.L.; Dow, W.C.; Miller, R.A. Lutetium Texaphyrin (PCI-0123): A Near-Infrared, Water-Soluble Photosensitizer. *Photochem. Photobiol.* **1996**, *63*, 892–897. [CrossRef]

54. Sessler, J.L.; Miller, R.A. Texaphyrins: New drugs with diverse clinical applications in radiation and photodynamic therapy. *Biochem. Pharmacol.* **2000**, *59*, 733–739. [CrossRef]

55. Du, K.; Mick, R.; Busch, T.; Zhu, T.C.; Finlay, J.; Yu, G.; Yodh, A.; Malkowicz, S.; Smith, D.; Whittington, R.; et al. Preliminary results of interstitial motexafin lutetium-mediated PDT for prostate cancer. *Lasers Surg. Med.* **2006**, *38*, 427–434. [CrossRef] [PubMed]

56. Rockson, S.G.; Lorenz, D.P.; Cheong, W.-F.; Woodburn, K.W. Photoangioplasty: An emerging clinical cardiovascular role for photodynamic therapy. *Circulation* **2000**, *102*, 591–596. [CrossRef] [PubMed]

57. Kogias, E.; Vougioukas, V.; Hubbe, U.; Halatsch, M.-E. Minimally Invasive Approach for the Treatment of Lateral Lumbar Disc Herniations. Technique and Results. *Minim. Invasive Neurosurg.* **2007**, *50*, 160–162. [CrossRef]

58. Wood, S.R.; Holroyd, J.A.; Brown, S.B. The Subcellular Localization of Zn(ll) Phthalocyanines and Their Redistribution on Exposure to Light. *Photochem. Photobiol.* **1997**, *65*, 397–402. [CrossRef] [PubMed]

59. Stuchinskaya, T.; Moreno, M.; Cook, M.J.; Edwards, D.R.; Russell, D.A. Targeted photodynamic therapy of breast cancer cells using antibody–phthalocyanine–gold nanoparticle conjugates. *Photochem. Photobiol. Sci.* **2011**, *10*, 822. [CrossRef]

60. Sekhejane, P.R.; Houreld, N.N.; Abrahamse, H. Multiorganelle Localization of Metallated Phthalocyanine Photosensitizer in Colorectal Cancer Cells (DLD-1 and CaCo-2) Enhances Efficacy of Photodynamic Therapy. *Int. J. Photoenergy* **2014**, *2014*, 1–10. [CrossRef]

61. Hunt, D.W.C. Rostaporfin (Miravant Medical Technologies). *IDrugs* **2002**, *5*, 180–186.

62. Kaplan, M.; Somers, R.H.; Greenburg, R.; Ackler, J. Photodynamic therapy in the management of metastatic cutaneous adenocarcinomas: Case reports from phase 1/2 studies using tin ethyl etiopurpurin (SnET2). *J. Surg. Oncol.* **1998**, *67*, 121–125. [CrossRef]

63. Selman, S.H.; Keck, R.W.; Hampton, J.A. Transperineal Photodynamic Ablation of the Canine Prostate. *J. Urol.* **1996**, *156*, 258–260. [CrossRef]

64. Agostinis, P.; Berg, K.; Cengel, K.A.; Foster, T.H.; Girotti, A.W.; Gollnick, S.O.; Hahn, S.M.; Hamblin, M.R.; Juzeniene, A.; Kessel, D.; et al. Photodynamic therapy of cancer: An update. *CA Cancer J. Clin.* **2011**, *61*, 250–281. [CrossRef] [PubMed]

65. Reiners, J.J.; Agostinis, P.; Berg, K.; Oleinick, N.L.; Kessel, D. Assessing autophagy in the context of photodynamic therapy. *Autophagy* **2010**, *6*, 7–18. [CrossRef] [PubMed]

66. Kruger, C.; Abrahamse, H. Utilisation of Targeted Nanoparticle Photosensitiser Drug Delivery Systems for the Enhancement of Photodynamic Therapy. *Molecules* **2018**, *23*, 2628. [CrossRef]

67. Redmond, R.W.; Gamlin, J.N. A compilation of singlet oxygen yields from biologically relevant molecules. *Photochem. Photobiol.* **1999**, *70*, 391–475. [CrossRef]

68. Kitamura, N.; Kohtani, S.; Nakagaki, R. Molecular aspects of furocoumarin reactions: Photophysics, photochemistry, photobiology, and structural analysis. *J. Photochem. Photobiol. C Photochem. Rev.* **2005**, *6*, 168–185. [CrossRef]

69. Fracarolli, L.; Rodrigues, G.B.; Pereira, A.C.; Júnior, N.S.M.; Silva-Junior, G.J.; Bachmann, L.; Wainwright, M.; Bastos, J.K.; Braga, G.U. Inactivation of plant-pathogenic fungus Colletotrichum acutatum with natural plant-produced photosensitizers under solar radiation. *J. Photochem. Photobiol. B Boil.* **2016**, *162*, 402–411. [CrossRef]

70. Chobot, V.; Vytlačilová, J.; Kubicová, L.; Opletal, L.; Jahodář, L.; Laakso, I.; Vuorela, P. Phototoxic activity of a thiophene polyacetylene from Leuzea carthamoides. *Fitoterapia* **2006**, *77*, 194–198. [CrossRef]

71. Lima, B.; Agüero, M.B.; Zygadlo, J.; Tapia, A.; Solís, C.; De Arias, A.R.; Yaluff, G.; Zacchino, S.; Feresin, G.E.; Schmeda-Hirschmann, G. Antimicrobial activity of extracts, essential oil and metabolites obtained from tagetes mendocina. *J. Chil. Chem. Soc.* **2009**, *54*, 68–72. [CrossRef]

72. Jin, Q.; Lee, J.W.; Jang, H.; Choi, J.E.; Kim, H.S.; Lee, N.; Hong, J.T.; Lee, M.K.; Hwang, B.Y. Dimeric sesquiterpene and thiophenes from the roots of Echinops latifolius. *Bioorg. Med. Chem. Lett.* **2016**, *26*, 5995–5998. [CrossRef]

73. Postigo, A.; Funes, M.; Petenatti, E.; Bottai, H.; Pacciaroni, A.; Sortino, M. Antifungal photosensitive activity of Porophyllum obscurum (Spreng.) DC.: Correlation of the chemical composition of the hexane extract with the bioactivity. *Photodiagn. Photodyn. Ther.* **2017**, *20*, 263–272. [CrossRef] [PubMed]

74. Ibrahim, S.R.M.; Abdallah, H.M.; El Halawany, A.M.; Mohamed, G.A. Naturally occurring thiophenes: Isolation, purification, structural elucidation, and evaluation of bioactivities. *Phytochem. Rev.* **2015**, *15*, 197–220. [CrossRef]

75. Park, K.; Lee, J.-H. Photosensitizer effect of curcumin on UVB-irradiated HaCaT cells through activation of caspase pathways. *Oncol. Rep.* **2007**, *17*, 537–540. [CrossRef] [PubMed]

76. Lin, H.-Y.; Lin, J.-N.; Ma, J.-W.; Yang, N.-S.; Ho, C.-T.; Kuo, S.-C.; Way, T.-D. Demethoxycurcumin induces autophagic and apoptotic responses on breast cancer cells in photodynamic therapy. *J. Funct. Foods* **2015**, *12*, 439–449. [CrossRef]

77. Randazzo, W.; Aznar, R.; Sánchez, G. Curcumin-Mediated Photodynamic Inactivation of Norovirus Surrogates. *Food Environ. Virol.* **2016**, *8*, 244–250. [CrossRef]

78. Lee, H.-J.; Kang, S.-M.; Jeong, S.-H.; Chung, K.-H.; Kim, B.-I. Antibacterial photodynamic therapy with curcumin and Curcuma xanthorrhiza extract against Streptococcus mutans. *Photodiagnosis Photodyn. Ther.* **2017**, *20*, 116–119. [CrossRef]

79. Bhavya, M.; Hebbar, H.U. Efficacy of blue LED in microbial inactivation: Effect of photosensitization and process parameters. *Int. J. Food Microbiol.* **2019**, *290*, 296–304. [CrossRef]

80. Morten, A.G.; Martinez, L.J.; Holt, N.; Sik, R.H.; Reszka, K.; Chignell, C.F.; Tonnesen, H.H.; Roberts, J.E. Photophysical Studies on Antimalariai Drugs. *Photochem. Photobiol.* **2008**, *69*, 282–287. [CrossRef]

81. Inbaraj, J.J.; Kukielczak, B.M.; Bilski, P.; Sandvik, S.L.; Chignell, C.F. Photochemistry and Photocytotoxicity of Alkaloids from Goldenseal (Hydrastis canadensis L.) 1. Berberine. *Chem. Res. Toxicol.* **2001**, *14*, 1529–1534. [CrossRef]

82. Flors, C.; Prat, C.; Suau, R.; Najera, F.; Nonell, S. Photochemistry of Phytoalexins Containing Phenalenone-like Chromophores: Photophysics and Singlet Oxygen Photosensitizing Properties of the Plant Oxoaporphine Alkaloid Oxoglaucine. *Photochem. Photobiol.* **2005**, *81*, 120. [CrossRef]

83. Lorente, C.; Thomas, A.H. Photophysics and photochemistry of pterins in aqueous solution. *Acc. Chem. Res.* **2006**, *39*, 395–402. [CrossRef] [PubMed]

84. Phillipson, J.D.; Roberts, M.F.; Zenk, M.H. *The Chemistry and Biology of Isoquinoline Alkaloids*; Springer Science & Business Media: Berlin, Germany, 2012.

85. Vignoni, M.; Erra-Balsells, R.; Epe, B.; Cabrerizo, F.M. Intra- and extra-cellular DNA damage by harmine and 9-methyl-harmine. *J. Photochem. Photobiol. B Boil.* **2014**, *132*, 66–71. [CrossRef] [PubMed]

86. Reid, L.O.; Roman, E.A.; Thomas, A.H.; Dántola, M.L. Photooxidation of Tryptophan and Tyrosine Residues in Human Serum Albumin Sensitized by Pterin: A Model for Globular Protein Photodamage in Skin. *Biochemistry* **2016**, *55*, 4777–4786. [CrossRef] [PubMed]

87. Yañuk, J.G.; Denofrio, M.P.; Rasse-Suriani, F.A.O.; Villarruel, F.D.; Fassetta, F.; Einschlag, F.S.G.; Erra-Balsells, R.; Epe, B.; Cabrerizo, F.M. DNA damage photo-induced by chloroharmine isomers: Hydrolysis versus oxidation of nucleobases. *Org. Biomol. Chem.* **2018**, *16*, 2170–2184. [CrossRef]

88. Daub, M.E.; Herrero, S.; Chung, K.-R. Photoactivated perylenequinone toxins in fungal pathogenesis of plants. *FEMS Microbiol. Lett.* **2005**, *252*, 197–206. [CrossRef]

89. Montoya, S.C.N.; Comini, L.R.; Sarmiento, M.; Becerra, C.; Albesa, I.; Argüello, G.A.; Cabrera, J.L. Natural anthraquinones probed as Type I and Type II photosensitizers: Singlet oxygen and superoxide anion production. *J. Photochem. Photobiol. B Boil.* **2005**, *78*, 77–83. [CrossRef]

90. Comini, L.R.; Montoya, S.C.N.; Sarmiento, M.; Cabrera, J.L.; Argüello, G.A. Characterizing some photophysical, photochemical and photobiological properties of photosensitizing anthraquinones. *J. Photochem. Photobiol. A Chem.* **2007**, *188*, 185–191. [CrossRef]

91. Mastrangelopoulou, M.; Grigalavicius, M.; Berg, K.; Ménard, M.; Theodossiou, T.A. Cytotoxic and Photocytotoxic Effects of Cercosporin on Human Tumor Cell Lines. *Photochem. Photobiol.* **2018**, *95*, 387–396. [CrossRef]

92. Panno, M.L.; Giordano, F.; Palma, M.G.; Bartella, V.; Rago, V.; Maggiolini, M.; Sisci, D.; Lanzino, M.; De Amicis, F.; Ando, S. Evidence that bergapten, independently of its photoactivation, enhances p53 gene expression and induces apoptosis in human breast cancer cells. *Curr. Cancer Drug Targets* **2009**, *9*, 469–481. [CrossRef]

93. Panno, M.L.; Giordano, F.; Rizza, P.; Pellegrino, M.; Zito, D.; Giordano, C.; Mauro, L.; Catalano, S.; Aquila, S.; Sisci, D.; et al. Bergapten induces ER depletion in breast cancer cells through SMAD4-mediated ubiquitination. *Breast Cancer Res. Treat.* **2012**, *136*, 443–455. [CrossRef]

94. Kim, S.-M.; Lee, J.H.; Sethi, G.; Kim, C.; Baek, S.H.; Nam, D.; Chung, W.-S.; Shim, B.S.; Ahn, K.S.; Kim, S.-H. Bergamottin, a natural furanocoumarin obtained from grapefruit juice induces chemosensitization and apoptosis through the inhibition of STAT3 signaling pathway in tumor cells. *Cancer Lett.* **2014**, *354*, 153–163. [CrossRef] [PubMed]

95. Kim, S.-M.; Lee, E.-J.; Lee, J.H.; Yang, W.M.; Nam, D.; Lee, J.H.; Lee, S.-G.; Um, J.-Y.; Shim, B.S.; Ahn, K.S. Simvastatin in combination with bergamottin potentiates TNF-induced apoptosis through modulation of NF-κB signalling pathway in human chronic myelogenous leukaemia. *Pharm. Boil.* **2016**, *54*, 1–11. [CrossRef] [PubMed]

96. Ge, Z.-C.; Qu, X.; Yu, H.-F.; Zhang, H.-M.; Wang, Z.-H.; Zhang, Z.-T. Antitumor and apoptotic effects of bergaptol are mediated via mitochondrial death pathway and cell cycle arrest in human breast carcinoma cells. *Bangladesh J. Pharmacol.* **2016**, *11*, 489. [CrossRef]

97. Nagatani, T.; Matsuzaki, T.; Kim, S.; Baba, N.; Ichiyama, S.; Miyamoto, H.; Nakajima, H. Treatment of cutaneous T-cell lymphoma (CTCL) by extracorporeal photochemotherapy. *J. Dermatol. Sci.* **1990**, *1*, 226. [CrossRef]

98. Bethea, D.; Fullmer, B.; Syed, S.; Seltzer, G.; Tiano, J.; Rischko, C.; Gillespie, L.; Brown, D.; Gasparro, F.P. Psoralen photobiology and photochemotherapy: 50 years of science and medicine. *J. Dermatol. Sci.* **1999**, *19*, 78–88. [CrossRef]

99. McKenna, K.E. PUVA, Psoralens and Skin Cancer. *Skin Cancer UV Radiat.* **1997**, 416–424.

100. El-Domyati, M.; Moftah, N.H.; Nasif, G.A.; Abdel-Wahab, H.M.; Barakat, M.T.; Abdel-Aziz, R.T. Evaluation of apoptosis regulatory proteins in response to PUVA therapy for psoriasis. *Photodermatol. Photoimmunol. Photomed.* **2013**, *29*, 18–26. [CrossRef]

101. Holtick, U.; Wang, X.N.; Marshall, S.R.; Von Bergwelt-Baildon, M.; Scheid, C.; Dickinson, A.M. In Vitro PUVA Treatment Preferentially Induces Apoptosis in Alloactivated T Cells. *Transplantation* **2012**, *94*, e31–e34. [CrossRef]

102. Schmitt, I.M.; Chimenti, S.; Gasparro, F.P. Psoralen-protein photochemistry—A forgotten field. *J. Photochem. Photobiol. B Boil.* **1995**, *27*, 101–107. [CrossRef]

103. Van Aelst, B.; Devloo, R.; Zachee, P.; T'Kindt, R.; Sandra, K.; Vandekerckhove, P.; Compernolle, V.; Feys, H.B. Psoralen and Ultraviolet A Light Treatment Directly Affects Phosphatidylinositol 3-Kinase Signal Transduction by Altering Plasma Membrane Packing. *J. Boil. Chem.* **2016**, *291*, 24364–24376. [CrossRef]

104. Xia, W.; Gooden, D.; Liu, L.; Zhao, S.; Soderblom, E.J.; Toone, E.J.; Beyer, W.F.; Walder, H.; Spector, N. Photo-Activated Psoralen Binds the ErbB2 Catalytic Kinase Domain, Blocking ErbB2 Signaling and Triggering Tumor Cell Apoptosis. *PLoS ONE* **2014**, *9*, e88983. [CrossRef] [PubMed]

105. Ghosh, G.; Colón, K.L.; Fuller, A.; Sainuddin, T.; Bradner, E.; McCain, J.; Monro, S.M.A.; Yin, H.; Hetu, M.W.; Cameron, C.G.; et al. Cyclometalated Ruthenium(II) Complexes Derived from α-Oligothiophenes as Highly Selective Cytotoxic or Photocytotoxic Agents. *Inorg. Chem.* **2018**, *57*, 7694–7712. [CrossRef] [PubMed]

106. Zhang, P.; Jin, W.-R.; Shi, Q.; He, H.; Ma, Z.; Qu, H.-B. Two novel thiophenes from Echinops grijissi Hance. *J. Asian Nat. Prod. Res.* **2008**, *10*, 977–981. [CrossRef] [PubMed]

107. Galushko, S.; Shishkina, I.; Alekseeva, I. Relationship between retention parameters in reversed-phase high-performance liquid chromatography and antitumour activity of some pyrimidine bases and nucleosides. *J. Chromatogr. A* **1991**, *547*, 161–166. [CrossRef]

108. Wang, Y.D.; Johnson, S.; Powell, D.; McGinnis, J.P.; Miranda, M.; Rabindran, S.K. Inhibition of tumor cell proliferation by thieno[2,3-d]pyrimidin-4(1H)-one-based analogs. *Bioorg. Med. Chem. Lett.* **2005**, *15*, 3763–3766. [CrossRef]

109. Alagarsamy, V.; Meena, S.; Ramseshu, K.; Solomon, V.; Thirumurugan, K.; Dhanabal, K.; Murugan, M. Synthesis, analgesic, anti-inflammatory, ulcerogenic index and antibacterial activities of novel 2-methylthio-3-substituted-5,6,7,8-tetrahydrobenzo (b) thieno[2,3-d]pyrimidin-4(3H)-ones. *Eur. J. Med. Chem.* **2006**, *41*, 1293–1300. [CrossRef]

110. Starcevic, K.; Kralj, M.; Piantanida, I.; Šuman, L.; Pavelic, K.; Karminski-Zamola, G. Synthesis, photochemical synthesis, DNA binding and antitumor evaluation of novel cyano- and amidino-substituted derivatives of naphtho-furans, naphtho-thiophenes, thieno-benzofurans, benzo-dithiophenes and their acyclic precursors. *Eur. J. Med. Chem.* **2006**, *41*, 925–939. [CrossRef]

111. Galindo, M.A.; Romero, M.A.; Navarro, J.A. Cyclic assemblies formed by metal ions, pyrimidines and isogeometrical heterocycles: DNA binding properties and antitumour activity. *Inorg. Chim. Acta* **2009**, *362*, 1027–1030. [CrossRef]

112. Prachayasittikul, S.; Worachartcheewan, A.; Nantasenamat, C.; Chinworrungsee, M.; Sornsongkhram, N.; Ruchirawat, S.; Prachayasittikul, V. Synthesis and structure–activity relationship of 2-thiopyrimidine-4-one analogs as antimicrobial and anticancer agents. *Eur. J. Med. Chem.* **2011**, *46*, 738–742. [CrossRef]

113. Jin, W.; Shi, Q.; Hong, C.; Cheng, Y.; Ma, Z.; Qu, H. Cytotoxic properties of thiophenes from Echinops grijissi Hance. *Phytomedicine* **2008**, *15*, 768–774. [CrossRef]

114. Karunagaran, D.; Rashmi, R.; Kumar, T.R.S. Induction of Apoptosis by Curcumin and Its Implications for Cancer Therapy. *Curr. Cancer Drug Targets* **2005**, *5*, 117–129. [CrossRef] [PubMed]

115. Tønnesen, H.H.; De Vries, H.; Karlsen, J.; Van Henegouwen, G.B. Studies on Curcumin and Curcuminoids IX: Investigation of the Photobiological Activity of Curcumin Using Bacterial Indicator Systems. *J. Pharm. Sci.* **1987**, *76*, 371–373. [CrossRef]

116. Dahl, T.A.; McGowan, W.M.; Shand, M.A.; Srinivasan, V.S. Photokilling of bacteria by the natural dye curcumin. *Arch. Microbiol.* **1989**, *151*, 183–185. [CrossRef] [PubMed]

117. Haukvik, T.; Bruzell, E.; Kristensen, S.; Tønnesen, H.H. Photokilling of bacteria by curcumin in selected polyethylene glycol 400 (PEG 400) preparations. Studies on curcumin and curcuminoids, XLI. *Die Pharm.* **2010**, *65*, 600–606.

118. Nardo, L.; Andreoni, A.; Másson, M.; Haukvik, T.; Tønnesen, H.H. Studies on Curcumin and Curcuminoids. XXXIX. Photophysical Properties of Bisdemethoxycurcumin. *J. Fluoresc.* **2010**, *21*, 627–635. [CrossRef] [PubMed]

119. Bruzell, E.M.; Morisbak, E.; Tønnesen, H.H. Studies on curcumin and curcuminoids. XXIX. Photoinduced cytotoxicity of curcumin in selected aqueous preparations. *Photochem. Photobiol. Sci.* **2005**, *4*, 523. [CrossRef]

120. Nardo, L.; Andreoni, A.; Bondani, M.; Másson, M.; Haukvik, T.; Tønnesen, H.H. Studies on Curcumin and Curcuminoids. XLVI. Photophysical Properties of Dimethoxycurcumin and Bis-dehydroxycurcumin. *J. Fluoresc.* **2011**, *22*, 597–608. [CrossRef]

121. Nardo, L.; Andreoni, A.; Bondani, M.; Másson, M.; Tønnesen, H.H. Studies on curcumin and curcuminoids. XXXIV. Photophysical properties of a symmetrical, non-substituted curcumin analogue. *J. Photochem. Photobiol. B Boil.* **2009**, *97*, 77–86. [CrossRef]

122. Araújo, N.C.; Fontana, C.R.; Gerbi, M.E.M.; Bagnato, V.S. Overall-Mouth Disinfection by Photodynamic Therapy Using Curcumin. *Photomed. Laser Surg.* **2012**, *30*, 96–101. [CrossRef]

123. Rego-Filho, F.D.A.; De Araujo, M.T.; De Oliveira, K.T.; Bagnato, V.S. Validation of Photodynamic Action via Photobleaching of a New Curcumin-Based Composite with Enhanced Water Solubility. *J. Fluoresc.* **2014**, *24*, 1407–1413. [CrossRef]

124. Sreedhar, A.; Sarkar, I.; Rajan, P.; Pai, J.; Malagi, S.; Kamath, V.; Barmappa, R. Comparative evaluation of the efficacy of curcumin gel with and without photo activation as an adjunct to scaling and root planing in the treatment of chronic periodontitis: A split mouth clinical and microbiological study. *J. Nat. Sci. Boil. Med.* **2015**, *6*, 102–S109. [CrossRef] [PubMed]

125. MacRobert, A.J.; Komerik, N. Photodynamic Therapy as an Alternative Antimicrobial Modality for Oral Infections. *J. Environ. Pathol. Toxicol. Oncol.* **2006**, *25*, 487–504. [CrossRef] [PubMed]

126. Priyadarsini, K.I. Photophysics, photochemistry and photobiology of curcumin: Studies from organic solutions, bio-mimetics and living cells. *J. Photochem. Photobiol. C Photochem. Rev.* **2009**, *10*, 81–95. [CrossRef]

127. Maheshwari, R.K.; Singh, A.K.; Gaddipati, J.; Srimal, R.C. Multiple biological activities of curcumin: A short review. *Life Sci.* **2006**, *78*, 2081–2087. [CrossRef] [PubMed]

128. Yance, D.R.; Sagar, S.M. Targeting Angiogenesis with Integrative Cancer Therapies. *Integr. Cancer Ther.* **2006**, *5*, 9–29. [CrossRef] [PubMed]

129. Salvioli, S.; Sikora, E.; Cooper, E.L.; Franceschi, C. Curcumin in Cell Death Processes: A Challenge for CAM of Age-Related Pathologies. *Evidence-Based Complement Altern. Med.* **2007**, *4*, 181–190. [CrossRef]

130. Vallianou, N.; Evangelopoulos, A.; Schizas, N.; Kazazis, C. Potential anticancer properties and mechanisms of action of curcumin. *Anticancer Res.* **2015**, *35*, 645–651.

131. Yang, J.-Y.; Zhong, X.; Yum, H.-W.; Lee, H.-J.; Kundu, J.K.; Na, H.-K.; Surh, Y.-J. Curcumin Inhibits STAT3 Signaling in the Colon of Dextran Sulfate Sodium-treated Mice. *J. Cancer Prev.* **2013**, *18*, 186–191. [CrossRef]

132. Dovigo, L.N.; Pavarina, A.C.; Carmello, J.C.; Machado, A.L.; Brunetti, I.L.; Bagnato, V.S. Susceptibility of clinical isolates of Candida to photodynamic effects of curcumin. *Lasers Surg. Med.* **2011**, *43*, 927–934. [CrossRef]

133. Bernd, A. Visible light and/or UVA offer a strong amplification of the anti-tumor effect of curcumin. *Phytochem. Rev.* **2013**, *13*, 183–189. [CrossRef]

134. Chan, W.-H.; Wu, H.-J. Anti-apoptotic effects of curcumin on photosensitized human epidermal carcinoma A431 cells. *J. Cell. Biochem.* **2004**, *92*, 200–212. [CrossRef] [PubMed]

135. Araújo, N.C.; Fontana, C.R.; Bagnato, V.S.; Gerbi, M.E.M. Photodynamic Effects of Curcumin Against Cariogenic Pathogens. *Photomed. Laser Surg.* **2012**, *30*, 393–399. [CrossRef]

136. Benyhe, S. Morphine: New aspects in the study of an ancient compound. *Life Sci.* **1994**, *55*, 969–979. [CrossRef]

137. Li, W.; Shao, Y.; Hu, L.; Zhang, X.; Chen, Y.; Tong, L.; Li, C.; Shen, X.; Ding, J. BM6, a new semi-synthetic vinca alkaloid, exhibits its potent in vivo anti-tumor activities via its high binding affinity for tubulin and improved pharmacokinetic profiles. *Cancer Boil. Ther.* **2007**, *6*, 787–794. [CrossRef] [PubMed]

138. Huang, M.; Gao, H.; Chen, Y.; Zhu, H.; Cai, Y.; Zhang, X.; Miao, Z.; Jiang, H.; Zhang, J.; Shen, H.; et al. Chimmitecan, a Novel 9-Substituted Camptothecin, with Improved Anticancer Pharmacologic Profiles In vitro and In vivo. *Clin. Cancer Res.* **2007**, *13*, 1298–1307. [CrossRef] [PubMed]

139. Sun, Y.; Xun, K.; Wang, Y.; Chen, X. A systematic review of the anticancer properties of berberine, a natural product from Chinese herbs. *Anti-Cancer Drugs* **2009**, *20*, 757–769. [CrossRef]

140. Eom, K.S.; Kim, H.-J.; So, H.-S.; Park, R.; Kim, T.Y. Berberine-induced apoptosis in human glioblastoma T98G cells is mediated by endoplasmic reticulum stress accompanying reactive oxygen species and mitochondrial dysfunction. *Boil. Pharm. Bull.* **2010**, *33*, 1644–1649. [CrossRef]

141. Diogo, C.V.; Machado, N.G.; Barbosa, I.A.; Serafim, T.L.; Burgeiro, A.; Oliveira, P.J. Berberine as a Promising Safe Anti-Cancer Agent- Is there a Role for Mitochondria? *Curr. Drug Targets* **2011**, *12*, 850–859. [CrossRef]

142. Tan, W.; Lu, J.-J.; Huang, M.; Li, Y.; Chen, M.; Wu, G.; Gong, J.; Zhong, Z.; Xu, Z.; Dang, Y.; et al. Anti-cancer natural products isolated from chinese medicinal herbs. *Chin. Med.* **2011**, *6*, 27. [CrossRef]

143. Burgeiro, A.A.C.; Gajate, C.; Dakir, E.H.; Villa-Pulgarin, J.A.; Oliveira, P.J.; Mollinedo, F. Involvement of mitochondrial and B-RAF/ERK signaling pathways in berberine-induced apoptosis in human melanoma cells. *Anti-Cancer Drugs* **2011**, *22*, 507–518. [CrossRef]

144. Youn, M.-J.; So, H.-S.; Cho, H.-J.; Kim, H.-J.; Kim, Y.; Lee, J.-H.; Sohn, J.S.; Kim, Y.K.; Chung, S.-Y.; Park, R. Berberine, a Natural Product, Combined with Cisplatin Enhanced Apoptosis through a Mitochondria/Caspase-Mediated Pathway in HeLa Cells. *Boil. Pharm. Bull.* **2008**, *31*, 789–795. [CrossRef] [PubMed]

145. Hur, J.-M.; Hyun, M.-S.; Lim, S.; Lee, W.-Y.; Kim, N. The combination of berberine and irradiation enhances anti-cancer effects via activation of p38 MAPK pathway and ROS generation in human hepatoma cells. *J. Cell. Biochem.* **2009**, *107*, 955–964. [CrossRef] [PubMed]

146. Andreazza, N.L.; Vevert-Bizet, C.; Bourg-Heckly, G.; Sureau, F.; Salvador, M.J.; Bonneau, S. Berberine as a Photosensitizing Agent for Antitumoral Photodynamic Therapy: Insights into its Association to Low Density Lipoproteins. *Int. J. Pharm.* **2016**, *510*, 240–249. [CrossRef] [PubMed]

147. Bhattacharyya, R.; Gupta, P.; Bandyopadhyay, S.K.; Patro, B.S.; Chattopadhyay, S. Coralyne, a protoberberine alkaloid, causes robust photosenstization of cancer cells through ATR-p38 MAPK-BAX and JAK2-STAT1-BAX pathways. *Chem. Interact.* **2018**, *285*, 27–39. [CrossRef] [PubMed]

148. Martín, J.P.; Labrador, V.; Freire, P.F.; Molero, M.L.; Hazen, M. Ultrastructural changes induced in HeLa cells after phototoxic treatment with harmine. *J. Appl. Toxicol.* **2004**, *24*, 197–201. [CrossRef] [PubMed]

149. Arnason, J.T.; Towers, G.H.N.; Abramowski, Z.; Campos, F.; Champagne, D.; McLachlan, D.; Philogène, B.J.R. Berberine: A naturally occurring phototoxic alkaloid. *J. Chem. Ecol.* **1984**, *10*, 115–123. [CrossRef]

150. Cheng, L.-L.; Wang, M.; Zhu, H.; Li, K.; Zhu, R.-R.; Sun, X.-Y.; Yao, S.-D.; Wu, Q.-S.; Wang, S.-L. Characterization of the transient species generated by the photoionization of Berberine: A laser flash photolysis study. *Spectrochim. Acta Part A Mol. Biomol. Spectrosc.* **2009**, *73*, 955–959. [CrossRef]

151. Jantova, S.; Letašiová, S.; Brezová, V.; Cipak, L.; Lábaj, J. Photochemical and phototoxic activity of berberine on murine fibroblast NIH-3T3 and Ehrlich ascites carcinoma cells. *J. Photochem. Photobiol. B Boil.* **2006**, *85*, 163–176. [CrossRef]

152. Dave, H.; Ledwani, L. A review on anthraquinones isolated from Cassia species and their applications. *Indian J. Nat. Prod. Resour.* **2012**, *3*, 291–319.

153. Seigler, D.S. *Plant Secondary Metabolism*; Springer Science & Business Media: Berlin, Germany, 1998.
154. Gutiérrez, I.; Bertolotti, S.G.; Biasutti, M.; Soltermann, A.T.; García, N.A. Quinones and hydroxyquinones as generators and quenchers of singlet molecular oxygen. *Can. J. Chem.* **1997**, *75*, 423–428. [CrossRef]
155. Pawłowska, J.; Tarasiuk, J.; Wolf, C.R.; Paine, M.J.I.; Borowski, E. Differential Ability of Cytostatics From Anthraquinone Group to Generate Free Radicals in Three Enzymatic Systems: NADH Dehydrogenase, NADPH Cytochrome P450 Reductase, and Xanthine Oxidase. *Oncol. Res. Featur. Preclin. Clin. Cancer Ther.* **2003**, *13*, 245–252. [CrossRef] [PubMed]
156. Singh, A. *Herbal Drugs as Therapeutic Agents*; CRC Press: Boca Raton, FL, USA, 2014.
157. Montoya, S.C.N.; Comini, L.; Vittar, B.R.; Fernández, I.M.; Rivarola, V.A.; Cabrera, J.L. Phototoxic effects of Heterophyllaea pustulata (Rubiaceae). *Toxicon* **2008**, *51*, 1409–1415. [CrossRef] [PubMed]
158. Comini, L.; Fernandez, I.; Vittar, N.R.; Montoya, S.N.; Cabrera, J.L.; Rivarola, V.A. Photodynamic activity of anthraquinones isolated from Heterophyllaea pustulata Hook f. (Rubiaceae) on MCF-7c3 breast cancer cells. *Phytomedicine* **2011**, *18*, 1093–1095. [CrossRef] [PubMed]
159. Vittar, N.B.R.; Awruch, J.; Azizuddin, K.; Rivarola, V.A. Caspase-independent apoptosis, in human MCF-7c3 breast cancer cells, following photodynamic therapy, with a novel water-soluble phthalocyanine. *Int. J. Biochem. Cell Boil.* **2010**, *42*, 1123–1131. [CrossRef]
160. Pirillo, J.; De Simone, B.C.; Russo, N. Photophysical properties prediction of selenium- and tellurium-substituted thymidine as potential UVA chemotherapeutic agents. *Theor. Chem. Accounts* **2015**, *135*, 8. [CrossRef]
161. Mazzone, G.; Alberto, M.E.; De Simone, B.C.; Marino, T.; Russo, N. Can Expanded Bacteriochlorins Act as Photosensitizers in Photodynamic Therapy? Good News from Density Functional Theory Computations. *Molecules* **2016**, *21*, 288. [CrossRef] [PubMed]
162. Mansoori, B.; Mohammadi, A.; Doustvandi, M.A.; Mohammadnejad, F.; Kamari, F.; Gjerstorff, M.F.; Baradaran, B.; Hamblin, M.R. Photodynamic therapy for cancer: Role of natural products. *Photodiagnosis Photodyn. Ther.* **2019**, *26*, 395–404. [CrossRef] [PubMed]
163. Pandey, R.K.; Goswami, L.N.; Chen, Y.; Gryshuk, A.; Missert, J.R.; Oseroff, A.; Dougherty, T.J. Nature: A rich source for developing multifunctional agents. tumor-imaging and photodynamic therapy. *Lasers Surg. Med.* **2006**, *38*, 445–467. [CrossRef]

9

Overcoming Resistance to Platinum-Based Drugs in Ovarian Cancer by Salinomycin and its Derivatives—An In Vitro Study

Marcin Michalak [1], Michał Stefan Lach [2,3,4,*], Michał Antoszczak [5], Adam Huczyński [5] and Wiktoria Maria Suchorska [2,4,*]

[1] Department of Radiation Therapy and Gynecologic Oncology, Greater Poland Cancer Centre, Garbary 15, 61–866 Poznań, Poland; marcin.michalak@wco.pl

[2] Radiobiology Lab, Greater Poland Cancer Centre, Garbary 15, 61–866 Poznań, Poland

[3] The Postgraduate School of Molecular Medicine, Medical University of Warsaw, Księcia Trojdena 2a, 02–109 Warsaw, Poland

[4] Department of Electroradiology, Poznań University of Medical Sciences, Garbary 15, 61–866 Poznań, Poland

[5] Department of Medical Chemistry, Faculty of Chemistry, Adam Mickiewicz University, Uniwersytetu Poznańskiego 8, 61–614 Poznań, Poland; michant@amu.edu.pl (M.A.); adhucz@amu.edu.pl (A.H.)

* Correspondence: michal.lach@wco.pl (M.S.L.); wiktoria.suchorska@wco.pl (W.M.S.); (M.S.L. & W.M.S.)

Abstract: Polyether ionophore salinomycin (SAL) and its semi-synthetic derivatives are recognized as very promising anticancer drug candidates due to their activity against various types of cancer cells, including multidrug-resistant populations. Ovarian cancer is the deadliest among gynecologic malignancies, which is connected with the development of chemoresistant forms of the disease in over 70% of patients after initial treatment regimen. Thus, we decided to examine the anticancer properties of SAL and selected SAL derivatives against a series of drug-sensitive (A2780, SK-OV-3) and derived drug-resistant (A2780 CDDP, SK-OV-3 CDDP) ovarian cancer cell lines. Although SAL analogs showed less promising IC_{50} values than SAL, they were identified as the antitumor agents that significantly overcome the resistance to platinum-based drugs in ovarian cancer, more potent than unmodified SAL and commonly used anticancer drugs—5-fluorouracil, gemcitabine, and cisplatin. Moreover, when compared with SAL used alone, our experiments proved for the first time increased selectivity of SAL-based dual therapy with 5-fluorouracil or gemcitabine, especially towards A2780 cell line. Looking closer at the results, SAL acted synergistically with 5-fluorouracil towards the drug-resistant A2780 cell line. Our results suggest that combinations of SAL with other antineoplastics may become a new therapeutic option for patients with ovarian cancer.

Keywords: salinomycin; anticancer activity; overcoming drug resistance; tumor specificity; synergy; 5-fluorouracil; gemcitabine; amides/esters; ovarian cancer

1. Introduction

Despite developing new therapeutic strategies and extensive knowledge about tumor biology, ovarian cancer (OvCa) remains a leading cause of mortality among gynecologic malignancies; asymptomatic early stages and lack of ambiguous biomarkers enabling detection of the disease lead to late diagnosis, mostly at stage III and IV [1,2]. Five-year overall survival for advanced OvCa is approximately 30% [3]. Most of the patients respond well to radical surgery and either neoadjuvant or adjuvant chemotherapy. However, 75% of patients develop recurrence [4]. Prognosis for patients with the recurrent disease is poor, especially for those diagnosed with the recurrence earlier than six months after completion of the initial platinum-based therapy [5]. This state is called platinum-resistance in opposition to platinum-sensitive patients who develop recurrence more than six months after completion of the initial therapy. The intrinsic and acquired resistance to platinum-based chemotherapy is the main reason for OvCa treatment failure [6,7].

A few theories have been proposed to explain the development of chemoresistance in human malignancies. The most likely one is related to cancer stem cell theory [8]. According to this concept, a malignant tumor consists of two populations of cells, namely cancer stem cells (CSCs) and differentiated cells. Self-renewal, repopulation, and resistance to irradiation and cytotoxic drugs are typical of the first narrow population. Contrary to that, differentiated cancer cells are sensitive to treatment and form a bulk population of the tumor cells. CSCs, similarly to pluripotent stem cells, have active developmental signaling pathways, such as Hedgehog, Notch, and Wnt/β-catenin. The latter two seem to be particularly responsible for OvCa platinum resistance [9,10]. Unfortunately, there is no single universal marker capable of distinguishing CSCs from the differentiated cancer cells. Such a marker could help to develop a highly specific targeted therapy against CSCs, which would improve OvCa patient outcome. Therefore, the main focus of OvCa therapies should be the elimination of CSCs. One of the molecules exhibiting anticancer potential and selective properties against CSCs is salinomycin (SAL, **1**, Figure 1).

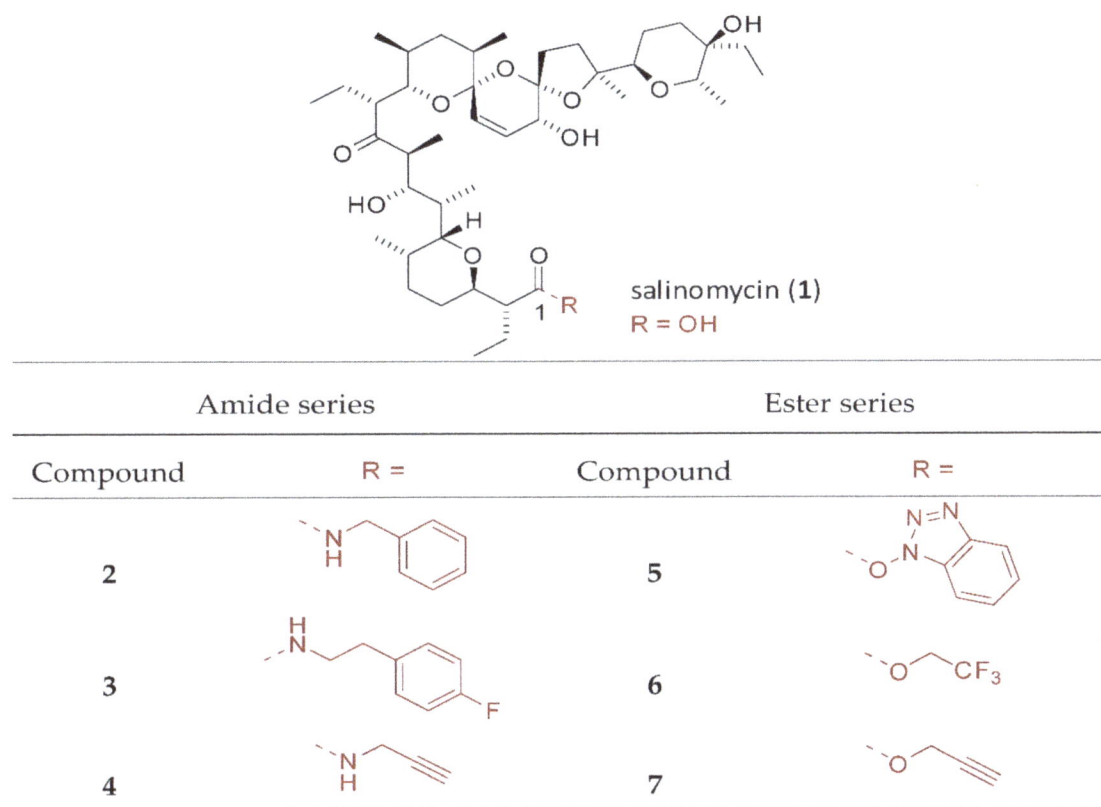

Figure 1. Structure of salinomycin and its derivatives studied in this work.

This is a monocarboxylic polyether antibiotic naturally synthesized by *Streptomyces albus* (strain no. 80614) [11]. SAL was identified in 2009 as the most active agent among 16,000 compounds tested towards breast CSCs [12]. Since then, SAL has been found effective against many other types of cancer cells and CSCs, including those displaying multidrug resistance (MDR) and has been used in a small group of patients with advanced carcinoma of the head, neck, breast, and ovary [13]. SAL acts as a sensitizer of malignant cells to radiotherapy or chemotherapy, i.e., colchicine, doxorubicin, and etoposide [14–17].

2. Results

2.1. Derivation of Cisplatin-Resistant Cell Lines

To test the usefulness of SAL and its derivatives in overcoming cisplatin-resistance, chemoresistant OvCa sub-cell lines were established. MTT and RT-qPCR followed the cell exposure to cisplatin to confirm derivation of stable phenotype of the resistant cell lines. A2780 CDDP and SK-OV-3 CDDP lines responded with morphological changes and increased IC_{50} against cisplatin as compared with their parental population (Figure 2A,B). Both resistant cell lines showed also enhanced expression of ABCB1, ABCG2, and ABCC2 versus control (Figure 2C,D). ABCB4 expression boosted significantly in SK-OV-3 CDDP cell line but only slightly in A2780 CDDP cell line.

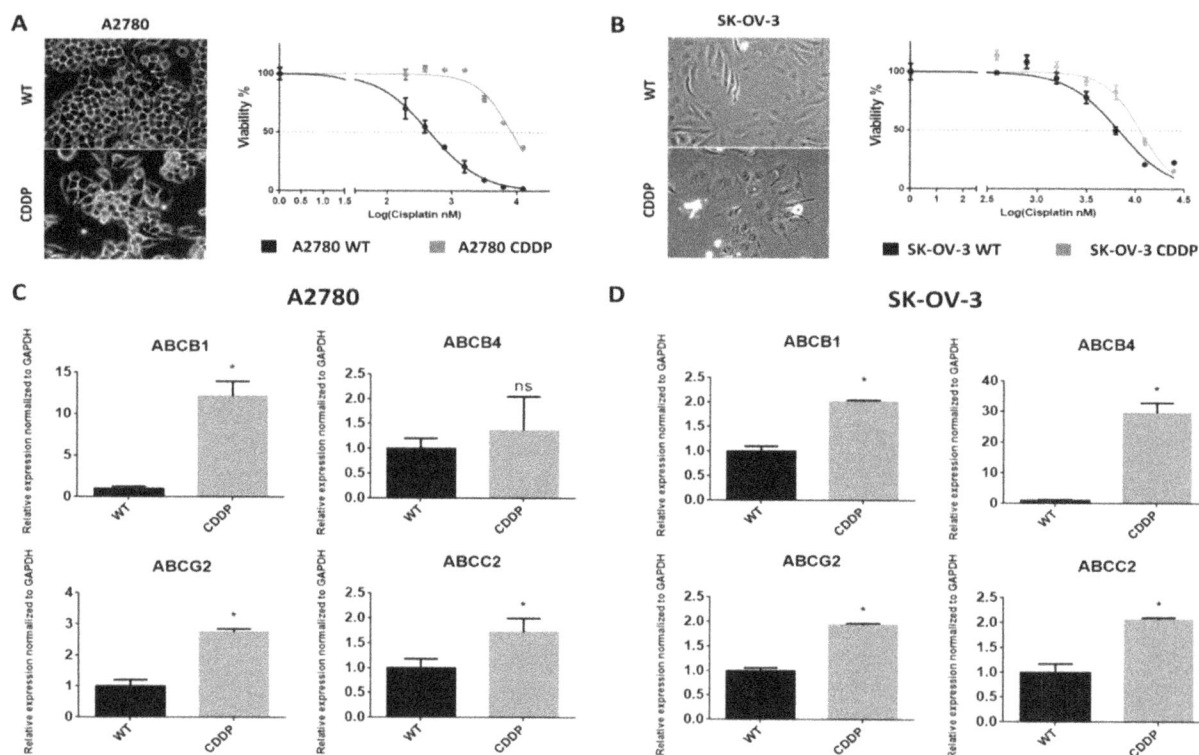

Figure 2. Overview of cisplatin-resistant ovarian cancer cell lines (A2780, SK-OV-3). (**A,B**) Morphological changes of both drug-resistant cancer sub-lines represent enlargement and slight spindle-like shape. Survival curves indicate increased IC_{50} for both resistant variants (RI = 18.08 for A2780; RI = 1.56 for SK-OV-3). The pictures were taken under 200× magnification. (**C,D**) RT-qPCR analysis of A2780 and SK-OV-3 revealed significantly increased expression of ABC drug transporters in derived resistant variants.

2.2. In Vitro Activity of Cytotoxic Drugs, Salinomycin, and Its Derivatives Against OvCa Cells

It was clearly proven that chemical modification of SAL and other polyether ionophores may not only increase the biological activity of resulting derivatives but also reduce their general toxicity [18–21]. Furthermore, SAL with a modified C1 carboxyl group (amides or esters) transports cations by a biomimetic mechanism, while chemically unmodified SAL transports cations through biological membranes via an electroneutral mechanism [22,23]. This change in ionophoretic properties may result in better biological properties of **SAL** analogs than of those with a native structure.

We devised a library of SAL derivatives based on the most active SAL amides and esters obtained in our previous studies by a chemical modification of C1 carboxyl group, i.e., amides **2** and **3**, as well as esters **5** and **6**, respectively (Figure 1) [18–20]. To expand structural diversity at C1 position and to better determine the structure-activity relationship (SAR), we additionally analyzed propargyl amide **4** and propargyl ester **7** (Figure 1), as these structures had shown promising bioactivity [19].

Data gathered in Table 1 indicate that all tested compounds exhibited biological activity against malignant cells. The effect towards ovarian A2780 cell line was distinctly better than that against metastatic ovarian SK-OV-3 cell line. Briefly, the most effective was chemically unmodified SAL, the activity of which was higher against A2780 cell line and comparable against SK-OV-3 cell line than that of reference anticancer drug—cisplatin (CDDP) (Table 1). In OvCa cell lines A2780, SK-OV-3 as well as their platinum-resistant sub-lines, all semi-synthetic derivatives of SAL (both from amide and ester series) needed significantly higher IC_{50} values to induce comparable biological effects than SAL itself (Table 1). The most active SAL analog was 4-fluorophenethyl amide **3** (Figure 1) but still its activity was one order of magnitude lower than that of unmodified SAL (Table 1). As expected, cisplatin-resistant sub-lines were more resistant to CDDP than both cisplatin-sensitive variants; thus, the anticancer activity of compounds **3** and **5** (Figure 1) was higher than that exhibited by CDDP towards A2780 CDDP cell line (Table 1).

However, to the best of our knowledge, there are no reports describing the effects of a dual therapy using SAL and 5-fluorouracil (5FU) or gemcitabine (GEM) towards OvCa cells. Therefore, we decided to check if SAL shows desired results when combined with these commonly used anticancer drugs. For this purpose, we prepared 1:1 molar mixtures of SAL and 5FU/GEM (**1** + 5FU and **1** + GEM, respectively) and tested their activity towards OvCa cell lines (Table 1). Interestingly, in both cases we witnessed a strong interaction between SAL and either 5FU or GEM. IC_{50} values for **1** + 5FU and **1** + GEM against all OvCa cell lines reached a low micromolar concentration range and were significantly lower than those exhibited by individual components (**1** and 5FU) and reference anticancer drug—CDDP (Table 1). More promising (lower) IC_{50} values were only obtained for GEM (Table 1), which is recommended for treatment of recurrent OvCa.

To determine the real therapeutic potential of novel anticancer drug candidates, it is necessary to check their effects (selectivity) towards normal cells. Judging by IC_{50} values, the tests performed in normal diploid human MRC-5 cell line suggested that all SAL derivatives were significantly less toxic towards non-malignant human cells than the chemically unmodified SAL (Table 1).

Table 1. The IC_{50} values estimated for ovarian cancer cell lines (A2780, SK-OV-3, both drug-sensitive and drug-resistant variants) and normal diploid human MRC-5 cell line after 72 h exposure to salinomycin (**SAL, 1**), its 1:1 molar mixtures with cytotoxic drugs (5-fluorouracil **5FU**, gemcitabine **GEM**), and salinomycin amides and esters (analogs **2–7**).

Compound		A2780		A2780 CDDP		SK-OV-3		SK-OV-3 CDDP		MRC-5	
		IC_{50} (µM)	CI 95%	IC_{50} (µM)	CI 95%	IC_{50} (µM)	CI 95%	IC_{50} (µM)	CI 95%	IC_{50} (µM)	CI 95%
SAL	1	0.11	0.08-0.13	0.29	0.27-0.29	4.01	3.13-5.11	3.72	3.24-4.25	10.15	5.14-20.01
salinomycin amides	2	27.05	24.25-30.18	24.90	19.98-31.04	183.45	156.43-215.24	140.60	119.40-165.71	213.33	186.19-244.52
	3	8.49	6.74-10.68	6.48	4.71-8.89	79.08	71.25-87.76	69.40	61.88-77.84	66.19	57.31-83.54
	4	14.38	11.99-17.23	12.54	9.58-16.40	91.17	81.42-102.07	58.53	53.22-64.37	98.96	88.13-111.13
salinomycin esters	5	25.50	20.44-31.79	7.74	6.04-9.94	205.88	188.71-224.65	103.41	82.63-129.38	58.81	47.05-73.53
	6	13.41	10.58-17.01	50.16	39.26-64.08	125.33	117.36-133.85	91.58	83.78-100.11	110.46	98.87-123.41
	7	37.31	27.95-49.56	45.74	35.49-57.05	179.72	146.77-219.90	94.56	85.65-104.41	160.96	96.41-268.69
1:1 molar mixtures	1 + 5FU	0.16	0.14-0.19	0.14	0.14-0.15	3.65	2.96-4.49	3.45	2.91-4.11	1.93	0.83-4.49
	1 + GEM	0.018	0.01-0.03	0.024	0.01-0.04	1.17	1.07-1.29	1.07	1.07-1.29	1.93	1.09-3.43
reference anticancer drugs	5FU	3.62	2.15-6.00	1.62	1.23-2.08	20.23	8.85-46.23	36.38	16.85-78.46	13.38	7.23-24.75
	GEM	0.007	0.006-0.007	0.02	0.01-0.02	0.002	0.00007-0.01	0.003	0.00003-0.02	0.04	0.01-0.012
	CDDP	0.47	0.40-0.50	8.33	7.40-9.37	4.03	3.48-4.61	6.72	5.96-7.56	15.7	12.9 -19.27

2.3. Salinomycin and Its Derivatives Overcome Cisplatin Resistance and are More Selective Against Cisplatin-Resistant OvCa Cells

To assess the effectiveness of the studied drugs in overcoming acquired cisplatin resistance, we calculated the resistance index (RI), based on the IC_{50} of derived cell lines (Figure 3A). The RI indicates how many more times a resistant sub-line (either A2780 CDDP or SK-OV-3 CDDP) is chemoresistant as compared with its parental cell line (either A2780 or SK-OV-3, respectively). An RI between 0 and 2 indicates that the cells are sensitive to the tested compound. An RI in the range from 2 to 10 means that the cells show moderate sensitivity to a drug. An RI above 10 indicates strong drug resistance [24]. None of the cancer cell lines developed strong resistance to the tested agents under the combinatory treatment of SAL with either 5FU or GEM (Figure 3A). Contrary to GEM, both **1** + 5FU and **1** + GEM co-treatments were capable of efficiently overcoming the drug resistance of OvCa cells, as manifested by considerably lower values of RI (Figure 3A).

Deeper analysis of RI parameters revealed that cancer cell line A2780, in opposition to SK-OV-3, developed some resistance to SAL (Figure 3A). This finding may indicate possible treatment failure on SAL clinical application. On the other hand, almost no SAL derivatives (except for **6** and **7**) developed even mild resistance during our experiments in both OvCa cell lines (Figure 3A). Generally, A2780 and SK-OV-3 cell lines turned out more sensitive to amide analogs of SAL (compounds **2–4**) than the corresponding ester derivatives (compounds **6–7**). The only exception to this rule was ester **5** (RI = 0.30 and RI = 0.50 for A2780 and SK-OV-3 cell line, respectively) (Figure 3A).

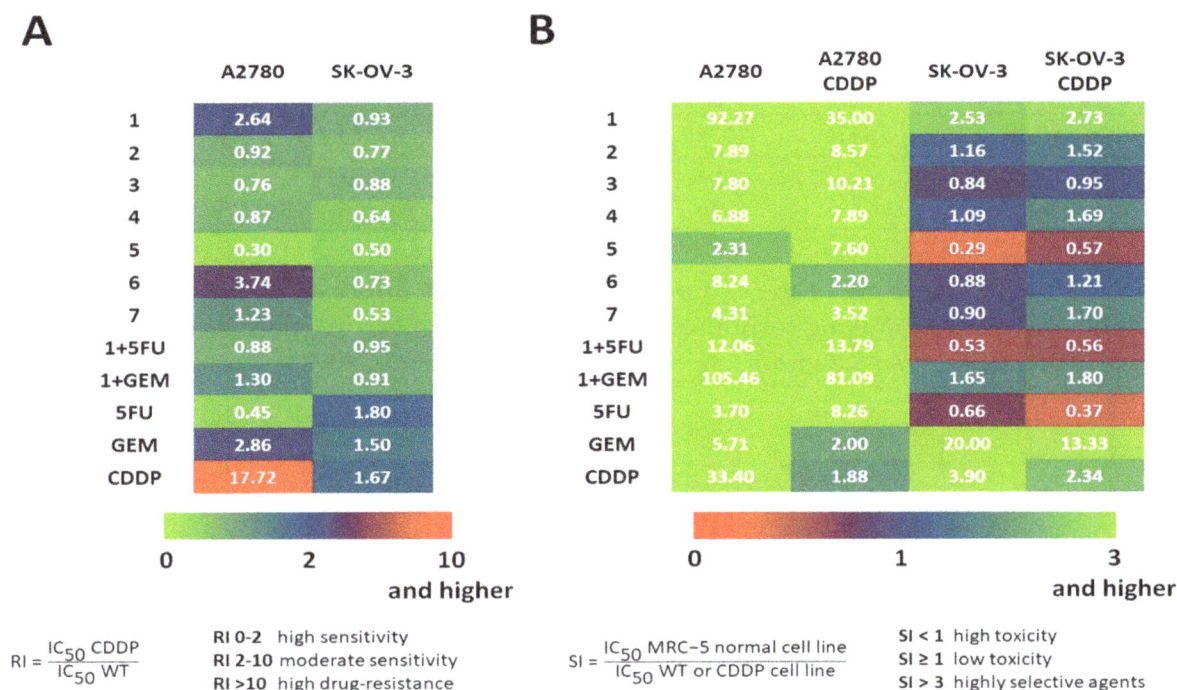

Figure 3. Calculated values of (**A**) the resistance indexes (RI), and (**B**) selectivity indexes (SI) of the tested compounds.

Further, to establish therapeutic potential of the tested anticancer agents, we used the difference in the antiproliferative activity towards the OvCa cell lines and the corresponding normal cell line to calculate the values of the selectivity index (SI) (Figure 3B). The SI is an important pharmaceutical parameter that facilitates the estimation of possible future clinical development; higher values of SI indicate greater anticancer specificity, and the compounds displaying an SI above 3.0 are considered highly selective agents [21,25]. Therefore, our study clearly proved that normal cells were less sensitive to SAL used alone or its combinations with other cytotoxic agents (5FU or GEM) than to amide and ester derivatives of SAL (Figure 3B).

Selectivity of SAL as well as its amide and ester analogs was very promising, especially in non-resistant and resistant to cisplatin A2780 cell lines (Figure 3B). However, the highest values of SI were noted for SAL and its 1:1 molar mixture with GEM (**1** + GEM, Figure 3B), and this effect decreased with time of exposure to the anticancer agents. On the other hand, SAL turned out more selective against SK-OV-3 cell line and its platinum-resistant variant than all analyzed amide and ester derivatives (Figure 3B). A combinatory treatment of OvCa cells involving SAL and GEM (**1** + GEM, Figure 3B) yielded very high SI values. The combination of the cytotoxic agents (regardless of their mechanism of anticancer action), either 5FU or GEM, with SAL was more effective than SAL or its derivatives used alone (Table 1 and Figure 3).

As OvCa cells seemed highly sensitive to the action of both **1** + 5FU and **1** + GEM (Table 1 and Figure 3), we decided to determine the exact effect (addictive, synergistic, or antagonistic) of the specific compound combinations. Using the 1:1 molar mixtures of SAL and 5FU or GEM, we performed standard viability assays and subjected the results to the analysis and determination of values of the combination indexes (CI) (Table 2). As previously described for a pair of drugs [26,27], CI > 1.3 indicates antagonism, CI = 1.1–1.3 indicates moderate antagonism, CI = 0.9–1.1 indicates additive effect, CI = 0.8–0.9 indicates slight synergism, CI = 0.6–0.8 indicates moderate synergism, CI = 0.4–0.6 indicates synergism, and CI = 0.2–0.4 indicates strong synergism. Interestingly, the results presented in Table 2 indicated that SAL in combination with 5FU acted synergistically (CI = 0.56) in A2780 CDDP cell line, whereas in SK-OV-3 and SK-OV-3 CDDP cell lines, they only showed an additive effect (CI = 1.09 and CI = 1.02, respectively).

Table 2. Calculated combination index (CI) values of simultaneously delivered salinomycin (**SAL, 1**) and cytotoxic drugs (5-fluorouracil **5FU**, gemcitabine **GEM**) in the 1:1 molar mixtures.

Combination of Compounds	A2780	A2780 CDDP	SK-OV-3	SK-OV-3 CDDP
1+5FU	1.57	0.56	1.09	1.02
1+GEM	2.86	1.60	691	360

After a primary screening of the compounds, SAL and its amides indicated in both OvCa cell lines variants the most promising response. To confirm their effect, Western blot analysis for B-cell lymphoma 2 (Bcl2), Bcl2 associated X protein (Bax), and caspase-3 (CASP3) was performed (Figure 4).

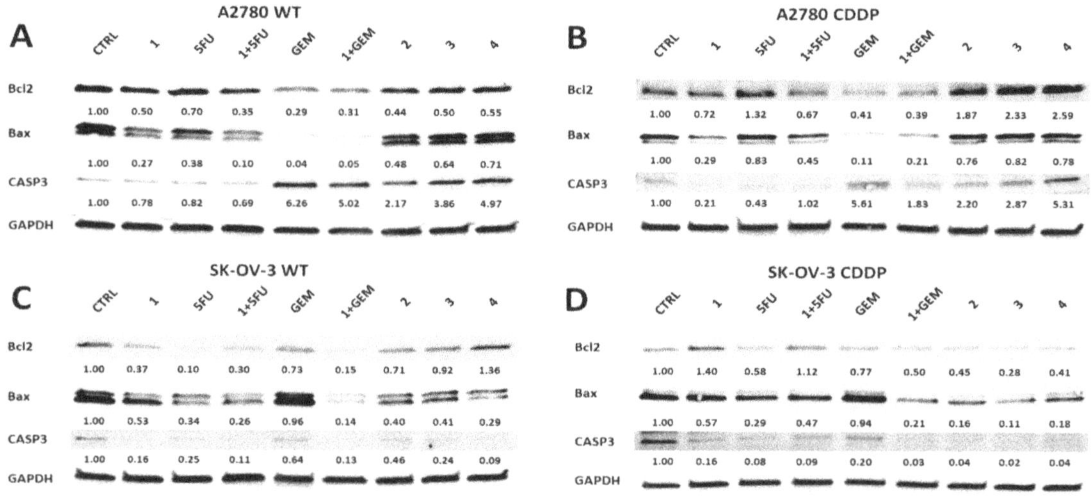

Figure 4. Western blot analysis of OvCa cell lines exposed to IC_{50} values of selected compounds for 72 h (**A–D**). The expression of anti-apoptotic (Bcl2) and apoptotic proteins (Bax and CASP3) was evaluated. The numbers describe the quantified level of band intensity normalized to expression of reference protein GAPDH and the control population.

In A2780 cells, the Bcl2 decreased in all groups in comparison with the control (Figure 4A). The lowest expression was observed in the GEM and 1 + GEM variant, but their effect was similar. The proapoptotic protein Bax also represented similar trends of expression as Bcl2. Interestingly, full form of caspase-3 (CASP3) was decreased in cells treated with SAL, 5FU, and their combination, but GEM and its combination with SAL, as well as amide derivatives of SAL, caused the enhanced expression of that protein. The antagonistic effect of combined SAL with 5FU or GEM was observed by decreasing expression of CASP3. In case of the A2780 CDDP variant, Bcl2 expression in cells treated with SAL, 1 + 5FU, GEM, and 1 + GEM was decreased (Figure 4B). Surprisingly, the SAL amides (3–5) caused increased Bcl2 expression. It is worth mentioning that a combination of 5FU with SAL caused downregulation of Bcl2. In all tested compounds the expression of Bax was inhibited in comparison with the control. Among them, a combination of SAL with 5FU caused decreased expression of Bax compared to 5FU alone. A similar effect onto Bax expression was observed in the GEM and its combination with SAL. In A2780 CDDP cell line, CASP3 expression in SAL and 5FU was decreased, and their combination caused a similar effect in comparison to control. However, the expression of that protein in GEM, 1 + GEM, 3, 4, and 5 variants was enhanced in comparison with the control. The combination of SAL with 5FU caused the enhanced expression of the full form of CASP3, which confirmed synergistic action of these compounds. On the other hand, the antagonistic effect was observed in GEM and its combination with SAL, where the cytotoxic effect was enhanced in only GEM-treated cells.

In SK-OV-3 cell line, Bcl2 expression was decreased in all studied compounds, except amide 4, compared to control (Figure 4C). Among them, SAL, 5FU, and 1+GEM showed the lowest expression. All tested compounds indicated decreased expression of Bax in comparison with control. The combination of SAL and 5FU did not cause the upregulation of these proteins exciding the level of compounds tested alone. The GEM indicated the highest expression level of Bax among tested molecules. Amide derivatives of SAL did not indicate increased expression of Bax in comparison with SAL. The similar tendencies of CASP3 expression were observed, excluding compound 2 and 3, which exhibited its higher expression in comparison with SAL. These observations confirmed the antagonistic effect in studied combinations of antineoplastic agents with SAL. In the case of SK-OV-3 CDDP cell line exposed to distinct molecules, the expression of Bcl2 only in SAL and SAL combined with 5FU was upregulated in comparison with the control (Figure 4D). Only the combination of SAL with GEM caused enhanced downregulation of Bcl-2 compared to exposition to them alone. Bax expression in those cells was decreased in comparison with the control. Among tested variants, 1 + 5FU exceeded the level of its expression compared to 5FU, but not to SAL alone. Again, GEM used separately induced its highest expression among all exposed compounds. The amide derivatives of SAL indicated lower expression of Bax in comparison with SAL. The presence of Bax downregulation in cells exposed to a combination of antineoplastics with SAL confirmed their antagonism. The expression of CASP3 and the action of compounds co-cultured with SK-OV-3 CDDP cells was similar to that of Bax. These results confirmed earlier estimated effects of combined SAL with 5FU or GEM in studied cell lines.

3. Discussion

One of the major problems in ovarian cancer (OvCa) treatment is development of chemoresistant residual cancer cells. Cancer stem cell (CSC)-targeted therapies should thus be developed [5]. One of the promising compounds in this respect is salinomycin (SAL). Its short-lasting side effects and low solubility in aqueous solutions may be avoided by some chemical modifications. These modifications provide new SAL molecules with improved stability and unaffected selective properties against CSCs, particularly effective in overcoming chemoresistant forms of the disease [28,29]. However, the synthesis of selective SAL derivatives is complicated due to the presence of multiple functional groups and a sensitive tricyclic 6-6-5 bis-spiroketal ring system in SAL structure [20,29,30].

In this study, we derived cisplatin-resistant cell lines A2780 CDDP and SK-OV-3 CDDP and evaluated the antiproliferative activity of selected amides and esters of SAL, as well as SAL used alone or in combination with other commonly used cytostatic agents, such as 5-fluorouracil (5FU) and gemcitabine (GEM), against these OvCa cells. To confirm the observed effect, Western blot analysis of proteins related to apoptosis (Bcl2, Bax and CASP3) was also performed.

We obtained resistant variants of cancer cell lines, as confirmed by increased IC_{50} against cisplatin estimated by MTT assay. These variants also showed elevated expression of genes related to drug transporters. ABCB1, ABCB4, ABCG2, and ABCC2 are well-described markers of drug resistance development in many cancers [31–35]. These proteins are characteristic of side populations of cells that represent stem-cell-like features, and in some cancers, they are recognized as markers of CSCs. They are responsible for active efflux of many anticancer agents causing treatment failure [35–37].

Our experiments provided interesting data regarding the activity of SAL and its derivatives against platinum resistance developed in OvCa cell lines in vitro. Creation of platinum-resistant OvCa cell line (SK-OV-3) did not induce the resistance of cancer cells to the action of SAL and its derivatives. This indicated that different molecular mechanisms are responsible for either platinum or SAL resistance, and additionally SAL could be identified as an effective agent in overcoming the platinum resistance of OvCa cells. However, A2780 CDDP variant exhibited moderate sensitivity to SAL and its 2,2,2-trifluoroethyl ester derivative (compound 6, Figure 1). This phenomenon could be related to the increased expression of ABCB1 and ABCG2 in resistant variants of A2780 cancer cell line. A study by the Boesch group revealed that in OvCa cell lines (A2780, IGROV1), selected ABCB1 and ABCG2 positive cells exhibited protective mechanisms against ionophore antibiotics, including SAL [38]. Contrary to that, a study in 2010 demonstrated that SAL treatments restored doxorubicin sensitivity in human doxorubicin-resistant epithelial OvCa cell line (A2780/ADR) exposed to doxorubicin either alone or in combination with SAL by inhibition of ABCB1 functionality [39]. Disparate results of these studies might be related to distinct co-activation of a group of genes in the same chromosomal region, where ABCB1 activation occurs by various cytotoxic agents [31].

Our experiments did not confirm the high anticancer activity of SAL derivatives reported recently in primary acute lymphoblastic leukemia (ALL) cells [20,40], which may be caused by a different type of malignancies and their adverse biology; ALL represents a hematological malignancy, while OvCa represents a malignant solid tumor. Until now, there have been only limited data showing the effects of SAL and its derivatives on OvCa cells. The recent data indicated that SAL itself affects a wide spectrum of mechanisms against OvCa biology, such as inhibition of the epithelial-mesenchymal transition (EMT) process (responsible for the development of metastatic disease), eradication of the CSC population ($CD44^+CD117^+$), and inhibition of the NF-kB signaling pathway (upregulation of proteins related to that pathway correspond with poor clinical prognosis in OvCa) [41–44]. Our study, for the first time, demonstrates that the combination of SAL with cytostatic agents (5FU and GEM) is more effective than SAL used alone or its amide and ester derivatives. 5FU is not commonly used in OvCa treatment—a few clinical trials revealed no significant improvement in clinical outcomes in advanced OvCa patients receiving 5FU combined with cisplatin or leucovorin [45–47]. Of note is that SAL acted synergistically with 5FU towards drug-resistant A2780 OvCa cell line. A similar effect was presented in studies concerning colorectal and hepatocellular carcinoma, which indicated the neutral or synergistic effect of the combination of SAL and 5FU [48,49]. In case of GEM, which is mostly used as a secondary line of chemotherapy after the development of resistant disease in OvCa, we did not observe the synergistic effect of combined SAL and GEM in both OvCa cell lines, as was found over their action in pancreatic carcinoma cell lines [50,51]. We think that one of the causes was their high molar ratio 1:1 used in our study versus 5 µM concentration of SAL and 5 µg·mL^{-1} applied in the pancreatic cancer cell lines [51]. The differences between the observed effects of these two nucleoside analogs in combination with SAL might be related to a disturbance of their cellular uptake by an ion imbalance caused by SAL. The concentrative nucleoside transporters (CNT) and equilibrative nucleoside transporters (ENT) are mostly engaged in the transport of GEM, while for 5FU, only ENT proteins are involved [52–55]. The mechanism of nucleoside transport by CNT proteins is Na$^+$-dependent, whereas in the case of ENT, they are mediated by facilitated diffusion [53,54]. SAL is responsible for the transport of potassium and sodium cations, which could lead to disturbance of the GEM uptake through CNT transporters (indicating high affinity to GEM), decreasing its activity against cancer cells [29,54,55].

The effect of combination of SAL with GEM or 5FU was confirmed by Western blot analysis of proteins related to apoptosis (Bcl2, Bax, and CASP3). Besides the same IC_{50} effect at distinct concentrations of studied compounds, SAL amide derivatives (3–5) caused enhanced expression of CASP3 in A2780 and A2780 CDDP cell lines, which could suggest different or more effective induction of apoptosis by these molecules. We did not observe a similar effect in SK-OV-3 cells, which could be related to intrinsic resistance mechanisms due to their metastatic origin. However, there is a lack of detailed mechanistic studies explaining the differences between SAL and amide derivatives against OvCa cell biology; thus, their further detailed characterization of action should be performed. On the other hand, for SAL used alone, we obtained similar findings as the Parajuli group, where the A2780 CDDP variant was tested, and a decrease of the Bcl2, Bax, and CASP3 was noted at similar doses that we used in our study; however, in their study, only after 1 μM of SAL, caspases were significantly increased [44,56]. They also indicated that the cause of apoptosis is related to activation of death receptor 5 (DR5) pathway, which was observed even at low doses of SAL (0.5 μM) [56]. In contrast, the Kaplan group observed induction of apoptosis by upregulation of CASP3 in OVCAR3 cell line even at 0.1 μM of SAL [57].

In summary, all findings mentioned above corresponded well with our results. Potent anticancer activity of SAL, lack of SAL resistance in platinum-resistant OvCa cell lines, and reversible SAL resistance imply the possible application of SAL in overcoming either primary or acquired platinum resistance (in platinum-resistant cell lines/patients). Further analyses of the SAL treatment used alone or in combination with other anticancer drugs, such as 5FU and GEM, will require identification of the most effective combination of SAL and the cytotoxic agent, and the mode of their administration (synchronous or sequential). Our results may contribute to the development of anticancer therapy based on SAL, which may give hope for heavily treated OvCa patients. Further studies should focus on discovering the mechanisms of action for SAL and its derivatives.

4. Materials and Methods

4.1. Chemical Part

4.1.1. Isolation of Salinomycin

Salinomycin sodium salt was isolated from commercially available veterinary premix SACOX® following acidic extraction, using the previously described procedure [18,19]. Briefly, isolated sodium salt of salinomycin was dissolved in CH_2Cl_2 and stirred vigorously with a layer of aqueous sulfuric acid (pH = 1.0). The organic layer containing salinomycin (SAL, **1**, Figure 1) was washed with distilled water. Then, CH_2Cl_2 was evaporated under reduced pressure to dryness giving SAL as clear oil. After three cycles of evaporation with *n*-pentane, this oil was transformed into white amorphous solid. Spectroscopic data for SAL were closely matched previously published data [22].

4.1.2. Synthesis of Salinomycin Derivatives

All SAL amides and esters (compounds **2–7**, Figure 1) obtained by a chemical modification of the C1 carboxyl group were prepared according to the procedures we described previously [18,19]. Spectroscopic data of all the compounds matched those found in the reference literature [18,19].

4.2. Biological Part

4.2.1. Cell Culture and Derivation of Cisplatin-Resistant Cell Lines

In this study, OvCa cell lines A2780 and SK-OV-3 (ATCC, Manassas, VA, USA) and human fetal lung fibroblasts cell line (MRC-5 pd19; ECACC, Salisbury, United Kingdom) were used to evaluate the antiproliferative activity of the tested compounds. OvCa cell lines were cultivated in RPMI 1640 containing 25 mM HEPES and 5 mM L-glutamine with 10% fetal bovine serum (FBS) (all provided from Biowest, Nuaillé, France) and 1% penicillin-streptomycin (Merck KGaA, Darmstadt, Germany). MRC-5 pd19 was cultured in DMEM supplemented with 10% FBS, 2 mM L-glutamine (all provided from Biowest, Nuaillé, France), 1% penicillin-streptomycin and 1% non-essential amino acids (NEAA) (both provided from Merck KGa, Darmstadt, Germany). To generate the cisplatin-resistant cell lines (A2780 CDDP; SK-OV-3 CDDP), increasing doses of cisplatin (CDDP) (Teva Pharmaceutical Industries Ltd. Petach Tikwa, Israel) were added to the culture medium, starting from the concentration of 100 ng mL^{-1}. Then, the cells were exposed to CDDP (3 cycles of 3 days each). After that, the cell culture medium was replaced with the fresh one without drugs for the next 3 days or one week until the cells recovered. After the 3 cycles, the dose of cisplatin was doubled until the concentration of 1000 ng· mL^{-1} was achieved. Then, to maintain a resistant phenotype, 1000 ng·mL^{-1} of **CDDP** was added once per 2 weeks for 3 days.

4.2.2. Isolation of RNA and RT-qPCR

The cells (2.5×10^5) were washed twice in Dulbecco's phosphate buffered saline (DPBS, Biowest, Nuaillé, France) and suspended in TRI reagent (Sigma-Aldrich, St. Louis, MO, USA). Next, RNA was isolated using Direct-zol RNA MiniPrep (Zymoresearch, Irvine, CA, USA) according to the manufacturer's instructions. Then 1 µg of RNA was collected to synthesize cDNA using iScript kit (BioRAD, Hercules, CA, USA). The cDNA was diluted 20 times, and 2.5 µL was added to the reaction mix composed of FastStart Essential DNA Probes Mix and specific probes (both provided by Roche Molecular Systems, Inc, Basel, Switzerland). The RT-qPCR reaction was performed as previously described [58]. The tested genes related to drug resistance included: ATP-binding cassette subfamily B member 1 (ABCB1), ATP-binding cassette subfamily B member 4 (ABCB4), ATP-binding cassette subfamily G member 2 (ABCG2), and ATP-binding cassette subfamily C member 2 (ABCC2). Relative gene expression level was determined using reference gene glyceraldehyde 3-phosphate dehydrogenase (GAPDH). The primers and molecular probes used in this study are listed in Table S1 (Supplementary Material).

4.2.3. Cell Viability Assay

For the evaluation of cell proliferation inhibition, we used the MTT (3-(4,5-dimethylthiazol-2-yl)-2,5-diphenyltetrazolium bromide) assay as previously described [59]. Briefly, A2780 WT and CDDP (2000 cells/well), SK-OV-3 WT and CDDP (800 cells/well), and MRC-5 pd19 (3000 cells/well) were seeded onto a 96-well plate for overnight until the cells attached. Next, the cells were exposed to the estimated concentrations of SAL, its derivatives, and anticancer drugs for 72 h (Table S2, Supplementary Material). Then the cell culture medium was replaced with the fresh one containing 0.5 mg·mL^{-1} of MTT (Affymetrix, Santa Clara, MA, USA) and left for 2 h at 37 °C. After that, the medium was replaced with DMSO (VWR, Darmstadt, Germany) and left at 37 °C for 10 min until the crystals were dissolved. The measurement was performed with a plate reader, Multiskan FC (Thermofisher, San Jose CA, USA) at 570 and 690 nm. Then, IC$_{50}$ and mean 95% CI were determined using GraphPad Prism 6 (Graph Pad Software, San Diego, CA, USA). The values of resistance index (RI), selectivity index (SI), and combination index (CI) were calculated as described previously [20,60].

4.2.4. Western Blot Analysis

After 72 h of exposure to IC$_{50}$ concentration of selected compounds, the OvCa cell lines were lysed using RIPA lysing buffer (Sigma Aldrich, St. Louis, MO, USA). For analysis, 10 µg of protein was used, calculated using Pierce™ BCA Protein Assay Kit (Thermofisher, San Jose, CA, USA) according to the manufacturer's instructions. The procedure was performed as previously described [52]. Briefly, after electrophoresis, proteins were transferred onto polyvinylidene difluoride (PVDF) membrane. After 2 h of blocking with non-fat milk (Sigma Aldrich, St. Louis, MO, USA), the membrane was incubated overnight at 4 °C with primary antibodies: anti-Bcl-2 (dilution 1:500; sc-509, Santa Cruz, Dallas, TX, USA), anti-Bax (dilution 1:500; sc-7480, Santa Cruz, Dallas, TX, USA), anti-CASP3 (full-form)(dilution 1:1000; no. ab49822, Abcam, Cambridge, UK), and reference protein GAPDH (dilution 1:500; no. sc-47724, Santa Cruz, Dallas, TX, USA). On the next day, after washes, the membranes were incubated with appropriate secondary antibodies conjugated with horseradish peroxidase (HRP) (dilution 1:1000; no. 7076 and 7074, Cell Signaling Technology, Leiden, Netherlands). Then the protein bands were visualized using WesternBright™ Quantum kit (Advansta, San Jose, CA, USA) and documented using the ChemiDoc Touch Imaging System (Bio-Rad Laboratories Ltd., Hercules, CA, USA). The intensity was measured using Image Lab Software (ver 6.0.1, Bio-Rad Laboratories Ltd., CA, USA). All buffers and equipment used during Western blot analysis were provided from Bio-Rad Laboratories Ltd., CA, USA.

4.2.5. Statistical Analysis

The statistical analysis of genes expression (Student's t-test) was performed using GraphPadPrism 6 package (Graph Pad Software, San Diego, CA, USA). The data were deemed significant at $p < 0.05$. All experiments were repeated at least three times.

Author Contributions: Conceptualization, A.H., M.A. and M.M.; methodology, M.A., M.S.L; validation, A.H., M.S.L, M.A., M.M. and W.M.S.; formal analysis, M.M., M.A., A.H, M.S.L., W.M.S.; investigation, M.A, M.S.L and M.M.; resources, A.H., M.A. and M.M., M.S.L.; writing—original draft preparation, M.M, M.A. and M.S.L.; writing—review and editing, M.A, A.H, M.M, M.S.L., W.M.S; supervision, M.M., A.H., W.M.S.; funding acquisition, M.A., M.M. All authors have read and agreed to the published version of the manuscript.

Abbreviations

5FU	5-fluorouracil
ABCB1	ATP-binding cassette subfamily B member 1
ABCB4	ATP-binding cassette subfamily B member 4
ABCC2	ATP-binding cassette subfamily C member 2
ABCG2	ATP-binding cassette subfamily G member 2
ALL	Acute lymphoblastic leukemia
Bax	Bcl2 associated X protein
Bcl-2	B-cell lymphoma 2
CASP3	Caspase 3
CDDP	Cisplatin
CI	Combination index
CNT	Concentrative nucleoside transporters
CSCs	Cancer stem cells
DMEM	Dulbecco modified eagle medium
EMT	Epithelial-mesenchymal transition
ENT	Equilibrative nucleoside transporters
FBS	Fetal bovine serum
GAPDH	Glyceraldehyde 3-phosphate dehydrogenase
GEM	Gemcitabine
HRP	Horseradish peroxidase
MDR	Multidrug resistance

MTT	3-(4,5-dimethylthiazol-2-yl)-2,5-diphenyltetrazolium bromide
NEAA	Non-essential amino acids
OvCa	Ovarian cancer
P-gp	P-glycoprotein
PVDF	Polyvinylidene difluoride
RI	Resistance indexes
RT-qPCR	Reverse transcriptase quantitative polymerase chain reaction
SAR	Structure-activity relationship
SI	Selectivity indexes

References

1. Siegel, R.L.; Miller, K.D.; Jemal, A. Cancer statistics, 2017. *CA Cancer J. Clin.* **2017**, *67*, 7–30. [CrossRef]
2. Rosenthal, A.N.; Menon, U.; Jacobs, I.J. Screening for ovarian cancer. *Clin. Obstet. Gynecol.* **2006**, *49*, 433–447. [CrossRef]
3. Marcus, C.S.; Maxwell, G.L.; Darcy, K.M.; Hamilton, C.A.; McGuire, W.P. Current Approaches and Challenges in Managing and Monitoring Treatment Response in Ovarian Cancer. *J. Cancer.* **2014**, *5*, 25–30.
4. Cooke, S.L.; Brenton, J.D. Evolution of platinum resistance in high-grade serous ovarian cancer. *Lancet Oncol.* **2011**, *12*, 1169–1174. [CrossRef]
5. Rocconi, R.P.; Case, A.S.; Straughn, J.M.; Estes, J.M.; Partridge, E.E. Role of chemotherapy for patients with recurrent platinum-resistant advanced epithelial ovarian cancer: A cost-effectiveness analysis. *Cancer* **2006**, *107*, 536–543. [CrossRef]
6. Au, K.K.; Josahkian, J.A.; Francis, J.A.; Squire, J.A.; Koti, M. Current state of biomarkers in ovarian cancer prognosis. *Futur. Oncol.* **2015**, *11*, 3187–3195. [CrossRef] [PubMed]
7. Kurman, R.J.; Shih, I.M. The Dualistic Model of Ovarian Carcinogenesis. *Am. J. Pathol.* **2016**, *186*, 733–747. [CrossRef] [PubMed]
8. Zhan, Q.; Wang, C.; Ngai, S. Ovarian Cancer Stem Cells: A New Target for Cancer. *Therapy* **2013**, *2013*, 916819. [CrossRef] [PubMed]
9. Nagaraj, A.B.; Joseph, P.; Kovalenko, O.; Singh, S.; Armstrong, A.; Redline, R.; Resnick, K.; Zanotti, K.; Waggoner, S.; DiFeo, A. Critical role of Wnt/β-catenin signaling in driving epithelial ovarian cancer platinum resistance. *Oncotarget* **2015**, *6*, 23720–23734. [CrossRef] [PubMed]
10. McAuliffe, S.M.; Morgan, S.L.; Wyant, G.A.; Tran, L.T.; Muto, K.W.; Chen, Y.S.; Chin, K.T.; Partridge, J.C.; Poole, B.B.; Cheng, K.H.; et al. Targeting Notch, a key pathway for ovarian cancer stem cells, sensitizes tumors to platinum therapy. *Proc. Natl. Acad. Sci.* **2012**, *109*, E2939–E2948. [CrossRef] [PubMed]
11. Miyazaki, Y.; Shibuya, M.; Sugawara, H.; Kawaguchi, O.; Hirsoe, C. Salinomycin, a new polyether antibiotic. *J. Antibiot. (Tokyo).* **1974**, *27*, 814–821. [CrossRef] [PubMed]
12. Gupta, P.B.; Onder, T.T.; Jiang, G.; Tao, K.; Kuperwasser, C.; Weinberg, R.A.; Lander, E.S. Identification of Selective Inhibitors of Cancer Stem Cells by High-Throughput Screening. *Cell* **2009**, *138*, 645–659. [CrossRef] [PubMed]
13. Naujokat, C.; Steinhart, R. Salinomycin as a Drug for Targeting Human Cancer Stem Cells. *J. Biomed. Biotechnol.* **2012**, *2012*, 950658. [CrossRef] [PubMed]
14. Antoszczak, M. A medicinal chemistry perspective on salinomycin as a potent anticancer and anti-CSCs agent. *Eur. J. Med. Chem.* **2019**, *164*, 366–377. [CrossRef]
15. Antoszczak, M.; Huczyński, A. Salinomycin and its derivatives–A new class of multiple-targeted "magic bullets". *Eur. J. Med. Chem.* **2019**, *176*, 208–227. [CrossRef]
16. Kaushik, V.; Yakisich, J.; Kumar, A.; Azad, N.; Iyer, A. Ionophores: Potential Use as Anticancer Drugs and Chemosensitizers. *Cancers* **2018**, *10*, 360. [CrossRef]
17. Versini, A.; Saier, L.; Sindikubwabo, F.; Müller, S.; Cañeque, T.; Rodriguez, R. Chemical biology of salinomycin. *Tetrahedron* **2018**, *74*, 5585–5614. [CrossRef]
18. Antoszczak, M.; Maj, E.; Stefańska, J.; Wietrzyk, J.; Janczak, J.; Brzezinski, B.; Huczyński, A. Synthesis, antiproliferative and antibacterial activity of new amides of salinomycin. *Bioorg. Med. Chem. Lett.* **2014**, *24*, 1724–1729. [CrossRef]

19. Antoszczak, M.; Popiel, K.; Stefańska, J.; Wietrzyk, J.; Maj, E.; Janczak, J.; Michalska, G.; Brzezinski, B.; Huczyński, A. Synthesis, cytotoxicity and antibacterial activity of new esters of polyether antibiotic – salinomycin. *Eur. J. Med. Chem.* **2014**, *76*, 435–444. [CrossRef]

20. Urbaniak, A.; Delgado, M.; Antoszczak, M.; Huczyński, A.; Chambers, T.C. Salinomycin derivatives exhibit activity against primary acute lymphoblastic leukemia (ALL) cells in vitro. *Biomed. Pharmacother.* **2018**, *99*, 384–390. [CrossRef]

21. Huczyński, A.; Rutkowski, J.; Popiel, K.; Maj, E.; Wietrzyk, J.; Stefańska, J.; Majcher, U.; Bartl, F. Synthesis, antiproliferative and antibacterial evaluation of C-ring modified colchicine analogues. *Eur. J. Med. Chem.* **2015**, *90*, 296–301. [CrossRef] [PubMed]

22. Huczyński, A.; Janczak, J.; Antoszczak, M.; Wietrzyk, J.; Maj, E.; Brzezinski, B. Antiproliferative activity of salinomycin and its derivatives. *Bioorg. Med. Chem. Lett.* **2012**, *22*, 7146–7150. [CrossRef] [PubMed]

23. Antonenko, Y.N.; Rokitskaya, T.I.; Huczyński, A. Electrogenic and nonelectrogenic ion fluxes across lipid and mitochondrial membranes mediated by monensin and monensin ethyl ester. *Biochim. Biophys. Acta - Biomembr.* **2015**, *1848*, 995–1004. [CrossRef] [PubMed]

24. Harker, W.G.; Slade, D.L.; Dalton, W.S.; Meltzer, P.S.; Trent, J.M. Multidrug resistance in mitoxantrone-selected HL-60 leukemia cells in the absence of P-glycoprotein overexpression. *Cancer Res.* **1989**, *49*, 4542–4549. [PubMed]

25. Badisa, R.B.; Darling-Reed, S.F.; Joseph, P.; Cooperwood, J.S.; Latinwo, L.M.; Goodman, C.B. Selective cytotoxic activities of two novel synthetic drugs on human breast carcinoma MCF-7 cells. *Anticancer Res.* **2009**, *29*, 2993–2996.

26. Chou, T.C. Drug combination studies and their synergy quantification using the Chou-Talalay method. *Cancer Res.* **2010**, *70*, 440–446. [CrossRef]

27. Ichite, N.; Chougule, M.B.; Jackson, T.; Fulzele, S.V.; Safe, S.; Singh, M. Enhancement of Docetaxel Anticancer Activity by a Novel Diindolylmethane Compound in Human Non-Small Cell Lung Cancer. *Clin. Cancer Res.* **2009**, *15*, 543–552. [CrossRef]

28. Dewangan, J.; Srivastava, S.; Rath, S.K. Salinomycin: A new paradigm in cancer therapy. *Tumor Biol.* **2017**, *39*, 101042831769503. [CrossRef]

29. Piperno, A.; Marrazzo, A.; Scala, A.; Rescifina, A. Chemistry and biology of salinomycin and its analogues. salinomycin and its analogues. In *Targets In Heterocyclic Systems*; Attanasi, O.A., Merino, P., Spinelli, D., Eds.; Società Chimica Italiana: Rome, Italy, 2015; Volume 19, pp. 177–213.

30. Kocieński, P.J.; Brown, R.C.D.; Pommier, A.; Procter, M.; Schmidt, B. Synthesis of salinomycin. *J. Chem. Soc. Perkin Trans.* **1998**, *1*, 9–40. [CrossRef]

31. Genovese, I.; Ilari, A.; Assaraf, Y.G.; Fazi, F.; Colotti, G. Not only P-glycoprotein: Amplification of the ABCB1- containing chromosome region 7q21 confers multidrug resistance upon cancer cells by coordinated overexpression of an assortment of resistance-related proteins. *Drug Resist. Updat.* **2017**, *32*, 23–46. [CrossRef]

32. Comsa, E.; Nguyen, K.; Loghin, F.; Boumendjel, A.; Peuchmaur, M.; Andrieu, T.; Falson, P. Ovarian cancer cells cisplatin sensitization agents selected by mass cytometry target ABCC2 inhibition. *Future Med. Chem.* **2018**, *10*, 1349–1360. [CrossRef] [PubMed]

33. Rubiś, B.; Hołysz, H.; Barczak, W.; Gryczka, R.; Łaciński, M.; Jagielski, P.; Czernikiewicz, A.; Półrolniczak, A.; Wojewoda, A.; Perz, K.; et al. Study of ABCB1 polymorphism frequency in breast cancer patients from Poland. *Pharmacol. Reports* **2012**, *64*, 1560–1566. [CrossRef]

34. Duan, Z.; Brakora, K.A.; Seiden, M.V. Inhibition of ABCB1 (MDR1) and ABCB4 (MDR3) expression by small interfering RNA and reversal of paclitaxel resistance in human ovarian cancer cells. *Mol. Cancer Ther.* **2004**, *3*, 833–838. [PubMed]

35. Luqmani, Y.A. Mechanisms of drug resistance in cancer chemotherapy. *Med. Princ. Pract.* **2005**, *14* (Suppl. 1), 35–48. [CrossRef]

36. Januchowski, R.; Wojtowicz, K.; Sujka-kordowska, P.; Andrzejewska, M.; Zabel, M. MDR Gene Expression Analysis of Six Drug-Resistant Ovarian Cancer Cell Lines. *Biomed. Res. Int.* **2013**, *2013*, 241763. [CrossRef] [PubMed]

37. Eckford, P.D.; Sharom, F.J. ABC Efflux Pump-Based Resistance to Chemotherapy Drugs. *Chem. Rev.* **2009**, 2989–3011. [CrossRef] [PubMed]

38. Boesch, M.; Zeimet, A.G.; Rumpold, H.; Gastl, G.; Sopper, S.; Wolf, D. Drug Transporter-Mediated Protection of Cancer Stem Cells From Ionophore Antibiotics. *Stem Cells Transl. Med.* **2015**, *4*, 1028–1032. [CrossRef]

39. Riccioni, R.; Dupuis, M.L.; Bernabei, M.; Petrucci, E.; Pasquini, L.; Mariani, G.; Cianfriglia, M.; Testa, U. The cancer stem cell selective inhibitor salinomycin is a p-glycoprotein inhibitor. *Blood Cells Mol. Dis.* **2010**, *45*, 86–92. [CrossRef]

40. Antoszczak, M.; Urbaniak, A.; Delgado, M.; Maj, E.; Borgström, B.; Wietrzyk, J.; Huczyński, A.; Yuan, Y.; Chambers, T.C.; Strand, D. Biological activity of doubly modified salinomycin analogs – Evaluation in vitro and ex vivo. *Eur. J. Med. Chem.* **2018**, *156*, 510–523. [CrossRef]

41. Li, R.; Dong, T.; Hu, C.; Lu, J.; Dai, J.; Liu, P. Salinomycin repressed the epithelial-mesenchymal transition of epithelial ovarian cancer cells via downregulating Wnt/β-catenin pathway. *Onco. Targets. Ther.* **2017**, *10*, 1317–1325. [CrossRef]

42. Chung, H.; Kim, Y.H.; Kwon, M.; Shin, S.J.; Kwon, S.H.; Cha, S.D.; Cho, C.H. The effect of salinomycin on ovarian cancer stem-like cells. *Obstet. Gynecol. Sci.* **2016**, *59*, 261–268. [CrossRef] [PubMed]

43. Lee, H.; Shin, S.; Chung, H.; Kwon, S.; Cha, S.; Lee, J.; Cho, C.; Lee, J. Salinomycin reduces stemness and induces apoptosis on human ovarian cancer stem cell. *J. Gynecol. Oncol.* **2017**, *28*, e14. [CrossRef] [PubMed]

44. Parajuli, B.; Lee, H.G.; Kwon, S.; Cha, S.; Shin, S.; Lee, G.; Bae, I.; Cho, C. Salinomycin inhibits Akt/NF-κB and induces apoptosis in cisplatin resistant ovarian cancer cells. *Cancer Epidemiol.* **2013**, *37*, 512–517. [CrossRef] [PubMed]

45. Préfontaine, M.; Donovan, J.T.; Powell, J.L.; Buley, L. Treatment of Refractory Ovarian Cancer with 5-Fluorouracil and Leucovorin. *Gynecol. Oncol.* **1996**, *61*, 249–252. [CrossRef] [PubMed]

46. Burnett, A.F.; Barter, J.F.; Potkul, R.K.; Jarvis, T.; Barnes, W.A. Ineffectiveness of continuous 5-fluorouracil as salvage therapy for ovarian cancer. *Am. J. Clin. Oncol.* **1994**, *17*, 490–493. [CrossRef]

47. Braly, P.S.; Berek, J.S.; Blessing, J.A.; Homesley, H.D.; Averette, H. Intraperitoneal Administration of Cisplatin and 5-Fluorouracil in Residual Ovarian Cancer: A Phase II Gynecologic Oncology Group Trial. *Gynecol. Oncol.* **1995**, *56*, 164–168. [CrossRef]

48. Wang, F.; Dai, W.; Wang, Y.; Shen, M.; Chen, K.; Cheng, P.; Zhang, Y.; Wang, C.; Li, J.; Zheng, Y.; et al. The synergistic in vitro and in vivo antitumor effect of combination therapy with salinomycin and 5-fluorouracil against hepatocellular carcinoma. *PLoS ONE* **2014**, *9*, e97414. [CrossRef]

49. Klose, J.; Eissele, J.; Volz, C.; Schmitt, S.; Ritter, A.; Ying, S.; Schmidt, T.; Heger, U.; Schneider, M.; Ulrich, A. Salinomycin inhibits metastatic colorectal cancer growth and interferes with Wnt/β-catenin signaling in CD133+ human colorectal cancer cells. *BMC Cancer* **2016**, *16*, 896. [CrossRef]

50. Berg, T.; Nøttrup, T.J.; Roed, H. Gemcitabine for recurrent ovarian cancer—A systematic review and meta-analysis. *Gynecol Oncol.* **2019**, *155*, 530–537. [CrossRef]

51. Zhang, G.N.; Liang, Y.; Zhou, L.J.; Chen, S.P.; Chen, G.; Zhang, T.P.; Kang, T.; Zhao, Y.P. Combination of salinomycin and gemcitabine eliminates pancreatic cancer cells. *Cancer Lett.* **2011**, *313*, 137–144. [CrossRef]

52. Hagmann, W.; Jesnowski, R.; Löhr, J.M. Interdependence of gemcitabine treatment, ransporter expression, and resistance in human pancreatic carcinoma cells. *Neoplasia.* **2010**, *12*, 740–747. [CrossRef] [PubMed]

53. Pastor-Anglada, M.; Pérez-Torras, S. Emerging Roles of Nucleoside Transporters. *Front Pharmacol.* **2018**, *9*, 606. [CrossRef] [PubMed]

54. Mackey, J.R.; Yao, S.Y.; Smith, K.M.; Karpinski, E.; Baldwin, S.A.; Cass, C.E.; Young, J.D. Gemcitabine transport in xenopus oocytes expressing recombinant plasma membrane mammalian nucleoside transporters. *J Natl Cancer Inst.* **1999**, *91*, 1876–1881. [CrossRef] [PubMed]

55. Hung, S.W.; Marrache, S.; Cummins, S.; Bhutia, Y.D.; Mody, H.; Hooks, S.B.; Dhar, S.; Govindarajan, R. Defective hCNT1 transport contributes to gemcitabine chemoresistance in ovarian cancer subtypes: Overcoming transport defects using a nanoparticle approach. *Cancer Lett.* **2015**, *359*, 233–240. [CrossRef]

56. Parajuli, B.; Shin, S.J.; Kwon, S.H.; Cha, S.D.; Chung, R.; Park, W.J.; Lee, H.G.; Cho, C.H. Salinomycin induces apoptosis via death receptor-5 up-regulation in cisplatin-resistant ovarian cancer cells. *Anticancer Res.* **2013**, *33*, 1457–1462.

57. Kaplan, F.; Teksen, F. Apoptotic effects of salinomycin on human ovarian cancer cell line (OVCAR-3). *Tumour Biol.* **2016**, *37*, 3897–3903. [CrossRef]

58. Lach, M.S.; Kulcenty, K.; Jankowska, K.; Trzeciak, T.; Richter, M.; Suchorska, W.M. Effect of cellular mass on chondrogenic differentiation during embryoid body formation. *Mol. Med. Rep.* **2018**, *18*, 2705–2714. [CrossRef]

59. Blaszczak, W.; Lach, M.; Barczak, W.; Suchorska, W. Fucoidan Exerts Anticancer Effects Against Head and Neck Squamous Cell Carcinoma In Vitro. *Molecules* **2018**, *23*, 3302. [CrossRef]

In Vitro and In Vivo Anti-Breast Cancer Activities of Some Newly Synthesized 5-(thiophen-2-yl)thieno-[2,3-d]pyrimidin-4-one Candidates

Abd El-Galil E. Amr [1,2,*], **Alhussein A. Ibrahimd** [2], **Mohamed F. El-Shehry** [3,4], **Hanaa M. Hosni** [3], **Ahmed A. Fayed** [2,5] and **Elsayed A. Elsayed** [6,7]

[1]   Pharmaceutical Chemistry Department, Drug Exploration & Development Chair (DEDC), College of Pharmacy, King Saud University, Riyadh 11451, Saudi Arabia
[2]   Applied Organic Chemistry Department, National Research Center, Cairo, Dokki 12622, Egypt; alhusseina62@yahoo.com (A.A.I.); dr_ahmedfayed14@yahoo.com (A.A.F.)
[3]   Pesticide Chemistry Department, National Research Center, Dokki 12622, Cairo, Egypt; hanaanrc@yahoo.com (M.F.E.-S.); hanaahosni434@yahoo.com (H.M.H.)
[4]   Chemistry Department, Al-Zahrawy University College, Karbala 56001, Iraq
[5]   Respiratory Therapy Department, College of Medical Rehabilitation Sciences, Taibah University, Madinah Munawara, 22624, Saudi Arabia
[6]   Zoology Department, Bioproducts Research Chair, Faculty of Science, King Saud University, Riyadh 11451, Saudi Arabia; eaelsayed@ksu.edu.sa
[7]   Chemistry of Natural and Microbial Products Department, National Research Centre, Dokki 12622, Cairo, Egypt
*   Correspondence: aamr@ksu.edu.sa;

Academic Editor: Qiao-Hong Chen

Abstract: In this study, some of new thiophenyl thienopyrimidinone derivatives **2–15** were prepared and tested as anti-cancer agents by using thiophenyl thieno[2,3-d]pyrimidinone derivative **2** as a starting material, which was prepared from cyclization of ethyl ester derivative **1** with formamide. Treatment of **2** with ethyl- chloroacetate gave thienopyrimidinone *N*-ethylacetate **3**, which was reacted with hydrazine hydrate or anthranilic acid to afford acetohydrazide **4** and benzo[d][1,3]oxazin-4-one **5**, respectively. Condensation of **4** with aromatic aldehydes or phenylisothiocyanate yielded Schiff base derivatives **6,7**, and thiosemicarbazise **10**, which were treated with 2-mercaptoacetic acid or chloroacetic acid to give the corresponding thiazolidinones **8**, **9**, and phenylimino-thiazolidinone **11**, respectively. Treatment of **4** with ethylacetoacetate or acetic acid/acetic anhydride gave pyrazole **12** and acetyl acetohydrazide **13** derivatives, respectively. The latter compound **13** was reacted with ethyl cycno-acetate or malononitrile to give **14** and **15**, respectively. In this work, we have studied the anti-cancer activity of the synthesized thienopyrimidinone derivatives against MCF-7 and MCF-10A cancer cells. Furthermore, in vivo experiments showed that the synthesized compounds significantly reduced tumor growth up to the 8th day of treatment in comparison to control animal models. Additionally, the synthesized derivatives showed potential inhibitory effects against pim-1 kinase activities.

Keywords: thiopene; thienopyrimidinone; thiazolidinone; anticancer activity

1. Introduction

Cancer is a major health problem acting as a global killer, so synthesizing new compounds, which may act as potent antitumor agents, is a great target for chemists working in this field. In this study, we are interested in synthesizing and studying biological activities of thieno[2,3-d]pyrimidinone derivatives [1–11]. Thienopyrimidinones are very important moieties that act as keys for pharmacological and pharmaceutical properties. They are reported to cause antiviral [12], antimicrobial [13], antihypertensive [14], analgesic, and anti-inflammatory activities [15]. They also inhibit various protein kinase enzymes, such as CK2 involved in particular anticancer activity [16]. Additionally, the nitrogenous ring system was associated with some types of biological activities such as: anti-inflammatory [17], insecticidal [18], antimicrobial and antituberculosis [19,20] activities. On the other hand, thienopyrimidinones contain a thiophene ring fused with a pyrimidinone nucleus. In general, this system was thought to be interesting in development of pharmaceutical compounds [21,22], and was not only evaluated as cGMP phosphodiesterase inhibitors [23], anti-viral [24], anti-inflammatory [25], anti-microbial agents [26], but also as kinase inhibitors and potential anti-cancer agents [27,28]. In continuation to our previous work, and to extend our research [1–11], from the above points, we have studied the anticancer activity of the newly synthesized substituted thienopyrimidinone derivatives against MCF-7 and MCF-10A cancer cells. Furthermore, the work was extended to evaluate the effects of synthesized derivatives on the inhibition of tumor growth in an in vivo animal model. Finally, we evaluated the inhibitory effects of our synthesized compounds against pim-1 kinase activity as a possible mechanism of their action.

2. Results and Discussion

2.1. Chemistry

A series of thiophenyl thienopyrimidinone derivatives 2–15 were prepared and tested as anti-cancer agents. Cyclization of ethyl 5'-amino-[2,3'-bithiophene]-4'-carboxylate (1) with formamide gave the corresponding thiophenylthieno[2,3-d]pyrimidinone derivative (2), which was treated with ethylchloroacetate to give thienopyrimidinone N-ethylacetate 3. Reaction of 3 with hydrazine hydrate or anthranilic acid afforded the corresponding hydrazide 4 and benzooxazinone 5 derivatives, respectively (Scheme 1).

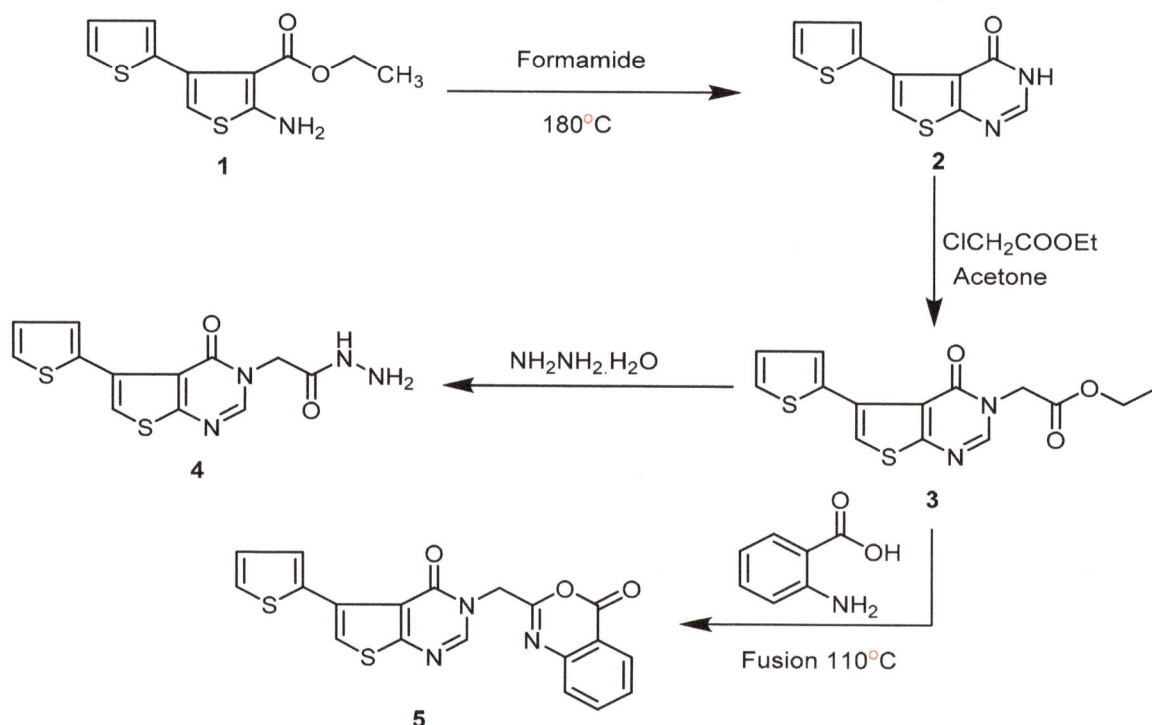

Scheme 1. Synthetic route for compounds 2–5.

Condensation of **4** with aromatic aldehydes, namely, 2,3-dimethoxybenzaldehyde or 4-chlorobenzaldehyde gave the corresponding Schiff base derivatives **6** and **7**, which were cyclized via reaction with 2-mercaptoacetic acid in dry benzene to give the corresponding thiazolidinone derivatives **8** and **9**, respectively. Treatment of **4** with phenylisothiocyanate gave thiosemicarbazide **10**, which was condensed with chloroacetic acid to afford phenyliminothiazolidinone derivative **11** (Scheme 2).

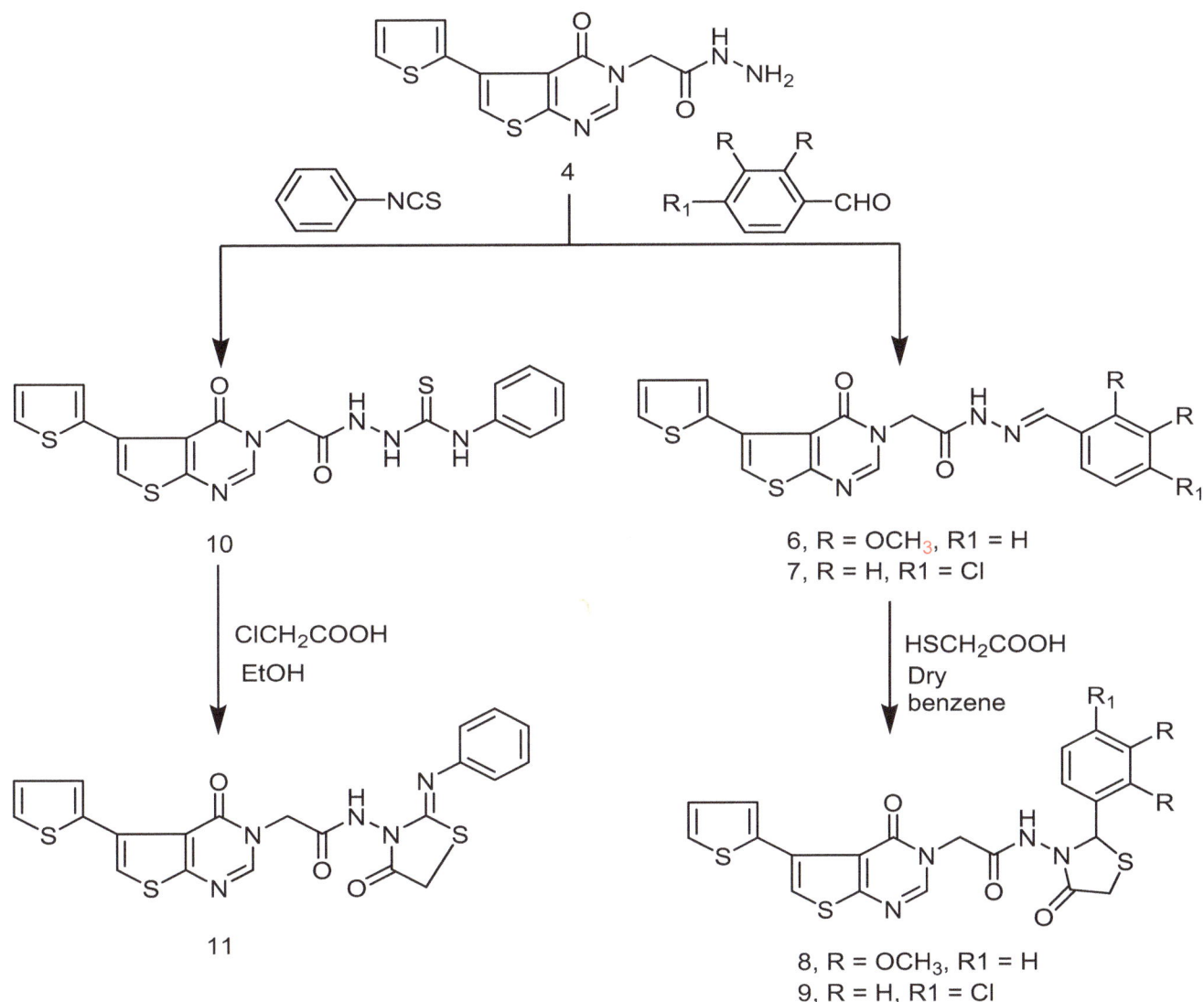

Scheme 2. Synthetic route for compounds **6–11**.

Finally, treatment of **4** with ethylacetoacetate or acetic acid/acetic anhydride gave the corresponding pyrazolyl derivative **12** and N-acetyl hydrazide **13**, respectively. The latter compound **13** was reacted with ethylcycnoacetate or malononitrile to give pyridine derivatives **14** and **15**, respectively (Scheme 3).

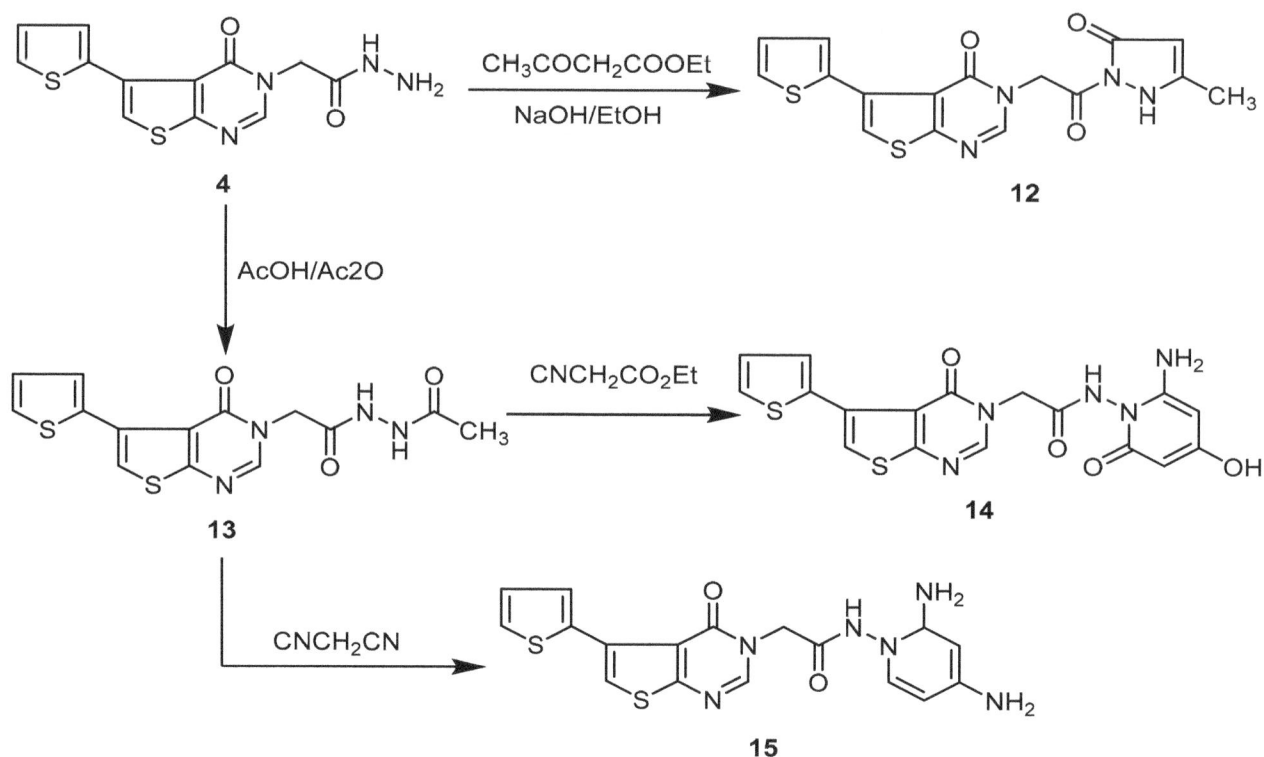

Scheme 3. Synthetic route for compounds **12–15**.

2.2. Biological Evaluation

MCF-7 cells were used to investigate the potential in vitro anti-proliferative potential of the synthesized compounds. With the exception of Cpd. **2** (data not shown), we found that all compounds have promising activities when used in μM concentration. On the other hand, Cisplatin and Milaplatin showed higher IC_{50} values (13.34 ± 0.11 and 18.43 ± 0.13 μM, respectively). DMSO at concentrations of 0.1% and 0.5%, had little or no toxicity, whereas higher concentrations inhibited the growth of MCF-7cells. Therefore, it seems DMSO could be solvents of choice acceptable to be used at concentrations < 0.5% (*v/v*) towards the examined cells and possibly for other cell lines. Also, the effect on cell viability was proportional to the concentration applied. From Figure 1, we can see that Cpd. **15, 14** and **8** (IC_{50}, 1.18 ± 0.032, 1.19 ± 0.042, 1.26 ± 0.052 μM, respectively) followed by **9** and **11** (IC_{50}, 2.37 ± 0.053 and 2.48 ± 0.054 μM respectively) produced the highest effect on cell viability. Secondly, compounds **12, 10** and **13**, showed moderate activities (IC_{50}, 3.36 ± 0.063, 3.55 ± 0.065 and 3.64 ± 0.074 μM, respectively). Compounds **7, 6, 5, 4** and **3** were the least active ones (IC_{50}, 4.33 ± 0.076, 4.52 ± 0.085, 4.76 ± 0.087, 4.87 ± 0.098 and 5.98 ± 0.099 μM, respectively). The order of activities can be arranged as **15 > 14 > 8 > 9 > 11 > 12 > 10 > 13 > 7 > 6 > 5 > 4 > 3**.

Results revealed that the substitution with pyridine moiety at the terminal NH improved the cytotoxic effect than the pyrimidone derivatives. In contrast, substitution with 5-membered di-heterocyclic ring system with aryl moiety decreased the obtained activities (methoxy phenyl > chlorophenyl). Attaching five membered pyrazolinone ring system bearing no aryl moiety at terminal NH (compound **12** decreased the activities than those containing aryl substitutions (compounds **9** and **11**). Compounds **10, 7** and **6** that contain aromatic *N*-substitution still have more potent activity. The increased effect of the aromatic ring may be attributed to ring aromaticity and electron resonance. On the other hand, aliphatic side chains (compounds **4** and **3**) or methylene bridges (Compound **5**) have less potent activities.

Additionally, results against non-tumorigenic MCF-10A proved that our derivatives have higher degrees of safety towards normal cells.

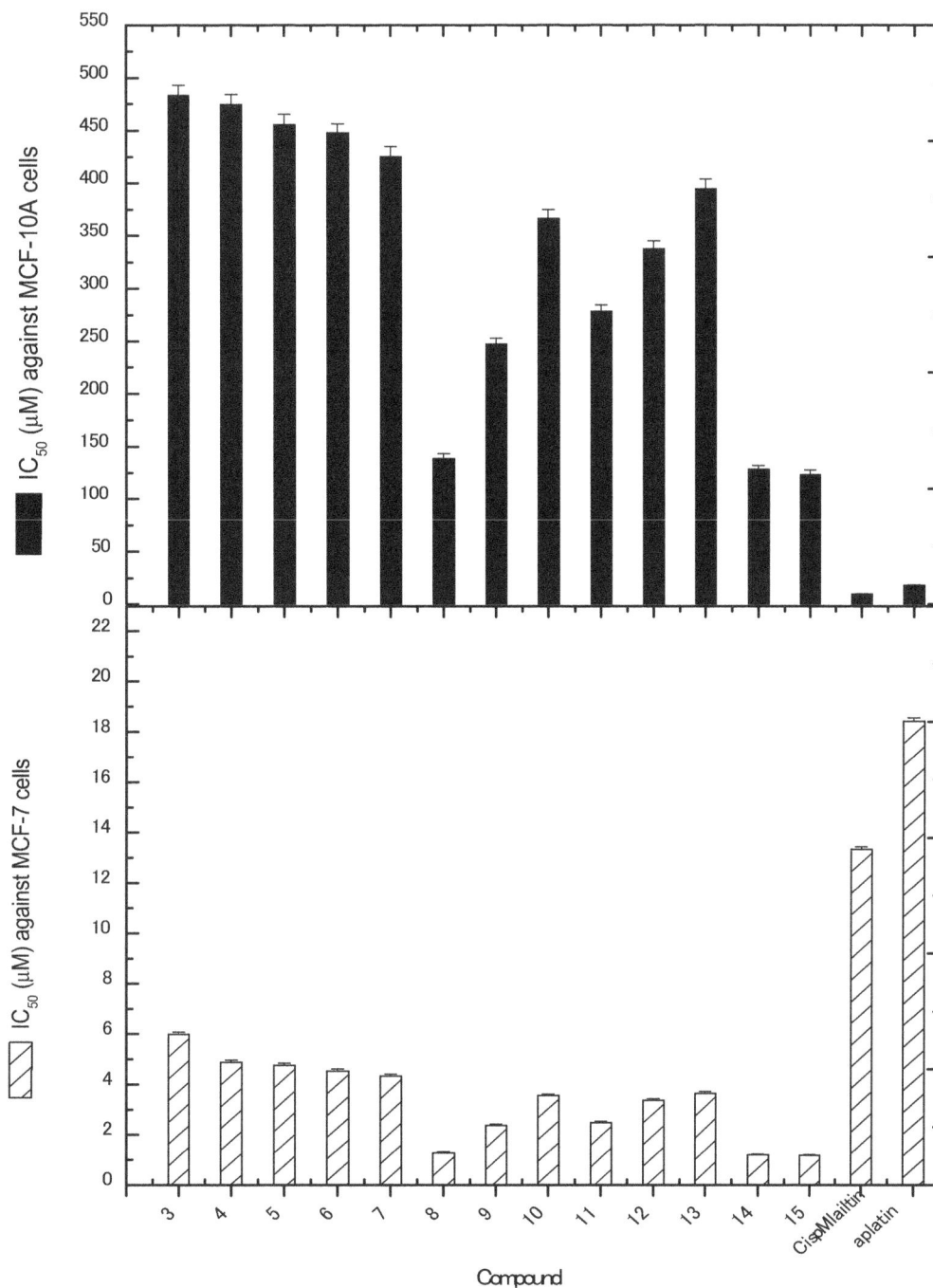

Figure 1. Obtained IC_{50} values for MCF-7 and MCF-10A cells.

In Vivo Xenograft Model

The in vivo anti-breast cancer activities of different synthesized derivatives were evaluated using a breast cancer mouse xenograft model. Figure 2 shows the increase in percentage of inhibition in tumor growth with treatment time when animals were exposed to different compounds. This was also compared with tumor development in control animals. It can be seen, that our derivatives reduced tumor growth starting day 2. The maximal effect was obtained after 8 days. Furthermore, the in vivo effect showed also the same inhibitory pattern obtained in the in vitro experiments. The average weight of each group of mice treated with drug and the control group summarized in Table 1.

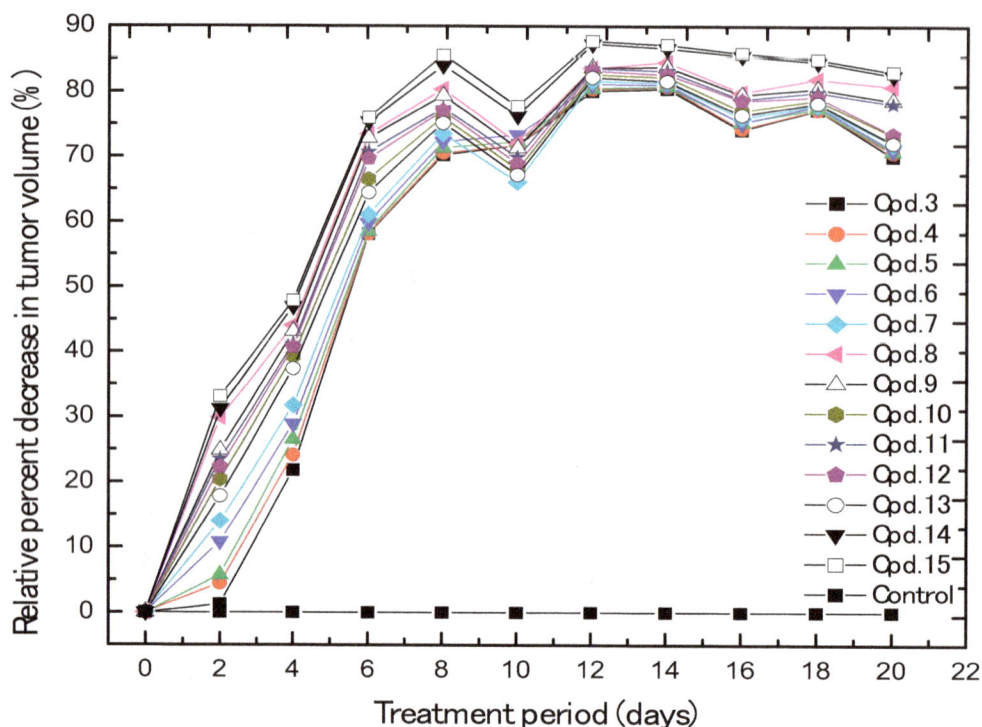

Figure 2. Relative percentage of decrease in tumor volume in response to prepared compounds.

Table 1. The average weight of each group of mice treated with drug and the control group.

Drugs	Average Weight of Animals in Grams after Days											
	0	2	4	6	8	10	12	14	16	18	20	22
Control	28	28	28	28	28.2	28.	28.3	28.4	28.4	28.4	28.4	28.4
3	28	28	28	28	28.2	27.9	27.8	27.7	27.7	27.6	27.7	27.7
4	24.2	24.2	24.1	24.0	23.9	23.9	23.7	23.7	23.6	23.6	23.6	236.
5	22.9	22.9	22.9	22.8	22.8	22.7	22.8	22.7	22.9	22.6	22.6	22.5
6	23.7	23.7	23.6	23.6	23.5	23.5	23.5	23.4	23.4	23.5	23.5	23.5
7	27.3	27.3	27.2	27.2	27.2	27.1	27.1	27.1	27.0	27.0	27.0	27.0
8	25.3	25.3	25.2	25.2	25.2	25.1	25.1	24.8	24.7	24.6	24.5	24.2
9	24.1	24.1	24.0	24.0	24.0	24.0	23.7	23.7	23.6	23.6	23.6	23.6
10	24.9	24.9	24.9	24.9	24.8	24.8	24.8	24.4	24.4	24.4	24.4	24.4
11	26.6	26.6	26.6	26.5	26.6	26.6	26.4	26.3	26.3	26.3	26.3	263.
12	27.4	27.4	27.4	27.3	27.3	27.3	27.2	27.2	27.2	27.1	27.1	27.1
13	25.4	25.4	25.4	25.4	25.4	25.3	25.3	25.3	25.3	25.3	25.3	25.3
14	26.5	26.4	26.3	26.2	26.1	25.9	25.9	25.9	25.8	25.8	25.7	25.7
15	26.1	26.1	26.1	25.8	25.8	25.7	25.7	25.6	25.6	25.5	25.5	25.2

The Provirus Integration in Maloney (Pim) kinases represents a family of constitutively active serine/threonine kinases and includes three subtypes (pim-1, pim-2 and pim-3). Pim kinases regulate many biological processes such as cell cycle, cell proliferation, apoptosis and drug resistance [29–32]. Being expressed in many types of solid and hematological cancers and almost absent in benign lesions, pim kinases proved to be a successful anti-cancer drug target of low toxicity [33–40]. Results obtained in Figure 3 showed that all synthesized compounds were showed potent inhibitory effects against pim-1 kinase.

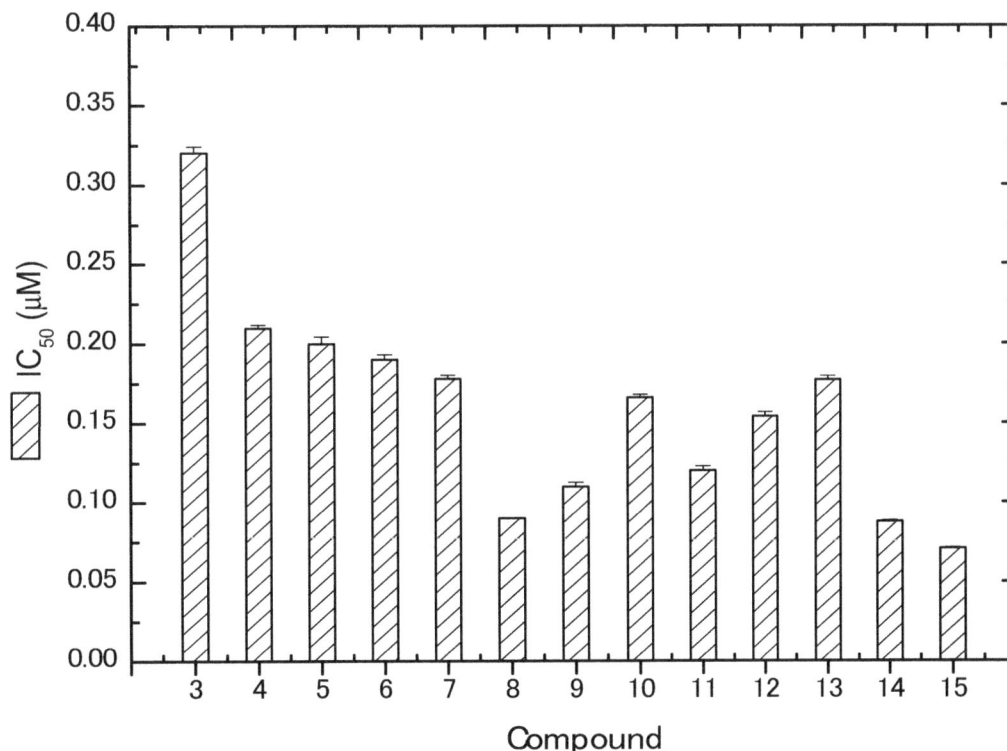

Figure 3. IC_{50} of the tested compounds against pim-1 Kinase.

3. Materials and Methods

3.1. Chemistry

"Melting points were determined in open glass capillary tubes with an Electro Thermal Digital melting point apparatus (model: IA9100) and are uncorrected. Elemental microanalyses were carried out in the microanalysis unit of NRC and were found within the acceptable limits of the calculated values. Infrared spectra (KBr) were recorded on a Nexus 670 FTIR Nicolet, Fourier Transform infrared spectrometer. ^{1}H- and ^{13}C NMR spectra were run in (DMSO-d_6) on Jeol 500 MHz instruments. Mass spectra were run on a MAT Finnigan SSQ 7000 spectrometer, using the electron impact technique (EI)."

Synthesis of 5-(thiophen-2-yl)thieno[2,3-d]pyrimidin-4(3H)-one **(2)**. A mixture of compound **1** (1 mmol, 253 mg) and formamide (20 mL) was heated at 180 °C in oil bath for 2 h. The formed solid was collected by filtration, washed with cold methanol, dried and crystallized from EtOH to give compound **2**. Yield 80%, M.p 192–194 °C; IR (KBr, cm^{-1}): ῡ 3323 (NH), 1659 (C=O). ^{1}H NMR (DMSO-d_6) δ_H: 7.11–7.72 (m, 4H, thiophene-H), 8.50 (s, 1H, CH-pyrimidine), 13.30 (s, 1H, NH, disappeared with D_2O). ^{13}C NMR: 119.98, 122.01, 122.17, 126.84, 127.75, 128.74, 131.26, 136.42, (8C, thiophene-C), 157.05 (1C, pyrimidine-C), 165.56 (C=O). Mass spectrum, m/z (EI, %): 234 (M^+, 100), 235 (M^+ + 1, 11), 236 (M^+ + 2, 9). Analysis for $C_{10}H_6N_2OS_2$ (234.29): Calculated: C, 51.27; H, 2.58; N, 11.96; S, 27.37. Found: C, 51.20; H, 2.50; N, 11.90; S, 27.30.

Synthesis of ethyl 2-(4-oxo-5-(thiophen-2-yl)thieno[2,3-d]pyrimidin-3(4H)-yl)acetate **(3)**. A mixture of **2** (1 mmol, 234 mg), ethylchloroacetate (1 mmol, 122 mg) and anhydrous potassium carbonate (8 mmol) in dry acetone (30 mL) was heated under reflux for 4h. The obtained solid was removed by filtration, the filtrate was concentrated, the precipitate solid was filtered off, dried, and crystallized from EtOH to give the ester derivative **3**. Yield 70%, m.p 135–137 °C. IR (KBr, cm^{-1}): ν 1753 (C=O, ester), 1655 (CO); ^{1}H NMR (DMSO-d_6), δ: 1.24 (t, 3H, CH_3), 4.20 (s, 2H, CH_2), 4.85 (q, 2H, CH_2-ethyl), 7.10–7.72 (m, 4H, thiophene-H), 8.50 (s, 1H, pyrimidine-H). ^{13}C-NMR (DMSO)-d_6 δc: 14.5 (CH_3), 40.2 (CH_2), 47.8 (CH_2), 119.9, 122.2, 126.9, 127.8, 128.7, 128.9, 131.3, 136.4 (8C, thiophene-C), 157.0 (1C, pyrimidine-C), 165.6,

168.3 (2C, 2CO). Mass spectrum, m/z (EI, %): 320 (M^+, 100), 321 ($M^+ + 1$, 18). Analysis for $C_{14}H_{12}N_2O_3S_2$ (320.38): Calculated: C, 52.49; H, 3.78; N, 8.74; S, 20.01. Found: C, 52.40; H, 3.70; N, 8.68; S, 19.86.

Synthesis of 2-(4-oxo-5-(thiophen-2-yl)thieno[2,3-d]pyrimidin-3(4H)-yl)acetohydrazide **(4)**. To a solution of **3** (1 mmol, 320 mg) in ethanol (50 mL), hydrazine hydrate (4 mmol, 85%) was added and refluxed for 8 h. The precipitated solid was collected by filteration, dried and crystallized from EtOH to give compound **4**. Yield 75%, m.p. 205–207 °C, IR (KBr, cm^{-1}): ν 3322 (NH), 3246 (NH_2), 1659 (C=O). ^{1}H-NMR (DMSO-d_6) δ: 3.39 (s, 2H, CH_2), 4.65 (s, 2H, NH_2, disappeared with D_2O), 7.10–7.65 (m, 4H, thiophene-H), 8.17 (s, 1H, pyrimidine-H), 12.58 (s, 1H, NH, disappeared with D_2O). ^{13}C-NMR (DMSOd$_6$) δc: 40.1 (CH_2), 120.5, 120.8, 126.6, 127.8, 128.7, 131.4, 133.5, 136.8 (8C, thiophene-C), 157.9 (1C, pyrimidine-C), 166.3, 169.4 (2C, 2CO). Mass spectrum, m/z (EI, %): 306 (M^+, 100), 307 ($M^+ + 1$, 14). Analysis for $C_{12}H_{10}N_4O_2S_2$ (306.36): Calculated: C, 47.05; H, 3.29; N, 18.29; S, 20.93. Found: C, 46.85; H, 3.20; N, 18.20; S, 20.85.

Synthesis of 2-((4-oxo-5-(thiophen-2-yl)thieno[2,3-d]pyrimidin-3(4H)-yl)methyl)-4H-benzo[d]-[1,3] oxazin-4-one **(5)**. A mixture of **3** (1 mmol, 320 mg) and anthranilic acid (1 mmol, 137 mg) was fused together at 110 °C in an oil bath for 3hr. The residue was boiled with ethanol, the formed solid was removed by filtration, the solid formed was filtered off, and crystallized from EtOH to give **5**. Yield 60%, m.p. 225–227 °C. IR (KBr, Cm^{-1}): ν 1750 (C=O), 1684 (C=O). ^{1}H-NMR (DMSO d$_6$) δ$_H$: 4.58 (s, 2H, CH_2), 7.10–7.54 (m, 4H, thiophene-H), 7.68-8.16 (m, 4H, Ph-H), 8.64 (s, 1H, pyrimidine-H). ^{13}C-MNR (DMSO-d_6) δ$_c$: 43.0 (CH_2), 120.0, 120.1, 121.3, 121.7, 126.7, 126.8, 127.7, 128.7, 131.3, 136.5, 136.6, 149.5, 149.7, 158.2 (14C, thiophene + Ph-C), 157.2 (1C, pyrimidine-C), 160.1, 165.6, 166.5 (3C, 3C=O). Mass spectrum, m/z (EI, %): 393 (M^+, 100). Analysis for $C_{19}H_{11}N_3O_3S_2$ (393.44): Calculated: C, 58.00; H, 2.82; N, 10.68; S, 16.30. Found: C, 57.90; H, 2.78; N, 10.60; S, 16.25.

Synthesis of hydrazone derivatives 6 and 7. To a mixture of **4** (1 mmol, 306 mg) and aromatic aldehydes, namely 3,4-dimethoxybenazaldehyed or 4-chlorobenzaldehyde (1 mmol) in ethanol (50 mL), few drops of piperidine were added and refluxed for 5 h, with stirring. After cooling, the formed solid was filtered off and recrystallized from dioxan to give the corresponding derivatives **6** and **7** respectively.

N'-(2,3-Dimethoxybenzylidene)-2-(4-oxo-5-(thiophen-2-yl)thieno[2,3-d]pyrimidin-3(4H)-yl)-acetohydrazide **(6)**. Yield 68%, m.p. 248–250 °C. IR (KBr, cm^{-1}): ν 3388 (NH), 1660 (C=O). ^{1}H-NMR (DMSO-d_6) δ$_H$: 3.72, 3.86 (2s, 6H, 2OCH$_3$), 4.11 (s, 2H, CH_2), 6.98-7.61 (m, 7H, thiophene + Ph-H), 8.60 (s, 1H, CH=N), 9.05 (s, 1H, pyrimidine-H), 10.51 (s, 1H, NH, disappeared with D_2O). ^{13}C-NMR (MDSO-d_6) δc: 44.1 (1C, CH_2), 56.1, 60.1 (2C, OCH$_3$), 114.3, 116.1, 119.5, 121.8, 124.0, 126.7, 127.7, 128.7, 129.3, 130.6, 131.3, 136.47, 149.07, 149.77 (14C, thiophene-C + Ph-C), 148.56 (1C, CH=N), 157.19 (1C, pyrimidine-C), 163.66, 169.74 (2C, 2C=O). Mass spectrum, m/z (EI, %): 454 (M^+, 100). Analysis for $C_{21}H_{18}N_4O_4S_2$ (454.52): Calculated: C, 55.49; H, 3.99; N, 12.33; S, 14.11. Found: C, 55.40; H, 3.90; N, 12.25; S, 13.96.

N'-(4-Chlorobenzylidene)-2-(4-oxo-5-(thiophen-2-yl)thieno[2,3-d]pyrimidin-3(4H)-yl)acetohydrazide **(7)**. Yield 65%, m.p. 250–252 °C. IR (KBr, Cm^{-1}): ν 3408 (NH), 1670 (CO), 1659 (CO). ^{1}H-NMR (DMSO-d_6) δH: 4.10 (s, 2H, CH_2), 7.10–7.80 (m, 9H, Ar-H + CH=N), 9.05 (s, 1H, pyrimidine-H), 10.56 (s, 1H, NH, disappeared with D_2O). ^{13}C-NMR (MDSO-d_6) δc: 44.1 (1C, CH_2), 145.2 (1C, CH=N), 119.5, 121.9, 124.0, 126.8, 127.8, 128.1, 129.3, 130.6, 131.3, 136.5, 149.1, 149.8 (14C, thiophene-C + Ph-C), 157.5 (1C, pyrimidine-C), 162.7, 169.9 (2C, 2C=O). Mass spectrum, m/z (EI, %): 428 (M^+, 100), 430 ($M^+ + 2$, 40). Analysis for $C_{19}H_{13}ClN_4O_2S_2$ (428.91): Calculated: C, 53.21; H, 3.06; N, 13.06; S, 14.95. Found: C, 53.12; H, 3.00; N, 13.00; S, 14.88.

Synthesis of thiazolidinone derivatives 8 and 9. To a stirred solution of **6** or **7** (1 mmol) in dry benzene (40 mL), thioglycollic acid (1 mmol, 92 mg) in dry benzene (10 mL) was added and refluxed for 12 h. The solvent was evaporated to dryness. The formed product was collected, and crystallized with dioxan to obtain the corresponding products **8** and **9**, respectively.

N-(2-(2,3-Dimethoxyphenyl)-4-oxothiazolidin-3-yl)-2-(4-oxo-5-(thiophen-2-yl)thieno[2,3-d]pyrimidin-3(4H)-yl)acetamide **(8)**. Yield 60%, m.p. 280–282 °C. IR (KBr, cm^{-1}): ν 3417 (NH), 1670, 1680, 1630 (3 C=O). ^{1}H-NMR (DMSO-d$_6$) δ$_H$: 3.65, 3.90 (2s, 6H, 2OCH$_3$), 4.66 (s, 2H, CH$_2$), 4.77 (s, 2H, CH$_2$), 5.86 (s, 1H, CH), 6.95-7.65 (m, 7H, thiophene + Ph-H), 8.49 (s, 1H, pyrimidine-H), 10.84 (s, 1H, NH, disappeared with D$_2$O). ^{13}C-NMR (DMSO-d$_6$) δ$_c$: 35.9, 47.4 (2C, 2CH$_2$), 56.5, 58.42 (2C, 2OCH$_3$), 59.2 (1C, CH), 113.4, 117.9, 118.9, 120.7, 121.8, 126.8, 127.5, 128.7, 130.7, 131.0, 136.5, 145.3, 149.5, 149.9 (14C, thiophene-C + Ph-C), 156.9 (1C, pyrimidine-C), 162.5, 165.4, 169.2 (3C, 3C=O). Mass spectrum, *m/z* (EI, %): 528 (M$^+$, 100), 529 (M$^+$ + 1, 30). Analysis for C$_{23}$H$_{20}$N$_4$O$_5$S$_3$ (528): Calculated: C, 52.26; H, 3.81; N, 10.60; S, 18.19. Found: C, 52.18; H, 3.75; N, 10.52; S, 18.10.

N-(2-(4-Chlorophenyl)-4-oxothiazolidin-3-yl)-2-(4-oxo-5-(thiophen-2-yl)thieno[2,3-d]-pyrimidin-3(4H)-yl)-acetamide **(9)**. Yield 75%, m.p. 175-177 °C. IR (KBr, cm^{-1}): ν 3417 (NH), 1720, 1630, 1660 (3C=O). ^{1}H-NMR (DMSO-d$_6$) δ$_H$: 3.81, 5.16 (2s, 4H, 2CH$_2$), 5.90 (s, 1H, CH), 7.08–7.72 (m, 8H, thiophene-H + Ph-H), 8.50 (s, 1H, pyrimidine-H), 10.92 (s, 1H, NH, disappeared with D$_2$O). ^{13}CNMR (DMSO-d$_6$) δc: 40.1, 48.2 (2C, 2CH$_2$), 65.2 (1C, CH), 120.0, 121.8, 127.7, 128.7, 129.3, 129.4, 131.3, 133.3, 135.0, 136.5, 143.5, 149.7 (14C, thiophene-C + Ph-C), 157.2 (1C, pyrimidine-C), 163.8, 165.6, 169.9 (3C, 3C=O). Mass spectrum, *m/z* (EI, %): 503 (M$^+$, 100), 505 (M$^+$ + 2, 34). Analysis for C$_{21}$H$_{15}$ClN$_4$O$_3$S$_3$ (503.01): Calculated: C, 50.14; H, 3.01; N, 11.14; S, 19.12. Found: C, 50.02; H, 3.00; N, 11.04; S, 19.06.

Synthesis of 2-(2-(4-oxo-5-(thiophen-2-yl)thieno[2,3-d]pyrimidin-3(4H)-yl)acetyl)-N-phenylhydrazine-1-carbothioamide **(10)**. A mixture of **4** (1mmol, 306 mg) and phenylisothiocynate (1 mmol, 135 mg) in dry dioxan (50 mL) was refluxed for 6 h. The obtained solid was filtered off, washed with ether, dried and recrystallized from ethanol to give thiosemicarbazide **10**. Yield 60%, m.p. 240–242 °C. IR (KBr, cm^{-1}): ν 3414-3323 (NH), 1680, 1660 (2CO). ^{1}H-NMR (DMSO-d$_6$) δ$_H$: 4.66 (s, 2H, CH$_2$), 6.95-7.58 (m, 9H, thiophene + Ph-H), 8.49 (s, 1H, pyrimidine-H), 8.70, 10.71, 12.78 (3s, 3H, 3NH, disappeared with D$_2$O). ^{13}CNMR (DMSO-d$_6$) δc: 40.16 (CH$_2$), 119.9, 121.8, 126.8, 127.9, 128.8, 129.1, 130.2, 131.3, 134.1, 136.5, 137.9, 149.9 (14C, thiophene + Ph-C), 156.5 (1C, pyrimimidine-C), 166.5, 169.1 (2C, 2C=O), 171.0 (1C, C=S). Mass spectrum, *m/z* (EI, %): 441 (M$^+$, 100), 442 (M$^+$ + 1, 26). Analysis for C$_{19}$H$_{15}$N$_5$O$_2$S$_3$ (441.54): Calculated: C, 51.68; H, 3.42; N, 15.86; S, 21.78. Found: C, 51.60; H, 3.40; N, 15.80; S, 21.70.

Synthesis of N-(4-oxo-2-(phenylimino)thiazolidin-3-yl)-2-(4-oxo-5-(thiophen-2-yl)thieno[2,3-d]-pyrimidin-3(4H)-yl)acetamide **(11)**. A mixture of **10** (1 mmol, 441 mg) and chloroacetic acid (1 mmol, 94 mg) in absolute ethanol (30 mL) was heated under reflux for 8 h. The solid formed was filtered off and crystallized with dioxane to give thiazole derivative **11**. Yield 60%, m.p. 255–257 °C. IR (KBr, cm^{-1}): ν 3420 (NH), 1720, 1630 (2C=O). ^{1}H-NMR (DMSO-d$_6$) δ$_H$: 3.76 (s, 2H, CH$_2$), 4.85 (s, 2H, CH$_2$), 6.95-7.65 (m, 9H, thiophene-H + Ph-H), 8.50 (s, 1H, pyrimidine-H), 11.10 (s, 1H, NH, disappeared with D$_2$O). ^{13}CNMR (DMSO-d$_6$) δc: 40.2 (CH$_2$), 56.8 (CH$_2$), 120.0, 122.0, 126.7, 128.7, 130.7, 131.3, 132.5, 136.4, (8C, thiophene-C), 145.2, 149.3, 150.8, 151.9 (6C, Ph-C), 156.6 (1C, pyrimidine-C), 158.1 (1C, C=N), 163.4, 165.7, 169.6 (3C, 3C=O). Mass spectrum, *m/z* (EI, %): 481 (M$^+$. 100), 482 (M$^+$ + 1, 24). Analysis for C$_{21}$H$_{15}$N$_5$O$_3$S$_3$ (481.56): Calculated: C, 52.38; H, 3.14; N, 14.54; S, 19.97. Found: C, 52.30; H, 3.10; N, 14.50; S, 19.90.

Synthesis of 3-(2-(3-methyl-5-oxo-2,5-dihydro-1H-pyrazol-1-yl)-2-oxoethyl)-5-(thiophen-2-yl)thieno-[2,3-d]pyrimidin-4(3H)-one **(12)**. A mixture of compound **4** (1 mmol, 306 mg) and ethylacetoacetate (1 mmol, 130 mg) in ethanolic sodium hydroxide (0.5 mmol/50 mL) was refluxed with stirring for 6 h. The precipitate was collected by filtration and crystallized from dioxane to give pyrazole derivative **12**. Yield 80%, m.p. 225–227 °C. IR (KBr, cm^{-1}): ν 3417 (NH), 1650, 1630 (2C=O). ^{1}H-NMR (DMSOd$_6$) δ$_H$: 1.70 (s, 3H, CH$_3$), 4.35 (s, 2H, CH$_2$), 5.65 (s, 1H, pyrazole-CH), 7.51–7.69 (m, 4H, thiophene-H), 8.46 (s, 1H, pyrimidine-H), 12.93 (s, 1H, NH, disappeared with D$_2$O). ^{13}C-NMR (DMSO-d$_6$) δc: 34.4 (CH$_3$), 47.0 (CH$_2$), 120.0, 123.8, 127.7, 128.7, 129.4, 130.9, 132.6, 136.5 (8C, thiophene), 98.3, 151.9 (2C, Pyrazole-C), 156.6 (1C, pyrimidine-C), 163.4, 166.5, 169.7 (3C, 3C=O). Mass spectrum, *m/z* (EI, %): 372

(M$^+$, 100), 373 (M$^+$ + 1, 18). Analysis for C$_{16}$H$_{12}$N$_4$O$_3$S$_2$ (372.42): Calculated: C, 51.60; H, 3.25; N, 15.04; S, 17.22. Found: C, 51.50; H, 3.20; N, 15.00; S, 17.16.

Synthesis of N'-acetyl-2-(4-oxo-5-(thiophen-2-yl)thieno[2,3-d]pyrimidin-3(4H)-yl)aceto-hydrazide (**13**). A solution of **4** (1 mmol, 306 mg) in a mixture of AcOH acid and Ac$_2$O (50 m, 1:1 *v/v*) was refluxed with stirring for 8 h. The reaction mixture was dropped onto iced-water. The obtained precipitate was filtered off, washed with water, and recrystallized from ethanol to give N-acetyl derivative **13**. Yield 70%, m.p. 235–237 °C. IR (KBr, cm^{-1}): ν 3369-3232 (NH, NH), 1732 (C=O). ^{1}H-NMR (DMSOd$_6$) δ$_H$: 1.86 (s, 3H, CH$_3$), 4.68 (s, 2H, CH$_2$), 7.10–7.70 (m, 4H, thiophene-H), 8.44 (s, 1H, pyrimidine-H), 10.70, 10.82 (2s, 2NH, disappeared with D$_2$O). ^{13}C-NMR (DMSO-d$_6$) δc: 20.1 (CH$_3$), 50.1 (CH$_2$), 119.9, 122.0, 122.2, 126.8, 127.8, 128.7, 131.3, 136.4 (8C, thiophene-C), 157.0 (1C, pyrimidine-C), 162.8, 165.6, 169.1 (3C, 3C=O). Mass spectrum, *m/z* (EI, %): 348 (M$^+$, 100), 349 (M$^+$ + 1, 16). Analysis for C$_{14}$H$_{12}$N$_4$O$_3$S$_2$ (348.40): Calculated: C, 48.27; H, 3.47; N, 16.08; S, 18.40. Found: C, 48.20; H, 3.40; N, 16.00; S, 18.32.

Synthesis of compounds 14 and 15. To a mixture of **13** (1 mmol, 348 mg) and ethylcyanoacetate or malononitrile (1 mmol) in EtOH (40 mL), a few drops of triethylamine were refluxed for 8 h, poured into iced-water. The precipitate was filtered off, and crystallized from EtOH to obtain compounds 14 and **15**, respectively.

N-(6-Amino-4-hydroxy-2-oxopyridin-1(2H)-yl)-2-(4-oxo-5-(thiophen-2-yl)thieno[2,3-d]-pyrimidin-3(4H)-yl)acetamide **(14)**. Yield 75%, m.p. 280–282 °C. IR (KBr, cm^{-1}): ν 3492-3196 (OH, NH$_2$, NH), 1420, 1680, 1653 (3 C=O). ^{1}H-NMR (DMSO-d$_6$) δ$_H$: 4.15 (s, 2H, CH$_2$), 4.95, 5.70 (2s, 2H, 2CH), 6.50 (s, 2H, NH$_2$, disappeared with D$_2$O), 7.15–7.74 (m, 4H, thiophene-H), 8.50 (s, 1H, pyrimidine-H), 10.25 (s, 1H, OH, disappeared with D$_2$O), 10.65 (s, 1H, NH, disappeared with D$_2$O). ^{13}C-NMR (DMSO-d$_6$) δc: 49.00 (CH$_2$), 116.1, 120.2, 121.8, 126.7, 127.9, 128.9, 131.3, 136.5 (8C, thiophene-C), 86.5, 100.2, 145.5, 158.7 (4C, pyridine-C), 156.2 (1C, pyrimidine-C), 164.1, 165.5, 169.5 (3C, 3CO). Mass spectrum, *m/z* (EI, %): 415 (M$^+$, 75). Analysis for C$_{17}$H$_{13}$N$_5$O$_4$S$_2$ (415.44): Calculated: C, 49.15; H, 3.15; N, 16.86; S, 15.43. Found: C, 49.05; H, 3.10; N, 16.80; S, 15.35.

N-(2,4-Diaminopyridin-1(2H)-yl)-2-(4-oxo-5-(thiophen-2-yl)thieno[2,3-d]-pyrimidin-3(4H)-yl)acetamide **(15)**. Yield 75%, m.p. 290–292 °C, IR (KBr, cm^{-1}). ν 3460-3345 (NH, NH2), 1680, 1653 (2C=O). ^{1}H-NMR (DMSO-d$_6$) δ$_H$: 4.13 (s, 2H, CH$_2$), 4.60 (s, 2H, NH$_2$, exchangeable with D$_2$O), 5.60–6.10 (m, 4H, 4CH), 7.10–8.72 (m, 4H, thiophene-H), 8.47 (s, 1H, pyrimidine-H), 9.12 (s, 2H, NH$_2$, disappeared with D$_2$O), 10.32 (s, 1H, NH, disappeared with D$_2$O). ^{13}C-NMR (DMSO-d$_6$) δc: 48.00 (CH$_2$), 115.1, 120.0, 121.8, 126.8, 127.7, 128.7, 131.3, 136.5 (8C, thiophene-C), 78.5, 105.1, 118.5, 139.7, 150.0 (5C, pyridine-C), 157.0 (1C, pyrimidine-C), 165.6, 169.3 (2C, 2CO). Mass spectrum, *m/z* (EI, %): 400 (M$^+$, 50). Analysis for C$_{17}$H$_{16}$N$_6$O$_2$S$_2$ (400.48): Calculated: C, 50.99; H, 4.03; N, 20.99; S, 16.01. Found: C, 50.90; H, 4.00; N, 20.90; S, 15.95.

3.2. Biological Evaluation

3.2.1. Cytotoxic Assay

"Human breast cancer cells (MCF-7) and normal non-tumorigenic MCF-10A cells were used throughout the work. Cells were obtained from ATCC, Gaithersburg, MD, USA. Standard MTT assay was used to explore the possible cytotoxic effects of the synthesized compounds [41,42]. Medium composition, cultivation conditions and assay performance were exactly the same as our previous work [43,44]. Cells were treated with varying concentrations (0–1 μM) of the compounds prepared in DMSO. After MTT addition, the absorbance of the dissolved formazan crystals was read at 570 nm [45]. The IC$_{50}$ values were obtained with linear regression equations using Origin® 6.1 software (Origin Lab Corporation, Northampton, MA, USA)".

3.2.2. Human Breast Cancer Xenograft Animal Model

"In this work, MCF-7 mouse xenograft model was used. The animal protocol was approved by the Institutional Animal Use Ethics and Care Committee of the University of Alabama at Birmingham (50-01-05-08B). Female athymic pathogen-free nude mice (nu/nu, 4–6 weeks) were purchased from Frederick Cancer Research and Development Center (Frederick, MD, USA). To establish MCF-7 human breast cancer xenografts, each of the female nude mice was first implanted with a 60-day (subcutaneously, s.c.) slow release estrogen pellet (SE-121, 1.7 mg 17α-estradiol/pellet; Innovative Research of America, Sarasota, FL, USA). After 24 h, grown cells were harvested, washed twice with serum-free medium, resuspended, and injected subcutaneously (5 million cells/0.2 mL) into the left inguinal area of the mice. During the experiment, animals were checked periodically and the percentages of tumor growth, as well as animal weights, were recorded. Every 48 h, the size of the tumor was recorded by measuring two perpendicular diameters of the tumor and tumor volume was calculated according to Wang et al. [46]".

"Treated animals and control groups (7–10 mice/group) received different compounds and vehicles, respectively. The tested compounds were dissolved in PEG400:ethanol:saline (57.1:14.3:28.6, *v/v/v*), and injected intraperitoneal (i.p.) at doses of 5 and 10 μM/kg/d, 3 d/wk for 3 weeks. The higher dose (10 μM/kg/d, 3 d/wk) inhibited MCF-7 xenograft tumor growth".

3.2.3. Pim-1 Kinase Inhibitory Activity

Materials and Methods

"The kinase inhibitory activity of the synthesized compounds was determined using the Kinexus compound profiling service, Canada. Compounds were tested at 50 nM concentration. The kinase used was cloned, expressed and purified using proprietary methods. Quality control testing is routinely performed to ensure compliance to acceptable standards. ^{33}P-ATP was purchased from PerkinElmer. All other materials were of standard laboratory grade".

Pim-1 Kinase Protein Assay

"The protein kinase target profiling was executed via employing a radioisotope assay format. All the assays were performed in a prepared radioactive working area. The protein kinase profiling assays were performed at room temperature for 20–30 min in a final volume of 25 μL according to the reported method [47]".

4. Conclusions

During the current work, different new **14** thiophenyl thienopyrimidinone derivatives were synthesized using variable cyclization and condensation routes. The synthesized derivatives showed promising potential biological potentials for their use in the pharmaceutical industry. They revealed higher in vitro cytotoxic activities against breast cancer cell line MCF-7 in comparison to known drugs, e.g., Cisplatin and Milaplatin. Furthermore, the prepared derivatives proved to be less toxic against the non-tumorigenic MCF-10A cell line. In vivo studies also showed potential reduction in tumor growth in animal models for all synthesized derivatives compared to control animals. Finally, mechanism of action studies showed that the newly synthesized derivatives exert their anticancer effects through the inhibition of pim-1 kinase enzymes.

Author Contributions: M.F.E.-S., A.A.I., A.A.F. and H.M.H. performed most of the experiments; A.E.-G.E.A. and M.A.A. analyzed the data; E.A.E. contributed to the anticancer activity assays; All authors read and approved the final manuscript.

Acknowledgments: The authors are grateful to the Deanship of Scientific Research, King Saud University for funding through Vice Deanship of Scientific Research Chairs.

References

1.   Amr, A.E.; Mohamed, A.M.; Mohamed, S.F.; Abdel-Hafez, N.A.; Hammam, A.G. Anticancer activities of some newly synthesized pyridine, pyrane and pyrimidine derivatives. *Bioorg. Med. Chem.* **2006**, *14*, 5481–5488. [CrossRef] [PubMed]

2.   Amr, A.E.; Abdalla, M.M. Anticancer activities of some synthesized 2,4,6-trisubstituted pyridine candidates. *Biomed. Res.* **2016**, *27*, 731–736.

3.   Mohamed, S.F.; Flefel, E.M.; Amr, A.E.; Abd El-Shafy, D.N. Anti-HSV-1 activity and mechanism of action of some new synthesized substituted pyrimidine, thiopyrimidine and thiazolopyrimidine derivatives. *Eur. J. Med. Chem.* **2010**, *45*, 1494–1501. [CrossRef] [PubMed]

4.   Ouf, N.H.; Amr, A.E. Synthesis and anti-inflammatory activity of some pyrimidines and thienopyrimidines using 1-(2-benzo[d][1,3]dioxol-5-yl)vinyl)-4-mercapto-6-methyl- pyrimidine-5-yl)- ethan-2-one as a starting material. *Mon. Chem.* **2008**, *139*, 579–585. [CrossRef]

5.   Abdel-Hafez, N.A.; Mohamed, A.M.; Amr, A.E.; Abdalla, M.M. Antiarrhythmic activities of some new synthesized tricyclic and tetracyclic thienopyridine derivatives. *Sci. Pharm.* **2009**, *77*, 539–553. [CrossRef]

6.   Abdulla, M.M.; Amr, A.E.; Al-Omar, M.A.; Hussain, A.A.; Shalaby, A.F.A. Anti- inflammatory activity and acute toxicity (LD$_{50}$) of some new synthesized pyridine-2-yl- phenyl)-2-methoxybenzamide and thieno[2,3-b]pyridine derivatives. *Life Sci. J.* **2013**, *10*, 286–297.

7.   Fayed, A.A.; Amr, A.E.; Al-Omar, M.A.; Mostafa, E.E. Synthesis and antimicrobial activity of some new substituted pyrido[3′,2′:4,5]thieno[3,2-d]pyrimidinone derivatives. *Russ. J. Bioorg. Chem.* **2014**, *40*, 308–313. [CrossRef]

8.   Ouf, N.H.; Sakran, M.I.; Amr, A.E. Anti-inflammatory activities of some newly synthesized substituted thienochromene and Schiff base derivatives. *Res. Chem. Intermed.* **2015**, *41*, 2521–2536. [CrossRef]

9.   Said, S.A.; El-Sayed, H.A.; Amr, A.E.; Abdalla, M.M. Selective and orally bioavailable CHK1 inhibitors of some synthesized substituted thieno[2,3-b]pyridine candidates. *Int. J. Pharm.* **2015**, *11*, 659–671.

10. Amr, A.E.; Al-Omar, M.A.; Abdalla, M.M. Biological evaluations of some synthesized pyrimidothieno[2,3-b]pyrimidine candidates as antiulcer agents. *Int. J. Pharm.* **2015**, *11*, 840–845. [CrossRef]

11. Amr, A.E.; Abdalla, M.M.; Ouf, N.H. Anti-angiogenic effects of some (5-hydroxy-4-methyl-2-((1-methyl-1H-indol-3-yl)methyl)thieno[2,3-d]pyrimidine derivatives. *J. Comput. Nanosci.* **2017**, *14*, 448–453. [CrossRef]

12. Nasr, M.N.; Gineinah, M.M. Pyrido[2,3-d]pyrimidines and pyrimido[5,4-5,6]pyrido[2,3-d] pyrimidines as new antiviral agents, synthesis and biologicalactivity. *Arch. Pharm. Pharm. Med. Chem.* **2002**, *335*, 289–295. [CrossRef]

13. Chambhare, R.V.; Khadse, B.G.; Bobde, A.S.; Bahekar, R.H. Synthesis and preliminary evaluation of some N-[5-(2-furanyl)-2-methyl-4-oxo-4H-thieno[2,3-d]pyrimidine-3-yl]- carboxamide and 3-substituted-5-(2-furanyl)-2-methyl-3H-thieno[2,3-d]pyrimidine-4-ones as antimicrobial agents. *Eur. J. Med. Chem.* **2003**, *38*, 89–100. [CrossRef]

14. Russell, R.K.; Press, J.B.; Rampulla, R.A.; McNally, J.J.; Falotico, R.; Keiser, J.A.; Bright, D.A.; Tobia, A. Thiophene systems. 9. Thienopyrimidinedione derivatives as potential antihypertensive agents. *J. Med. Chem.* **1988**, *31*, 1786–1793. [CrossRef]

15. Alagarsamy, V.; Meena, S.; Ramseshu, K.V.; Solomon, V.R.; Thirumurugan, K.; Dhanabal, K.; Murugan, M. Synthesis, analgesic, anti-inflammatory, ulcerogenic index and antibacterial activities of novel 2-methylthio-3-substituted-5,6,7,8-tetrahydrobenzo thieno [2,3-d]pyrimidin- 4(3h)-ones. *Eur. J. Med. Chem.* **2006**, *41*, 1293–1300. [CrossRef] [PubMed]

16. Petrie, C.R.; Cottam, H.B.; Mckernan, P.A.; Robins, R.K.; Revankar, G.R. Synthesis and biological activity of 6-azacadeguomycin and certain 3,4,6-trisubstituted pyrazolo-[3,4-d]pyrimidine ribonuleosi. *J. Med. Chem.* **1985**, *28*, 1010–1016. [CrossRef]

17. Mullican, M.D.; Wilson, M.W.; Connor, D.T.; Kostlan, C.R.; Schrier, D.J.; Dyer, R.D. Design of 5-(3,5-di-tert-butyl-4-hydroxyphenyl)-l,3,4-thiadiazoles-1,3,4-oxadiazoles, and 1,2,4-triazoles as orally-active, nonulcerogenic antiinflammatory agents. *J. Med. Chem.* **1993**, *36*, 1090–1099. [CrossRef] [PubMed]

18. Shi, W.; Qian, X.; Zhang, R.; Song, G. Synthesis and quantitative structure-activity relationships of new 2,5-disubstituted-1,3,4-oxadiazoles. *J. Agric. Food Chem.* **2001**, *49*, 124–130. [CrossRef] [PubMed]

19. Gaonkar, S.L.; Rai, K.M.L.; Prabhuswamy, B. Synthesis and antimicrobial studies of a new series of 2-{4-[2-(5-ethylpyridin-2-yl)ethoxy]phenyl}-5-substituted-1,3,4-oxadiazoles. *Eur. J. Med. Chem.* **2006**, *41*, 841–846. [CrossRef] [PubMed]

20. Patel, R.V.; Pate, P.K.; Kumari, P.; Rajani, D.P.; Chikhalia, K.H. Synthesis of benzimida zolyl-1,3,4-oxadiazol-2ylthio-n-phenyl (benzothiazolyl) acetamides as antibacterial, antifungal and antituberculosis agents. *Eur. J. Med. Chem.* **2012**, *53*, 41–51. [CrossRef] [PubMed]

21. Varvounis, G.; Giannopoulos, T. Synthesis, Chemistry, and Biological Properties of Thienopyrimidines. In *Advances in Heterocyclic Chemistry*; Alan, R.K., Ed.; Academic Press: Cambridge, MA, USA, 1996; pp. 193–283.

22. Litvinov, V.P. The Chemistry of Thienopyrimidines. In *Advances in Heterocyclic Chemistry*; Alan, R.K., Ed.; Academic Press: Cambridge, MA, USA, 2006; pp. 83–143.

23. Dumaître, B.; Dodic, N. Synthesis and cyclic GMP phosphodiesterase inhibitory activity of a series of 6-phenylpyrazolo[3,4-d]pyrimidines. *J. Med. Chem.* **1996**, *39*, 1635–1644. [CrossRef] [PubMed]

24. El-Sherbeny, M.A.; El-Ashmawy, M.B.; El-Subbagh, H.I.; El-Emam, A.A.; Badria, F.A. Synthesis, antimicrobial and antiviral evaluation of certain thienopyrimidine derivatives. *Eur. J. Med. Chem.* **1995**, *30*, 445–449. [CrossRef]

25. Rizk, O.H.; Shaaban, O.G.; El-Ashmawy, I.M. Design, synthesis and biological evaluation of some novel thienopyrimidines and fused thienopyrimidines as anti-inflammatory agents. *Eur. J. Med. Chem.* **2012**, *55*, 85–93. [CrossRef] [PubMed]

26. Aly, H.M.; Saleh, N.M.; Elhady, H.A. Design and synthesis of some new thiophene, thienopyrimidine and thienothiadiazine derivatives of antipyrine as potential antimicrobial agents. *Eur. J. Med. Chem.* **2011**, *46*, 4566–4572. [CrossRef] [PubMed]

27. Elrazaz, E.Z.; Serya, R.A.T.; Ismail, N.S.M.; Abou El Ella, D.A.; Abouzid, K.A.M. Thieno[2,3-d]pyrimidine based derivatives as kinase inhibitors and anticancer agents. *Future Journal of Pharmaceutical Sciences* **2015**, *1*, 33–41. [CrossRef]

28. Munchhof, M.J.; Beebe, J.S.; Casavant, J.M.; Cooper, B.A.; Doty, J.L.; Higdon, R.C.; Hillerman, S.M.; Soderstrom, C.I.; Knauth, E.A.; Marx, M.A.; et al. Design and SAR of thienopyrimidine and thienopyridine inhibitors of VEGFR-2 kinase activity. *Bioorg. Med. Chem. Lett.* **2004**, *14*, 21–24. [CrossRef] [PubMed]

29. Le, B.T.; Kumarasiri, M.; Adams, J.R.; Yu, M.; Milne, R.; Sykes, M.J.; Wang, S. Targeting Pim kinases for cancer treatment: Opportunities and challenges. *Future Med. Chem.* **2015**, *7*, 35–53. [CrossRef]

30. Narlik-Grassow, M.; Blanco-Aparicio, C.; Carnero, A. The PIM family of serine/threonine kinases in cancer. *Med. Res. Rev.* **2014**, *34*, 136–159. [CrossRef]

31. Nawijn, M.C.; Alendar, A.; Berns, A. For better or for worse: The role of PIM oncogenes in tumorigenesis. *Nat. Rev. Cancer* **2011**, *11*, 23–34. [CrossRef]

32. Cuypers, H.T.; Selten, G.; Quint, W.; Zijlstra, M.; Maandag, E.R.; Boelens, W.; van Wezenbeek, P.; Melief, C.; Berns, A. Murine leukemia virus induced T-cell lymphomagenesis: Integration of proviruses in a distinct chromosomal region. *Cell* **1984**, *37*, 141–150. [CrossRef]

33. Tursynbay, Y.; Zhang, J.; Li, Z.; Tokay, T.; Zhumadilov, Z.; Wu, D.; Xie, Y. PIM-1 kinase as cancer drug target: An update (Review). *Biomed. Rep.* **2016**, *4*, 140–146. [CrossRef] [PubMed]

34. Keane, N.A.; Reidy, M.; Natoni, A.; Raab, M.S.; O'Dwyer, M. Targeting the PIM kinases in multiple myeloma. *Blood Cancer J.* **2015**, *5*, e325. [CrossRef] [PubMed]

35. Foulks, J.M.; Carpenter, K.J.; Luo, B.; Xu, Y.; Senina, A.; Nix, R.; Chan, A.; Clifford, A.; Wilkes, M.; Vollmer, D.; et al. A small-molecule inhibitor of pim kinases as a potential treatment for urothelial carcinomas. *Neoplasia* **2014**, *16*, 403–412. [CrossRef] [PubMed]

36. Decker, S.; Finter, J.; Forde, A.J.; Kissel, S.; Schwaller, J.; Mack, T.S.; Kuhn, A.; Gray, N.; Follo, M.; Jumaa, H.; et al. PIM kinases are essential for chronic lymphocytic leukemia cell survival (PIM2/3) and CXCR4-mediated microenvironmental interactions (PIM1). *Mol. Cancer* **2014**, *13*, 1231–1245. [CrossRef] [PubMed]

37. Lu, J.; Zavorotinskaya, T.; Dai, Y.; Niu, X.H.; Castillo, J.; Sim, J.; Yu, J.; Wang, Y.; Langowski, J.L.; Holash, J.; et al. PIM2 is required for maintaining multiple myeloma cell growth through modulating TSC2 phosphorylation. *Blood* **2013**, *122*, 1610–1620. [CrossRef] [PubMed]

38. Drygin, D.; Haddach, M.; Pierre, F.; Ryckman, D.M. Potential use of selective and nonselective pim kinase inhibitors for cancer therapy. *J. Med. Chem.* **2012**, *55*, 8199–8208. [CrossRef] [PubMed]

39. Guo, S.; Mao, X.; Chen, J.; Huang, B.; Jin, C.; Xu, Z.; Qiu, S. Overexpression of Pim-1 in bladder cancer. *J. Exp. Clin. Cancer Res.* **2010**, *29*, 161–167. [CrossRef] [PubMed]

40. Brault, L.; Gasser, C.; Bracher, F.; Huber, K.; Knapp, S.; Schwaller, J. PIM serine/threonine kinases in the pathogenesis and therapy of hematologic malignancies and solid cancers. *Haematologica* **2010**, *95*, 1004–1015. [CrossRef] [PubMed]

41. Elsayed, E.A.; Sharaf-Eldin, M.A.; Wadaan, M. In vitro evaluation of cytotoxic activities of essential oil from Moringa oleifera seeds on HeLa, HepG2, MCF-7, CACO-2 and L929 cell lines. *Asian Pac. J. Cancer Prev.* **2015**, *16*, 4671–4675. [CrossRef]

42. Elsayed, E.A.; Farooq, M.; Dailin, D.; El-Enshasy, H.A.; Othman, N.Z.; Malek, R.; Danial, E.; Wadaan, M. In vitro and in vivo biological screening of kefiran polysaccharide produced by lactobacillus kefiranofaciens. *Biomed. Res.* **2017**, *28*, 594–600.

43. Amr, A.E.; Elsayed, E.A.; Al-Omar, M.A.; Badr Eldin, H.O.; Nossier, E.S.; Abdallah, M.M. Design, synthesis, anticancer evaluation and molecular modeling of novel estrogen derivatives. *Molecules* **2019**, *24*, 416. [CrossRef]

44. Amr, A.E.; El-Naggar, M.; Al-Omar, M.A.; Elsayed, E.A.; Abdalla, M.M. In vitro and in vivo anti-breast cancer activities of some synthesized pyrazolinyl-estran-17-one candidates. *Molecules* **2018**, *23*, 1572. [CrossRef]

45. McCauley, J.; Zivanovic, A.; Skropeta, D. Bioassays for anticancer activities. *Methods Mol. Biol.* **2013**, *1055*, 191–205.

46. Wang, H.; Yu, D.; Agrawal, S.; Zhang, R. Experimental therapy of human prostate cancer by inhibiting MDM2 expression with novel mixed-backbone antisense oligonucleotides: In vitro and in vivo activities and mechanisms. *Prostate* **2003**, *54*, 194–205. [CrossRef]

47. Naguib, B.H.; El-Nassan, H.B.; Abdelghany, T.M. Synthesis of new pyridothieno- pyrimidinone derivatives as Pim-1 inhibitors. *J. Enzyme Inhibit. Med. Chem.* **2017**, *32*, 457–467. [CrossRef]

Synthesis, Antiproliferative Activity and Molecular Docking Studies of Novel Doubly Modified Colchicine Amides and Sulfonamides as Anticancer Agents

Julia Krzywik [1,2], Witold Mozga [2], Maral Aminpour [3], Jan Janczak [4], Ewa Maj [5],
Joanna Wietrzyk [5], Jack A. Tuszyński [3,6] and Adam Huczyński [1,*]

[1] Department of Medical Chemistry, Faculty of Chemistry, Adam Mickiewicz University,
    Uniwersytetu Poznańskiego 8, 61–614 Poznań, Poland; julia.krzywik@amu.edu.pl
[2] TriMen Chemicals, Piłsudskiego 141, 92–318 Łódź, Poland; mozga@trimen.pl
[3] Department of Oncology, University of Alberta, Edmonton, AB T6G 1Z2, Canada;
    aminpour@ualberta.ca (M.A.); jack.tuszynski@gmail.com (J.A.T.)
[4] Institute of Low Temperature and Structure Research, Polish Academy of Sciences, PO Box 1410,
    50–950 Wrocław, Poland; j.janczak@intibs.pl
[5] Hirszfeld Institute of Immunology and Experimental Therapy, Polish Academy of Sciences, Rudolfa Weigla 12,
    53–114 Wrocław, Poland; ewa.maj@hirszfeld.pl (E.M.); joanna.wietrzyk@hirszfeld.pl (J.W.)
[6] DIMEAS, Politecnico di Torino, Corso Duca degli Abruzzi, 24, 10129 Torino, Italy
*   Correspondence: adhucz@amu.edu.pl;

Academic Editor: Qiao-Hong Chen

Abstract: Colchicine is a well-known compound with strong antiproliferative activity that has had limited use in chemotherapy because of its toxicity. In order to create more potent anticancer agents, a series of novel colchicine derivatives have been obtained by simultaneous modification at C7 (amides and sulfonamides) and at C10 (methylamino group) positions and characterized by spectroscopic methods. All the synthesized compounds have been tested in vitro to evaluate their cytotoxicity toward A549, MCF-7, LoVo, LoVo/DX and BALB/3T3 cell lines. Additionally, the activity of the studied compounds was investigated using computational methods involving molecular docking of the colchicine derivatives to β-tubulin. The majority of the obtained derivatives exhibited higher cytotoxicity than colchicine, doxorubicin or cisplatin against tested cancer cell lines. Furthermore, molecular modeling studies of the obtained compounds revealed their possible binding modes into the colchicine binding site of tubulin.

Keywords: anticancer agents; colchicine amide; colchicine sulfonamide; tubulin inhibitors; docking studies; crystal structure

1. Introduction

Microtubules, which are composed of α- and β-tubulin heterodimers, are involved in a large number of processes, such as intracellular transport, cell shape development, cell division and cell motility. During cell division microtubules form the mitotic spindle that in normal cells correctly separates the chromosomes into two daughter cells. In cancer cells the rate of mitosis is typically increased but chromosome segregation is imperfect leading to aneuploidy. Microtubules formed during mitosis are considered as an ideal target for anticancer drugs since no cell can divide without the force generated by microtubules. Therefore, many inhibitors of microtubule dynamics have been investigated for their potential use as cancer chemotherapy drugs [1–7]. One of these compounds is colchicine **1** (see Scheme 1), a well–known tropolone alkaloid isolated from *Colchicum autumnale*, which has been shown to exhibit very high cytotoxic effects. It binds to tubulin at the colchicine binding site and induces conformational change in the tubulin dimer making it incompetent for microtubule assembly. As a result, the cell cycle is blocked and apoptosis is induced [8–14]. Unfortunately, colchicine is too toxic to be useful as an antitumor agent [8,15–21]. Nevertheless, it has found use in therapy, e.g., for the treatment of familial Mediterranean fever, Behcet's disease or acute gout [22–27].

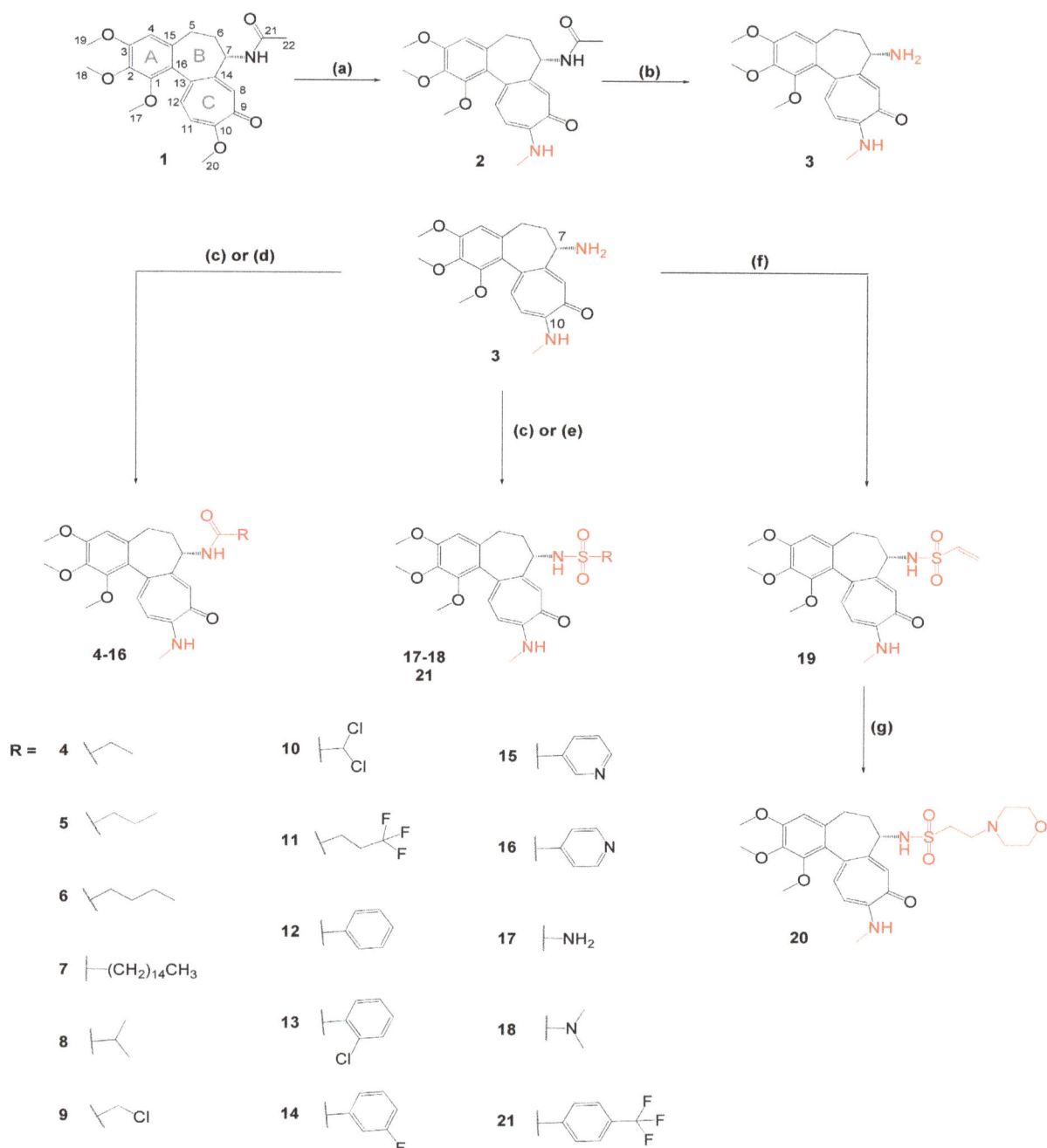

Scheme 1. Synthesis of doubly modified colchicine derivatives (**2–21**), changes at C7 and C10 positions are highlighted in red. Reagents and conditions: (**a**) NHCH$_3$/EtOH, reflux; (**b**) 2M HCl, reflux; (**c**) RC(O)Cl or RSO$_2$Cl, Et$_3$N, DCM, 0 °C to RT for **4, 8, 13, 15–16, 18** and **21**; (**d**) RCOOH, EDCI, DCM, RT for **5–7, 9–12** and **14**; (**e**) (1) *N*-(*tert*-butoxycarbonyl)-*N*-[4-(dimethylazaniumylidene)-1,4-dihydropyridin-1-ylsulfonyl]azanide, DCM, RT, (2) 4M HCl/EtOAc, RT for **17**; (**f**) ClCH$_2$CH$_2$SO$_2$Cl, Et$_3$N, DCM, 0 °C to RT; (**g**) morpholine, DCM, RT.

Therefore, over the past few decades much interest has been focused on structural modifications of **1** in the hope of improving its therapeutic index [28–31]. Numerous double-modified colchicine derivatives have been synthesized with the group at position C7 substituted by various amide and sulfonamide moieties as well as with replacement of the methoxy group at position C10 by a group containing either a nitrogen or a sulfur atom and their biological activities have been determined [28,29,32–36]. These results have shown that new derivatives may have lower toxicity with respect to normal cells while maintaining high antitumor activity. In addition, from the chemical point of view, such a change at position C10 allows obtaining compounds more resistant to acid hydrolysis [29,30,33]. We have decided to check various amide and sulfonamide moieties because they have long been valued for their rich biological and chemical profiles and have emerged as a promising class of compounds in drug discovery [37–41].

Herein, we report the synthesis, crystallographic and spectroscopic analysis of a series of structurally different derivatives of colchicine obtained by its modification at position C7 (various amide, sulfonamide or sulfamide moieties) and at position C10 (methylamino group). We also describe the results of in vitro antiproliferative activity evaluation of colchicine (**1**) and the obtained colchicine derivatives (**2–21**) against four human cancer cell lines and one normal murine embryonic fibroblast cell line. To acquire more knowledge about the molecular mechanism of action of the investigated compounds (**1–21**), we also present results of *in silico* molecular docking study of the colchicine binding site (CBS) of β-tubulin.

2. Results and Discussion

2.1. Chemistry

To investigate the effect of methylamino group at position C10 and, at the same time, various amide, sulfonamide and sulfamide moieties at position C7 of colchicine **1** on its antiproliferative activity, eighteen new derivatives (**4–21**) were synthesized. To facilitate the structure-activity relationship analysis (SAR) we designed compounds with different side chains at position C7: alkyl chains of various length, straight and branched (**4–8**), unsaturated alkyl chain (**19**), alkyl chains of various lengths containing halogen atoms (**9–11**), an aromatic group without or with substituents (**12–16, 21**), and compounds containing an amino group **17–18** and **20**.

The general route for the synthesis of colchicine derivatives **2–21** is depicted in Scheme 1. Colchicine (**1**) was treated with methylamine solution in ethanol to give 10-methylamino-10-demethoxycolchicine (**2**) with 80% yield, according to the method described earlier [42]. The replacement of water solution of methylamine by ethanol solution eliminated the work up after the reaction and permitted obtaining comparable final yields. Next, hydrolysis of **2** with 2M HCl yielded N-deacetyl-10-methylamino-10-demethoxycolchicine (**3**). Compounds **4–16, 18–19** and **21** were readily available from **3** by treatment with respective acid/ sulfonamide/ sulfamide chloride in the presence of triethylamine or with the corresponding carboxylic acid and carbodiimide as a condensing agent. Compound **17** was prepared using a N-(*tert*-butoxycarbonyl)-N-[4-(dimethylazaniumylidene)-1,4-dihydropyridin-1-ylsulfonyl]azanide and further modified by removal of the *tert*-butoxycarbonyl group from amine with HCl [43]. Vinylsulfonamide **19** was synthesized from 2-chloroethanesulfonyl chloride and **3** through sulfonylation and in situ β-elimination of HCl. Compound **19** was used as the Michael acceptor with an electron-deficient double bond for the reaction with morpholine to produce compound **20 [44,45]**. All synthesized compounds were isolated in pure form after column chromatography.

The purity and structures of the obtained compounds **2–21** were determined using the LC-MS, ^{1}H and ^{13}C NMR methods and are shown in the Supplementary Materials and discussed below. The characteristic signals of -OCH$_3$ group at position C10 of **1** in the ^{1}H NMR and ^{13}C NMR spectra were observed as a singlet at 4.0 ppm and at 56.5 ppm, respectively. These signals vanish after the reaction of colchicine with methylamine proving the substitution of the -OCH$_3$ group in the tropolone ring of **1**. After the introduction of -NHCH$_3$ at position C10 the signals of this group in the obtained derivatives (**2–21**) were visible approx. at 3.1 ppm as a doublet and approx. at 7.4 ppm as a quartet in ^{1}H NMR and approx. at 29.5 ppm in ^{13}C NMR. The chemical shifts of the amide moiety can be found in the range 7.9–9.7 ppm in ^{1}H NMR and in the range 164.2–175.2 ppm in ^{13}C NMR, depending on the substituent used. The ESI mass spectrometry confirmed the structure of the obtained compounds by the presence of an *m/z* signals assigned to the corresponding pseudomolecular ions of these compounds.

2.2. X-ray Crystal Analysis

Structural characterization of the colchicine derivatives is very important in order to understand their anticancer properties stemming from their interaction with tubulin as well as to enable structure–activity relationship analysis (SAR) and related investigation. Therefore, structural analyses of all crystals that were suitable for X-ray analysis of single crystals were performed. Crystals of **6**, **11**, **12**, **14**, **18** and **19** suitable for the X-ray single crystal analysis were obtained by recrystallization of the respective colchicine derivatives from acetonitrile, whereas crystals **15** and **16** from ethyl acetate solutions. All crystals were measured at room (295 K) and low (100 K) temperature. Details of the data collection parameters, crystallographic data and the final agreement parameters are listed in Supplementary Table S1. In the temperature range from 295 K to 100 K, no structural phase transitions were observed in the crystals studied, although for colchicine derivative **11** at low temperature some disorder of the -CF$_3$ group in the -CH$_2$-CH$_2$-CF$_3$ group at atom C21 could be observed. Colchicine derivatives **6**, **11**, **12**, **14**, **15**, and **16** crystallize in the P3$_2$21 space group of the trigonal system while derivative **18** crystallizes in the P2$_1$2$_1$2$_1$ space group of the orthorhombic system and derivative **19** crystallizes in the P2$_1$ space group of the monoclinic system. These space groups are chiral since the compounds contain an asymmetric carbon (C7) atom. The absolute configuration at the C7 atom is *S* in all structures. The molecular structures of all colchicine derivatives (**6**, **11**, **12**, **14**, **15**, **16**, **18** and **19**) are illustrated in Supplementary Figure S60. The planar phenyl A and tropolone C rings in all colchicine derivatives (**6**, **11**, **12**, **14**, **15**, **16**, **18** and **19**) are twisted around the C13–C16 bond with the torsion angle describing the twisting conformation C1–C16–C13–C12 between ~53° and ~56° at 100 K and they do not differ significantly from the values at room temperature (Table 1). Ring B in all colchicine derivatives exhibits a similar puckering pattern and the extent of its non-planarity is such that it adopts a conformation, which is close to the twist-boat with a flattening caused by the fusion of rings A and C (see Supplementary Figure S60). So the conformation of the fused A, B and C rings of colchicine skeleton in the investigated derivatives is quite similar to that in colchicine itself [46].

Table 1. Selected torsion angles (°) of colchicine derivatives **6**, **11**, **12**, **14**, **15**, **16**, **18** and **19** obtained by X-ray analysis and DFT computation for a comparison.

		6	11	12	14	15	16	18	19
C1–C16–C13–C12	100 K	53.1(4)	55.5(6)	53.7(3)	54.0(5)	53.6(4)	54.1(3)	56.1(4)	55.3(3)
	295 K	55.2(4)	55.5(6)	55.0(3)	54.4(4)	54.7(4)	55.0(3)	56.1(4)	55.9(4)
	DFT value	53.1	52.3	53.4	53.5	52.9	53.3	54.5	56.0
C17–O1–C1–C2	100 K	−79.0(4)	−86.4(6)	−89.3(3)	−90.6(5)	−87.3(4)	−86.8(4)	−108.6(3)	66.2(3)
	295 K	−86.5(4)	−86.4(6)	−86.4(4)	−87.4(5)	−87.8(4)	−86.4(4)	−106.8(3)	65.6(4)
	DFT value	−73.0	−70.7	−80.3	−80.0	−72.9	−79.4	−74.8	59.2
C18–O2–C2–C3	100 K	108.0(3)	105.2(6)	96.1(2)	95.5(4)	99.7(4)	94.5(3)	−77.5(4)	−102.7(3)
	295 K	106.9(4)	105.2(6)	98.7(3)	98.0(4)	101.4(4)	98.7(3)	−74.0(4)	−100.6(4)
	DFT value	70.1	68.8	82.1	82.3	71.1	81.1	−59.6	−77.2
C19–O3–C3–C4	100 K	−14.1(5)	−10.5(9)	8.6(4)	14.4(6)	−6.0(6)	7.4(6)	1.2(5)	7.7(4)
	295 K	−8.1(7)	−10.5(10)	6.9(6)	11.4(7)	−2.3(6)–3.8	6.9(6)	0.2(5)	6.8(5)
	DFT value	−4.0	−3.7	−2.0	−1.9		−1.9	0.7	3.1
C20–N1–C10–C11	100 K	7.7(5)	8.8(8)	4.6(3)	4.4(6)	5.0(5)	6.6(4)	−0.2(5)	4.7(4)
	295 K	6.8(6)	8.7(9)	7.5(4)	5.0(6)	5.2(5)	7.5(4)	−1.7(5)	4.0(7)
	DFT value	−0.9	−0.9	−1.4	−1.0	−1.2	−1.3	0.2	−1.6

The methoxy group -OCH$_3$ linked to the phenyl ring at C3 is almost coplanar with the ring in all structures of colchicine derivatives, whereas the other two methoxy groups linked at C1 and

C2 atoms of the phenyl ring have different orientations in some colchicine derivatives (Table 1). The *N*-methylamino group (-NHCH$_3$) linked to tropolone C ring at C10 atom is almost coplanar with the ring. The differences between the conformations of the investigated colchicine derivatives are illustrated in Figure 1 and Table 1. For clarity, the colchicine derivatives have been divided into two groups, according to the substituent in ring B at position C7; one group comprises the derivatives with a chain substituent (Figure 1a) and the other group comprises the derivatives with a substituent containing an aromatic ring (Figure 1b). Analysis of these results reveals a significant difference in the torsion angle C17-O1-C1-C2 in compounds 18 (~−109°) and 19 (~66°) or the difference between the calculated (~−103°) and measured (~−77°) torsion angle C18-O2 -C2-C3 in compound 19. These differences result from different approach to the description of the molecule conformations, the X-ray analysis values refer to the conformation of molecules in crystals, in which the intermolecular interactions play a significant role and leads crystallization and specific crystal packing, while the DFT values refer to a single isolated molecule in the gas state with the intermolecular interactions not taken into account.

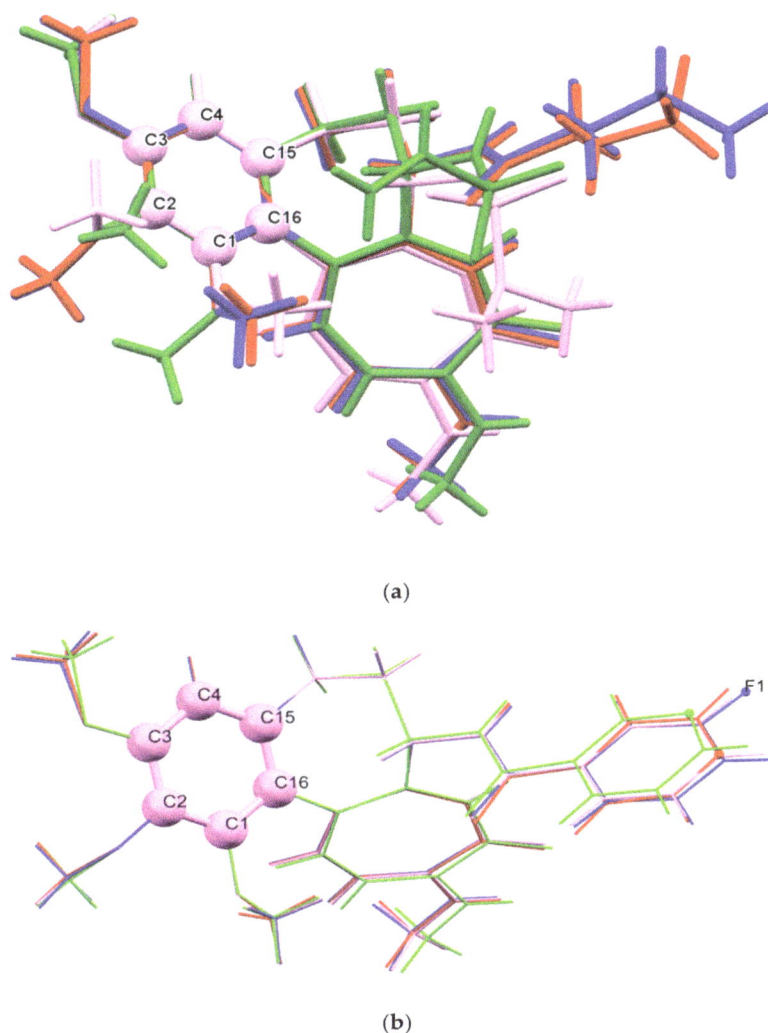

(a)

(b)

Figure 1. Comparison of the X-ray structure of (**a**) derivatives with a chain substituent at position C7: **6** (blue), **11** (red), **18** (pink) and **19** (green) and (**b**) derivatives with a substituent containing an aromatic ring at position C7: **12** (pink), **14** (blue), **15** (green) and **16** (red) showing the conformation of the colchicine skeleton. The molecules are overlapped one over another so that the ring C1-C2-C3-C4-C15-C16 is at the same position.

2.3. Molecular Electrostatic Potential Map Analysis

The role of the trimethoxyphenyl ring A of colchicine as well as that of the tropolone ring C in tubulin binding have been studied in great details. The tropolonoic ring C of the colchicine skeleton is found to be crucial for the interaction with tubulin [47,48]. The molecular electrostatic potential map (MESP) correlated with the electronic density in a molecule and is a powerful tool for analyzing interactions [49–51]. It was, therefore, calculated for all structurally characterized colchicine derivatives. Additionally, the gas-phase structures of all molecules were determined using the DFT optimization with the Gaussian09 program package [52]. All calculations were carried out by the DFT method using the Becke3-Lee–Yang–Parr correlation functional (B3LYP) [53–56] with the 6–31 + G basis set, starting from the X-ray geometry of molecules. The gas-phase optimized conformations of all colchicine derivatives are, in general, in good agreement with those obtained from the X-ray single crystal investigation, however the optimized torsion angle C18–O2–C2–C3 describing the orientation of the methoxy group is significantly smaller than that provided by the X-ray analysis (Table 1 and for more details see Supplementary Table S2).

The region of tubulin that interacts with colchicine is near the αβ-tubulin/dimer interface [57]. In order to better understand the interaction of the colchicine derivatives with tubulin, the molecular electrostatic potential was calculated for all structurally characterized colchicine derivatives as well as, for comparison, for colchicine itself. The three-dimensional MESP maps for colchicine derivatives and for colchicine itself were calculated on the basis of the DFT (B3LYP) optimized geometries of molecules and mapped onto the total electron density isosurface (0.008 eÅ^{-3}) for both molecules using the GaussView 5.0 program (Figure 2). The color coding of MESP is in the range of −0.05 (red) to 0.05 eÅ^{-1} (blue). For all colchicine derivatives, the regions of negative MESP are usually associated with the lone pair of electronegative atoms (O and N), whereas the regions of positive MESP are associated with the electropositive atoms (Figure 2).

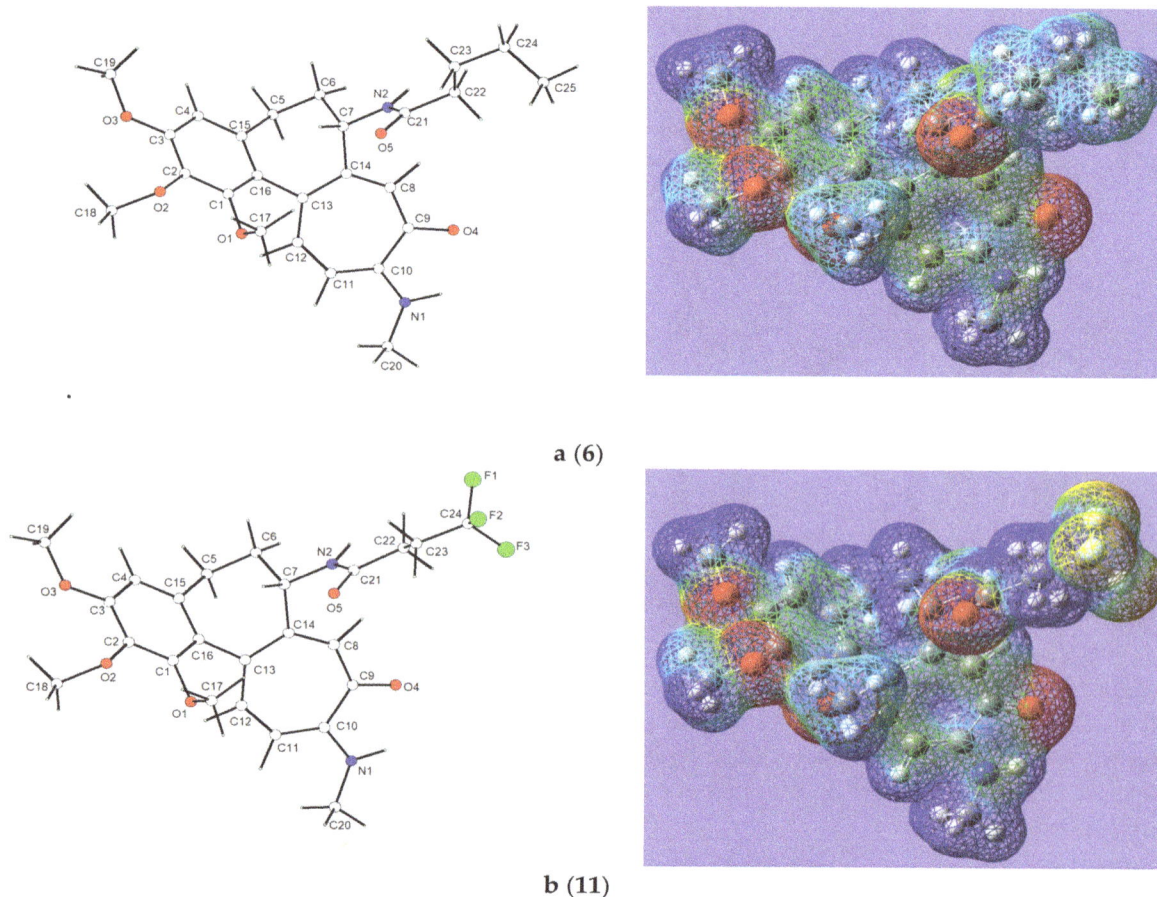

a (6)

b (11)

Figure 2. *Cont.*

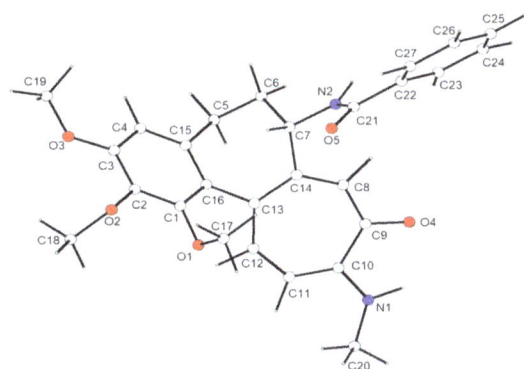 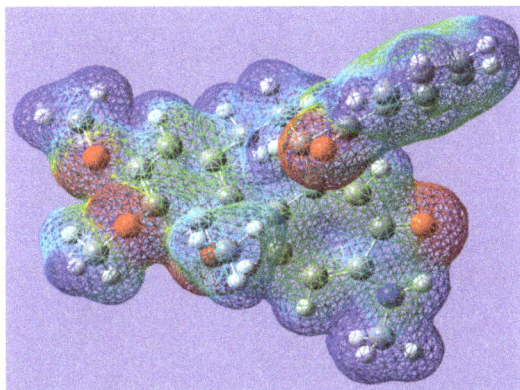

c (12)

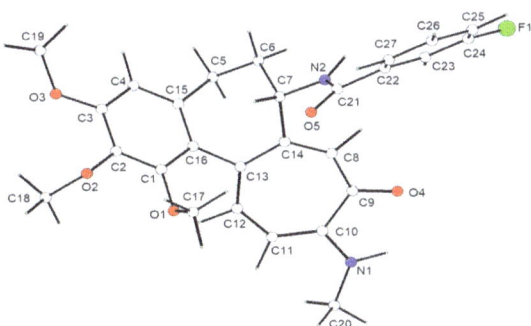 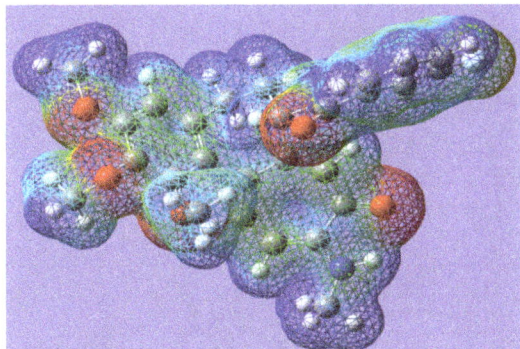

d (14)

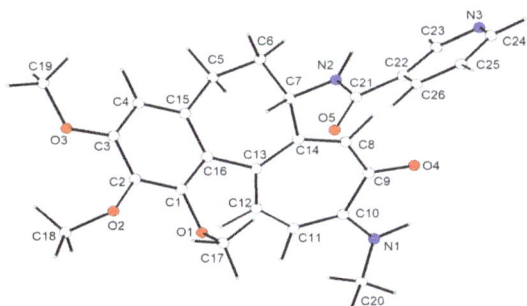 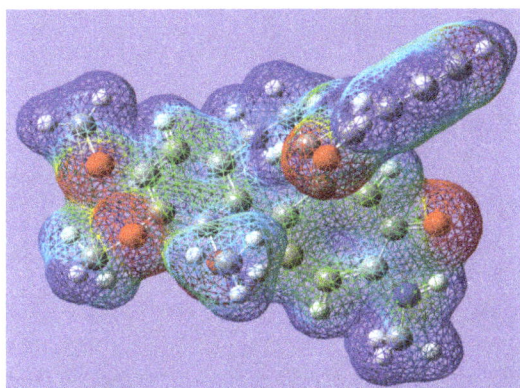

e (15)

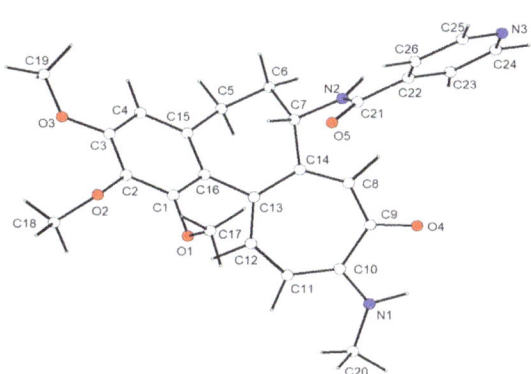 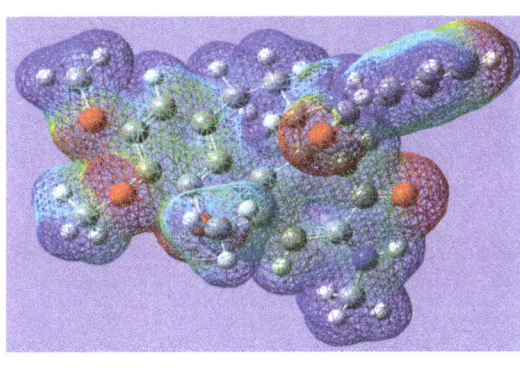

f (16)

Figure 2. *Cont.*

g (18)

h (19)

i (colchicine **1**)

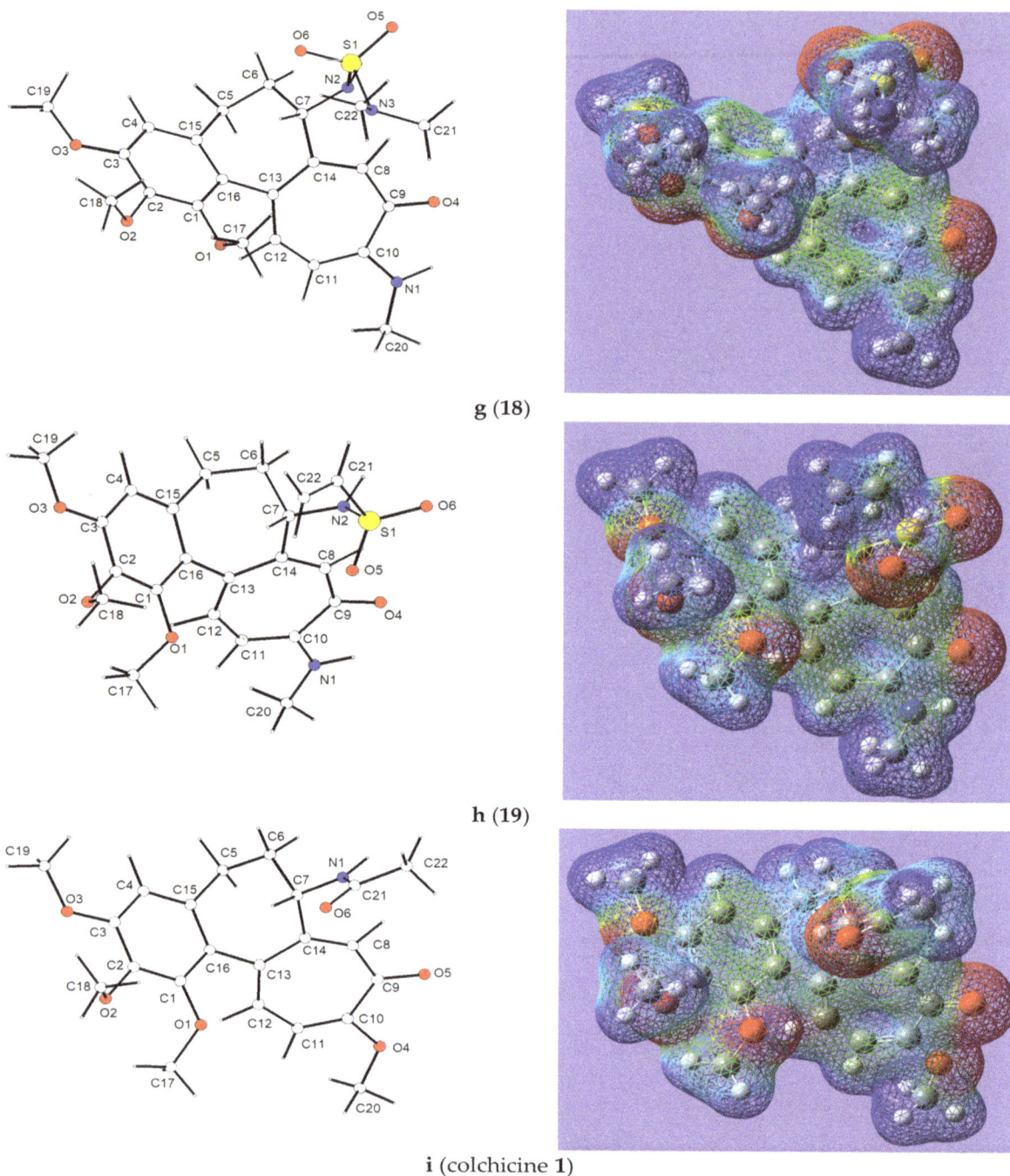

Figure 2. Optimized conformation (left) and three-dimensional molecular electrostatic potential map (right) for colchicine derivatives (**a–h**) and colchicine itself (**i**), for comparison. Color code: $-0.05\ \text{e\AA}^{-1}$ (red) to $+0.05\ \text{e\AA}^{-1}$ (blue).

The nucleophilic regions in colchicine derivatives are observed near oxygen atoms of all methoxy and carbonyl groups. In addition, significantly less negative value of MESP than that near the oxygen atoms spreads across the aromatic phenyl rings. The planar conformation of tropolone ring C, showing the alternating single and double C-C bonds, is manifested as partial delocalization of the π electrons resulting in a slightly negative value of MESP on both sides of the planar fragment of colchicine derivatives. The molecular electrostatic potential for colchicine itself was also calculated for comparison (Figure 2i). In all colchicine derivatives the methoxy (-OCH$_3$) substituent in the tropolone C ring is replaced by N-methylamino substituent (-NHCH$_3$), therefore, MESP maps show a less negative area near this group (Figure 2a–h) compared to the MESP map of colchicine itself (Figure 2i).

Additionally, the replacement in colchicine molecule of the -NHC(O)CH$_3$ group in ring B at C7 atom with various substituents modified the size of the molecule and the maps of electrostatic potential. This is particularly visible for derivatives **11**, **14** and **18**, **19** in which the -NHC(O)CH$_3$ group is replaced by -NHC(O)C$_2$H$_4$CF$_3$, -NHC(O)C$_6$H$_4$F in **11** and **14**, respectively, and in **18** and **19** by the substituents containing sulfonyl group (-SO$_2$R).

The DFT results, especially the three-dimensional molecular electrostatic potential map (MESP) providing information on the distribution of the electron density of molecules are useful for predictions of interactions between the tested compounds and homology modeled tubulin βI. The formation of guest-host complexes (colchicine derivatives as guest and tubulin as host) depends on the guest's fit into the host cavity and their interactions that result from the mutual matching of electrostatic interactions.

2.4. In Vitro Determination of Drug-Induced Inhibition of Human Cancer Cell Line Growth

The synthesized colchicine derivatives **2–21** and starting material **1** were evaluated for their in vitro antiproliferative effect on four human cancer cell lines, including one cell line displaying various levels of drug resistance and additionally one normal murine embryonic fibroblast cells.

The majority of new derivatives of **1** showed antiproliferative activity in the nanomolar range and were characterized by lower IC$_{50}$ values than unmodified colchicine **1**, as well as doxorubicin and cisplatin, commonly used as antitumor agents in cancer chemotherapy (Table 2). From the set of tested compounds, the ones most active against A549 tumor cell line were **2**, **4–6**, **8–14** and **18–19** (IC$_{50} \leq$ 15 nM), against MCF-7 tumor cell line-were **2**, **9–17** and **19** (IC$_{50} \leq$ 13 nM), against LoVo tumor cell line-were **2**, **4–6**, **8–16**, **18–19** (IC$_{50} \leq$ 11 nM) of which the lowest IC$_{50}$ values were shown by compounds **9–10** and **13** (IC$_{50}$ = 0.7–1.8 nM). Moreover, compound **13** was observed to be most active towards the LoVo/DX line (IC$_{50}$ = 9.6 nM), approx. 170 times more potent than unmodified colchicine **1** (IC$_{50}$ = 1646.6 nM). Compound **7** from amides and compound **20** from sulfonamides showed the weakest activity (the highest IC$_{50}$ values) against all cancer cell lines tested. The decrease in cytotoxicity of compound **7** could be related to an increase in hydrophobicity (high calculated octanol/water partition coefficient clog$P$ = 8.7, see Table 3). It is well known that high clog$P$ value and therefore low hydrophilicity are responsible for poor absorption and permeation to the colchicine binding pocket in β-tubulin. The high IC$_{50}$ value for compound **20** may be due to the presence of a morpholine ring which is a large volume substituent and can adopt different conformations. Although these compounds were the least potent out of the whole series of tested derivatives (**1–21**), their IC$_{50}$ values were in the micromolar range (see Table 2).

Table 2. Antiproliferative activity (IC$_{50}$) of colchicine (**1**) and its derivatives (**2–21**) compared with antiproliferative activity of standard anticancer drugs doxorubicin and cisplatin and the calculated values of the resistance index (RI) of tested compounds.

Compound	A549	MCF-7	LoVo	LoVo/DX		BALB/3T3
	IC$_{50}$ [nM]	IC$_{50}$ [nM]	IC$_{50}$ [nM]	IC$_{50}$ [nM]	RI	IC$_{50}$ [nM]
1	115.3 ± 23.6	22.6 ± 1.3	17.5 ± 2.5	1646.6 ± 314.0	93.9	115.3 ± 36.8
2	10.8 ± 1.3	8.6 ± 1.3	4.3 ± 1.3	271.3 ± 99.9	63.0	10.8 ± 1.3
3	16.9 ± 2.8	19.7 ± 1.7	14.0 ± 1.7	129.2 ± 11.8	9.2	19.7 ± 7.0
4	14.6 ± 2.4	14.6 ± 1.5	9.7 ± 1.5	271.8 ± 104.4	28.0	19.4 ± 4.1
5	14.1 ± 2.4	14.1 ± 1.4	9.6 ± 0.5	194.8 ± 51.9	20.2	16.4 ± 3.5
6	13.6 ± 1.4	15.9 ± 6.6	6.8 ± 3.9	102.3 ± 20.7	15.0	13.6 ± 2.3
7	613.8 ± 194.4	464.8 ± 186.7	62.4 ± 16.9	2435.7 ± 923.4	39.0	545.9 ± 104.4
8	11.7 ± 1.4	18.8 ± 9.9	7.0 ± 1.4	171.2 ± 41.3	24.3	28.1 ± 10.8
9	11.6 ± 2.8	9.2 ± 1.4	1.8 ± 0.4	62.4 ± 6.7	35.2	11.6 ± 2.3
10	8.6 ± 1.3	8.6 ± 1.2	1.5 ± 0.5	38.5 ± 21.6	25.8	10.7 ± 1.3
11	14.6 ± 2.1	12.7 ± 0.4	10.4 ± 1.3	289.6 ± 165.2	27.8	81.3 ± 20.4
12	13.0 ± 1.3	13.0 ± 1.3	8.5 ± 0.4	99.9 ± 10.0	11.8	13.0 ± 3.3
13	6.3 ± 3.2	9.2 ± 0.8	0.7 ± 0.1	9.6 ± 3.3	14.0	6.2 ± 1.6
14	10.7 ± 0.6	12.6 ± 1.3	8.6 ± 0.8	102.5 ± 24.9	12.0	12.6 ± 2.1
15	36.8 ± 12.1	13.0 ± 2.2	10.8 ± 1.3	832.1 ± 292.7	76.8	43.3 ± 29.7
16	17.3 ± 3.7	12.8 ± 0.9	10.8 ± 1.3	946.9 ± 260.5	87.4	52.0 ± 29.3

Table 2. *Cont.*

17	56.6 ± 14.7	10.3 ± 3.9	21.1 ± 17.5	6466.0 ± 264.2	306.0	100.1 ± 24.1
18	10.6 ± 0.6	15.5 ± 1.7	9.3 ± 1.1	540.2 ± 107.2	57.8	14.2 ± 13.2
19	11.4 ± 1.7	13.0 ± 4.3	8.4 ± 0.7	306.7 ± 144.9	36.7	8.3 ± 3.8
20	800.3 ± 130.0	150.0 ± 25.3	268.4 ± 94.0	44385.7 ± 23852.0	165.4	991.1 ± 280.5
21	85.5 ± 5.4	134.3 ± 41.5	73.5 ± 15.7	6122.0 ± 825.1	83.3	87.6 ± 13.5
Doxorubicin	141.7 ± 46.0	204.2 ± 47.8	99.4 ± 41.0	8732.0 ± 2540.7	87.9	149.0 ±126.8
Cisplatin	5741.0 ± 968.0	7139.8 ± 1218.7	7076.3 ± 1596.2	8336.5 ± 1119.2	1.2	5665.1 ± 31.8

The IC_{50} value is defined as the concentration of a compound at which 50% growth inhibition is observed. The IC_{50} values shown are mean ± SD. Human lung adenocarcinoma (A549), human breast adenocarcinoma (MCF-7), human colon adenocarcinoma cell line (LoVo) and doxorubicin-resistant subline (LoVo/DX), normal murine embryonic fibroblast cell line (BALB/3T3). The RI (Resistance Index) indicates how many times more chemoresistant is a resistant subline relative to its parental cell line. The RI was calculated for each compound using the formula: RI = (IC_{50} for LoVo/DX cell line)/(IC_{50} for LoVo cell line). When RI is 0–2, the cells are sensitive to the compound tested, RI in the range 2–10 means that the cells shows moderate sensitivity to the drug tested, RI above 10 indicates strong drug resistance.

Table 3. Computational predictions of interactions between tested compounds (**1–21**) and homology modeled tubulin βI. 3D representation and 2D layout of colchicine derivatives–tubulin protein complex, binding energy (BE), calculated octanol/water partition coefficient (clog*P*) and active residues are tabulated.

Compound	3D Representation of the Interactions	2D Representation of the Interactions	Binding Energy [kcal/mol]	clog*P*	Active Residues
1			−41.0	1.1	Ala179 Val180 **Cys674** **Leu688** Asn691 Ala749 **Lys785**
2			−39.3	1.6	Cys674 Ala683 **Leu688** **Lys785**
3			−4.0	0.9	Cys674 Lys687 **Leu688** **Asn691**
4			−43.4	1.9	Cys674 Ala683 **Leu688** Asn691 Met692 Ala749 **Lys785**

Table 3. *Cont.*

Compound	3D Representation of the Interactions	2D Representation of the Interactions	Binding Energy [kcal/mol]	clog*P*	Active Residues
5			−43.0	2.5	Ala179 Val180 **Cys674** **Leu688** Asn691 Ala749 **Lys785**
6			−37.2	3.0	Asn100 Ser177 Ala179 Leu681 **Lys687** Leu688 Asn691 **Lys785**
7			−53.7	8.7	Gln10 Asn100 Ser177 Thr178 Cys674 Leu681 Asn682 Ala683 **Lys687** **Leu688** Asn691 Ala749 **Lys785**
8			−32.3	2.7	Ser177 Leu681 Ala683 **Leu688** **Lys785**
9			−44.0	2.2	Ala179 Cys674 Ala683 Lys687 **Leu688** Asn691 Met693 Ala749 **Lys785**
10			−41.8	2.7	Ala179 Cys674 Ala683 **Leu688** Asn691 Asn782 **Lys785**

Table 3. *Cont.*

Compound	3D Representation of the Interactions	2D Representation of the Interactions	Binding Energy [kcal/mol]	clog*P*	Active Residues
11			−34.7	3.0	Ala179 Cys674 Leu681 Ala683 Lys687 **Leu688** Asn691 **Lys785**
12			−35.2	3.3	Ser177 Ala179 Leu681 Lys687 **Leu688** Asn691 **Lys785**
13			−40.1	3.9	Cys674 Leu681 Ala683 **Lys687** **Leu688** Asn691 **Lys785**
14			−34.3	3.4	Val176 Ser177 Thr178 Ala179 **Gln680** Leu688 **Lys785**
15			−43.9	2.0	**Asn100** **Ser177** Cys674 **Leu681** Asn682 Ala683 **Lys687** **Leu688** Asn691 **Lys785**
16			−38.3	2.0	Ser177 Thr178 Cys674 Leu681 Ala683 **Leu688** Asn691 **Lys785**

Table 3. *Cont.*

Compound	3D Representation of the Interactions	2D Representation of the Interactions	Binding Energy [kcal/mol]	clog*P*	Active Residues
17			−34.8	1.9	**Gln10** **Ser177** Thr178 Ala179 Asn682 Ala683 **Asp684** **Lys687** Asn691 Lys785
18			−54.6	2.5	**Gln10** Ala99 Asn100 **Gly142** **Gly143** **Thr144** **Ser177** Thr178 Ala179 Leu681
19			−23.4	2..8	**Ser177** Thr178 **Leu681** Ala683 Asp684 **Lys687** Asn691 **Lys785**
20			−59.6	2.4	Gly9 Gln10 Ala11 **Asp68** Ala99 **Asn100** Gly142 Gly143 Thr144 **Gly145** Ser177 Thr178 **Lys687**
21			−29.8	4.9	Ala179 Val180 **Cys674** **Leu688** Asn691 Ala749 **Lys785**

Legend:
- ◯ polar
- ◯ acidic
- ◯ basic
- ◯ greasy
- proximity contour
- ▸ sidechain acceptor
- ◂ sidechain donor
- ▸ backbone acceptor
- ◂ backbone donor
- ligand exposure
- ◯ solvent residue
- ◯ metal complex
- solvent contact
- metal/ion contact
- receptor exposure
- arene-arene
- arene-H
- arene-cation

Although the synthesized compounds are effective toward cancer cells, their potential is limited against cells with developed drug resistance. The data presented in Table 2 show that unmodified colchicine **1** and all of the colchicine derivatives **2–21** less effectively inhibited the proliferation of the doxorubicin-resistant subline LoVo/DX than the sensitive LoVo cell line. The calculated values of RI clearly confirmed that none of the tested amides and sulfonamides was able to overcome the drug resistance of LoVo/DX cell line (RI ranges from 11.8 to 306.0). It can be explained by the upregulated expression of efflux transporters in these cells, playing an important role in drug transport in many organs and determining the drug resistance of cancer cells. Because this type of resistance is one of the mechanisms of cancer resistance [58], compounds **1–2** and **4–21** are probably good substrates for such pumps. Increased efflux of compounds makes it impossible to reach their adequate concentrations in the cell and consequently to exert efficient cytotoxic effect. The only compound which showed RI < 10 was derivative **3**, having at position C7 a free amino group. Keeping in mind its good activity ($IC_{50} <$ 20 nM for three cancer cells, see Table 2) it can be still considered as a good starting point for the chase after antitumor agents active against drug resistant lines.

The selectivity index (SI) was calculated to evaluate the toxicity of the compounds studied against normal cells and to predict their therapeutic potential (see Figure 3). High SI values result from large differences between the cytotoxicity against cancer and normal cells and this means that cancer cells will be killed at a higher rate than normal ones. From the set of tested compounds with methylamino group at position C10 and alkyl chains at position C7 (**2, 4–8, 19**) the best selectivity index for A549, MCF-7 and LoVo cells (SI = 1.5–4.0) showed **8** with short and branched substituent (isobutyric acid derivative). The 4,4,4-trifluorobutyric acid derivative **11** (from compounds with alkyl chains of various lengths containing halogen atoms **9–11**) showed outstanding selectivity for three out of four cancer cells (SI = 5.6–7.8). It should be emphasized that compound **11** was the only compound with SI values greater than that of unmodified colchicine **1** for all tumor cell lines. Despite the fact that compounds **9**, **10,** and **13** stood out from the synthesized compounds in terms of IC_{50} values, their selectivity indices were high only for LoVo lines (SI = 6.5–9.1), they were very cytotoxic also to non-cancerous BALB/3T3 cells (IC_{50} = 6.2–11.6 nM). Among aryl amides and sulfonamides **12–16** and **21**, distinctive SI values were derived for colchicine derivatives containingnicotinic and isonicotinic amide residue (SI ranges 3.0 to 4.8). These results are noteworthy and suggest that extended and more detailed research of similar derivatives is necessary to determine the importance of ring aromaticity, its size or heteroatom type. Especially high SI values for MCF-7 were obtained for sulfamide **17** (SI = 9.8) and sulfonamide containing a morpholine ring **20** (SI = 6.6). These results deserve special attention and require further studies to determine whether the conversion of an amide bond to a sulfonamide bond with an appropriate substituent would allow obtaining compounds highly selective towards MCF7 cells, compared to colchicine **1**. As many as thirteen of the obtained derivatives exhibited SI ≥ 2 for LoVo cell line (see Figure 3). The results indicated that properly designed doubly modified (at C7 and C10 positions) colchicine derivatives can have greater selectivity towards cancer cells than the parental compound.

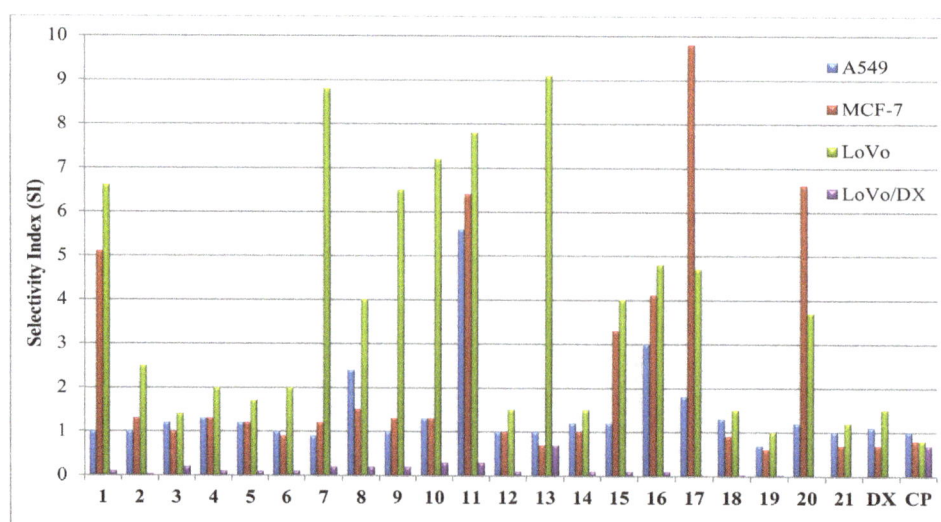

Figure 3. Comparison of selectivity index (SI) values of the tested compounds. The SI was calculated for each compound using the formula: SI = (IC_{50} for normal cell line BALB/3T3)/(IC_{50} for respective cancerous cell line). A favorable SI > 1.0 indicates a drug with efficacy against tumor cells greater than the toxicity against normal cells.

2.5. In Silico Determination of the Molecular Mode of Action

In the present study, computational investigation including molecular docking, molecular dynamics (MD) simulations, molecular mechanics generalized Born/surface area (MM/GBSA) binding free energy calculations and decomposition of pair-wise free energy on a per-residue basis were conducted to deeply explore the molecular basis for the binding of twenty novel double modified colchicine amides and sulfonamides to β-tubulin. The latter is one of the subunits of microtubules in the cytoskeleton structure of every eukaryotic cell, which is the target of many anticancer drugs. The twenty structures of colchicine derivatives described above were docked into the βI-tubulin (the most abundant isotype in most cancer tumors) colchicine binding site.

On the basis of our computational predictions, according to increasing binding energy, the compounds are ordered as follows: **20** (−59.6), **18** (−54.6), **7** (−53.7), **9** (−44.0), **15** (−43.9), **4** (−43.4), **5** (−43.1), **10** (−41.8), **1** (−41.1), **13** (−40.1), **2** (−39.3), **16** (−38.3), **6** (−37.2), **12** (−35.2), **17** (−34.9), **11** (−34.7), **14** (−34.3), **8** (−32.3), **21** (−29.8), **19** (−23.4), **3** (−4.0) kcal/mol with the binding energies in the parenthesis given in units of kcal/mol. Binding energies of these compounds are shown in Figure 4 and Table 3.

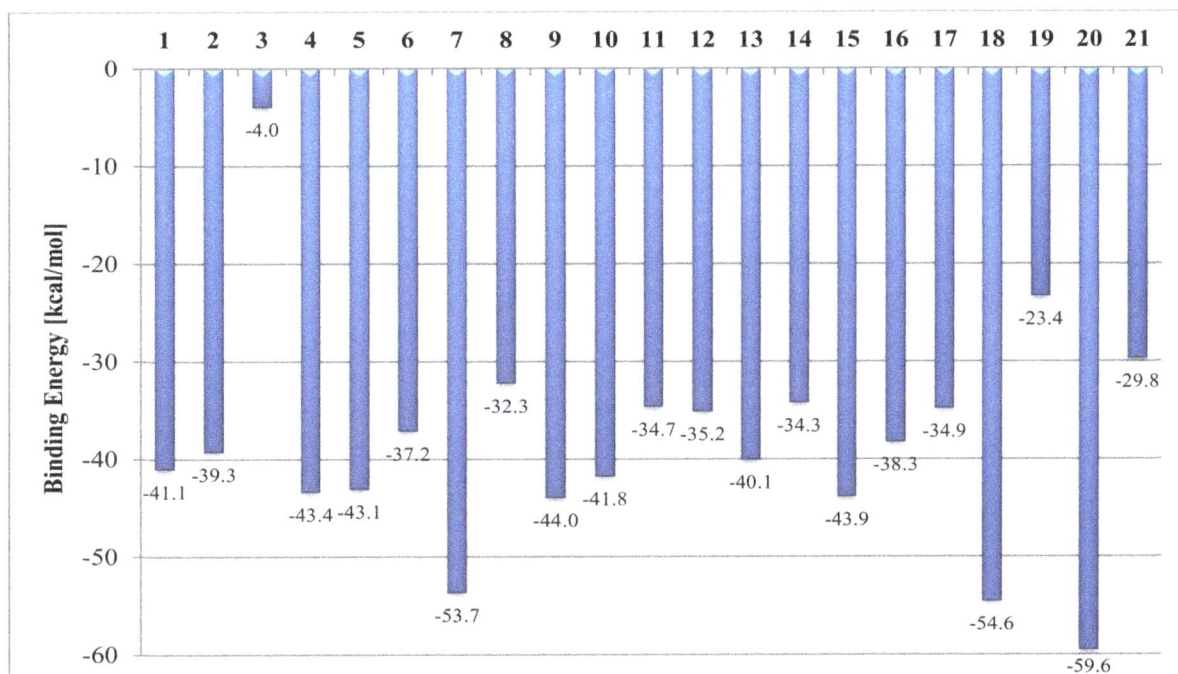

Figure 4. Comparison of binding energies of the tested compounds complexed with tubulin βI. Binding energies have been estimated using the MM/GBSA method.

In view of the calculated binding energies, we can conclude that there is no strong correlation (the lower the binding energy, the more biologically active the chemical compound) between *in silico* computer calculations (BE values, Figure 4) and in vitro activity results (IC_{50} values, Table 2).

The lowest binding energies, −59.6 and −53.7 kcal/mol, were shown by sulfonamide **20** (derivative with the morpholine ring) and amide **7** (derivative of palmitic acid), respectively. However, these compounds showed the weakest antiproliferative activity (highest IC_{50} values) among all compounds tested (**1–21**).

Compound **18** has the third lowest energy (−54.6 kcal/mol) and good cytotoxicity with IC_{50} from 9.3 to 15.5 nM for LoVo, A549 and MCF-7 cancer cells. The molecular-level computations indicate that **18** fits well to βI-tubulin and probably uses this binding site as a target. The majority of the other derivatives **2**, **4–6**, **8–17** exhibited binding energy less than −30.0 kcal/mol, so close to the energy of unmodified colchicine **1** (BE = −41.1 kcal/mol), which is a compound known to inhibit tubulin polymerization. These compounds bind to the active sites of βI-tubulin isotype and may therefore have a mechanism of action similar to **1** and may be colchicine binding site inhibitors, although their in vitro activities towards various cells characterized by an IC_{50} value (Table 2) were lower than that of colchicine **1**.

Derivative **3** showed the highest binding energy value (BE = −4.0 kcal/mol), therefore its antiproliferative activity is not exclusively the result of interaction with tubulin. This is an important finding because compound **3** was the only one which showed any possibility of breaking the drug resistance of the LoVo/DX line (RI = 9.2, see Table 2).

Therefore, we can see that the results only partly correlate with in vitro determined biological activity of these compounds as indicated though the corresponding IC_{50} values. This may be explained by several additional effects taking place in living cells compared to the computational simulations that focus only on the binding mode of the compounds to the target. Primarily off-target interactions involving efflux transporters with different affinities for the individual compounds and differences in solubility of these colchicine derivatives or their membrane permeability. Additionally, the lack of significant correlation may be due to the fact that in various cancer cells the expression of specific β-tubulin isotypes significantly varies [59]. We propose the inclusion of binding affinity calculations for these compounds with regard to not only other tubulin isotypes but also with respect to most important efflux transporters in order to minimize them and hence increase the activity of the drug in vitro and *in vivo*.

Schematic interactions of the compounds with CBS of βI-tubulin residues are shown in Table 3.

In 3D representation, the interacting residues predicted from pairwise per-residue binding free energy decomposition calculations (E < −2 kcal/mol) are shown in stick presentation and their carbons and the ribbon are colored as green. Tubulin is shown in cartoon representation. Hydrogen bonds and their directionality are represented as black dashed arrows. The structures are color-coded as follows: tubulin αI, brown; tubulin βI, beige. Compounds are displayed with sticks and the atoms are colored as O (red), C (gray), N (blue), S (yellow), Cl (green) and F (pink). Binding energy defines the affinity of binding for colchicine derivatives complexed with tubulin βI. Binding energies are predicted by MM/GBSA method. The last column contains information about the active residues with the binding free energy decomposition (E_{decomp}) less than −2 kcal/mol (the residues with E_{decomp} < −3 kcal/mol are highlighted in boldface). The last line contains the graphical key to help interpret the 2D part of the ligand interactions panel.

Derivative compounds are designed with different side chains at C7 position of colchicine **1**. Compounds **2**, **4–8** have alkyl chains of various lengths, straight and branched and compound **19** has an unsaturated alkyl chain. The second lowest binding energy compound **7** within all the compounds is in this group (BE = −53.6 kcal/mol). Compound **7** appears to be engaged in some interactions with α-tubulin (−3 < E_{decomp} < −2 kcal/mol). Most of the compounds in this group are bound through Lys785, Lys687 and Leu688 residues.

Compounds **9–11** were designed with alkyl chains of various length containing halogen atoms side chains at position C7 of colchicine **1**. In this group, the common binding residues with (−3 < E_{decomp} < −2 kcal/mol) are Ala179, Cys674, Asn691, while the strongest binding residues (E_{decomp} < −3 kcal/mol) are Leu688 and Lys785.

Compounds **12–16**, **21** were designed with an aromatic group side chain without or with substituents at C7 position of colchicine **1**. The same trend of strong binding of Leu688 and Lys785 residues with the compounds is seen in this group. The binding energies in this group are on the higher side compared to the other compounds.

As the last group, compounds **17–18** and **20** contain the sulfonamide moieties at position C7 of colchicine **1**. The strongest binding residues in this group belong to both α-tubulin (Gln10 and Ser177) in compound **17**, (Gln10, Gly142, Gly143, Thr144 and Ser177) in compound **18** and (Asp68 and Asn100) in compound **20** with (E_{decomp} < −3 kcal/mol) and β-tubulin (Asp684, Asn691, Lys785) in compound **17** and Lys687 in compound **20**. The lowest binding energy between all the compounds characterizes compounds **20** and **18**, which mainly bind to α-tubulin.

In the experimental part of the study, the highest IC_{50} values (the weakest activity) were found for compound **7** from the amides and compound **20** from the sulfonamides studied against all cancer cell lines tested. According to our computational analysis, although these compounds show the lowest binding energies, they do not bind to the CBS, which is located in β-tubulin and has the tendency to go beyond and also bind to α-tubulin.

3. Materials and Methods

3.1. General

All solvents, substrates and reagents were obtained from TriMen Chemicals (Poland) or Sigma Aldrich and were used without further purification. $CDCl_3$ and CD_2Cl_2 spectral grade solvents were stored over 3 Å molecular sieves for several days. TLC analysis was performed using pre-coated glass plates (0.2 mm thickness, GF-254, pore size 60 Å) from Agela Technologies and spots were visualized by UV-light. Products were purified by flash chromatography using high-purity grade silica gel (pore size 60 Å, 230–400 mesh particle size, 40–63 μm particle size) from SiliCycle Inc. Preparative HPLC was performed on LC-20AP Shimadzu with ELSD-LTII detector equipped with Phenomenex Luna C18 250 × 21 mm, 5 μm column eluted with 20 mL/min flow over 20 min of acetonitrile in water. Solvents were removed using a rotary evaporator.

3.2. Spectroscopic Measurements

NMR spectra were recorded on Bruker Avance DRX 500 (^{1}H NMR at 500 MHz and ^{13}C NMR at 126 MHz) magnetic resonance spectrometers. ^{1}H NMR spectra are reported in chemical shifts downfield from TMS using the respective residual solvent peak as internal standard ($CDCl_3$ δ 7.26 ppm, CD_2Cl_2 δ 5.32 ppm, $(CD_3)_2SO$ δ 2.50 ppm). ^{1}H NMR spectra are described as follows: chemical shift (δ, ppm), multiplicity (s = singlet, d = doublet, t = triplet, q = quartet, dd = doublet of doublets, dt = doublet of triplets, dq = doublet of quartets, m = multiplet), coupling constant (*J*) in Hz, and integration. ^{13}C NMR spectra are described in chemical shifts downfield from TMS using the respective residual solvent peak as internal standard ($CDCl_3$ δ 77.16 ppm, CD_2Cl_2 δ 53.84 ppm and $(CD_3)_2SO$ δ 39.52 ppm).

Electrospray ionization (ESI) mass spectra were obtained on a Waters Alliance 2695 separation module with a PDA 2996 UV detector and Waters Micromass ZQ 2000 mass detector equipped with Restek Ultra Biphenyl 50 × 3 mm, 3 μm column eluted with 0.3 mL/min flow of 3–100% gradient (over 6 min) of acetonitrile in water.

3.3. Synthesis

3.3.1. Synthesis of **2**

To a solution of **1** (1.0 equiv.) in EtOH, a methylamine (solution 33% in EtOH, 10.0 equiv.) was added. The mixture was stirred at reflux for 24 h and then concentrated under reduced pressure to dryness. The residue was purified using column flash chromatography (silica gel; DCM/MeOH) and next lyophilized from dioxane to give the pure product **2** as a yellow solid with a yield of 80%.

ESI-MS for $C_{22}H_{26}N_2O_5$ (*m/z*): $[M + H]^+$ 399, $[M + Na]^+$ 421, $[2M + H]^+$ 797, $[2M + Na]^+$ 819, $[M - H]^-$ 397, $[M + HCOO^-]^-$ 443.

^{1}H NMR (500 MHz, $CDCl_3$) δ 8.70 (d, *J* = 6.4 Hz, 1H), 7.58 (s, 1H), 7.46 (d, *J* = 11.1 Hz, 1H), 7.28–7.25 (m, 1H), 6.58 (d, *J* = 11.3 Hz, 1H), 6.52 (s, 1H), 4.73–4.64 (m, 1H), 3.93 (s, 3H), 3.88 (s, 3H), 3.61 (s, 3H), 3.08 (d, *J* = 5.4 Hz, 3H), 2.47–2.43 (m, 1H), 2.37–2.31 (m, 1H), 2.29–2.22 (m, 1H), 2.02–1.96 (m, 1H), 1.94 (s, 3H).

^{13}C NMR (126 MHz, $CDCl_3$) δ 175.11, 170.19, 155.23, 152.91, 151.61, 151.10, 141.51, 139.37, 134.66, 130.42, 126.93, 122.81, 108.28, 107.20, 61.46, 61.40, 56.16, 52.72, 37.06, 30.15, 29.53, 22.74.

3.3.2. Synthesis of 3

To a solution of compound 2 (1.0 equiv.) in dioxane, 2M HCl (10.0 equiv.) was added and the mixture was stirred at reflux. Reaction progress was monitored by LC-MS. Then the reaction mixture was neutralized with 4M NaOH to pH~10 and extracted four times with EtOAc. The organic layers were combined, washed with brine, dried over Na_2SO_4, filtered and evaporated under reduced pressure. The residue was purified using column flash chromatography (silica gel; DCM/MeOH) and next lyophilized from dioxane to give the pure product 3 as a yellow solid with a yield of 73%.

ESI-MS for $C_{20}H_{24}N_2O_4$ (m/z): $[M + H]^+$ 357, $[M + Na]^+$ 379, $[2M + Na]^+$ 735.

^1H NMR (500 MHz, CDCl$_3$) δ 7.61 (s, 1H), 7.33 (d, J = 11.1 Hz, 1H), 7.23–7.21 (m, 1H), 6.50 (s, 1H), 6.50 (d, J = 11.4 Hz, 2H), 3.87 (s, 3H), 3.87 (s, 3H), 3.75–3.72 (m, 1H), 3.59 (s, 3H), 3.05 (d, J = 5.5 Hz, 3H), 2.41–2.37 (m, 1H), 2.33–2.31 (m, 2H), 2.25 (s, 2H), 1.71–1.61 (m, 1H).

^{13}C NMR (126 MHz, CDCl$_3$) δ 175.57, 154.99, 153.25, 152.76, 150.59, 141.06, 138.73, 135.41, 129.74, 126.63, 123.68, 107.35, 106.94, 61.19, 60.84, 56.06, 54.01, 40.90, 30.69, 29.48.

3.3.3. General Procedure for the Synthesis of Colchicine Derivatives 4, 8, 13, 15–16, 18 and 21

Compounds 4, 8, 13, 15–16, 18 and 21 were obtained directly from compound 3. To a solution of compound 3 (1.0 equiv.) and Et_3N (3.0 equiv.) in DCM in an ice bath, the corresponding acid/sulfonyl/sulfamide chloride (1.1 equiv.) diluted with DCM was added slowly. Next the ice bath was removed and the reaction mixture was stirred at RT. Reaction progress was monitored by LC-MS. Then the reaction mixture was diluted with EtOAc, washed with H_2O, 1M K_2CO_3, brine and dried over Na_2SO_4. The residue was purified using column flash chromatography (silica gel; DCM/MeOH) and next lyophilized from dioxane to give respective compound.

Compound 4

Yellow solid, yield 86%.

ESI-MS for $C_{23}H_{28}N_2O_5$ (m/z): $[M + H]^+$ 413, $[M + Na]^+$ 435, $[2M + H]^+$ 825, $[2M + Na]^+$ 847, $[M-H]^-$ 411, $[M + HCOO^-]^-$ 457.

^1H NMR (500 MHz, CDCl$_3$) δ 8.46 (s, 1H), 7.53 (s, 1H), 7.44 (d, J = 11.1 Hz, 1H), 7.25–7.21 (m, 1H), 6.55 (d, J = 11.4 Hz, 1H), 6.50 (s, 1H), 4.72–4.65 (m, 1H), 3.91 (s, 3H), 3.86 (s, 3H), 3.61 (s, 3H), 3.06 (d, J = 5.4 Hz, 3H), 2.44–2.40 (m, 1H), 2.33–2.30 (m, 1H), 2.26–2.17 (m, 3H), 1.94–1.88 (m, 1H), 1.05 (t, J = 7.6 Hz, 3H).

^{13}C NMR (126 MHz, CDCl$_3$) δ 175.09, 173.89, 155.20, 152.86, 151.64, 151.09, 141.49, 139.23, 134.67, 130.33, 126.95, 122.94, 108.14, 107.20, 61.44, 56.14, 52.37, 37.20, 30.18, 29.53, 29.11, 9.72.

Compound 8

Yellow solid, yield 96%.

ESI-MS for $C_{24}H_{30}N_2O_5$ (m/z): $[M + H]^+$ 427, $[M + Na]^+$ 449, $[2M + H]^+$ 853, $[2M + Na]^+$ 875, $[M-H]^-$ 425, $[M + HCOO^-]^-$ 471.

^1H NMR (500 MHz, CDCl$_3$) δ 7.48 (d, J = 11.2 Hz, 1H), 7.45 (s, 1H), 7.31–7.28 (m, 1H), 6.67 (d, J = 7.3 Hz, 1H), 6.59 (d, J = 11.3 Hz, 1H), 6.53 (s, 1H), 4.75–4.63 (m, 1H), 3.94 (s, 3H), 3.89 (s, 3H), 3.63 (s, 3H), 3.10 (d, J = 5.4 Hz, 3H), 2.53–2.43 (m, 2H), 2.38–2.32 (m, 1H), 2.28–2.20 (m, 1H), 1.93–1.82 (m, 1H), 1.14 (t, J = 6.7 Hz, 6H).

^{13}C NMR (126 MHz, CDCl$_3$) δ 176.86, 175.21, 155.19, 152.85, 151.15, 141.56, 139.08, 134.55, 130.09, 126.97, 123.07, 107.91, 107.22, 61.51, 61.45, 56.13, 51.96, 37.56, 35.21, 30.19, 29.54, 19.70, 19.60.

Compound 13

Yellow solid, yield 86%.

ESI-MS for $C_{27}H_{27}ClN_2O_5$ (m/z): $[M + H]^+$ 495/497, $[M + Na]^+$ 517, $[2M + H]^+$ 989/991, $[M-H]^-$ 493/495, $[M + HCOO^-]^-$ 540.

^{1}H NMR (500 MHz, CD$_2$Cl$_2$) δ 8.12 (d, J = 7.5 Hz, 1H), 7.60 (s, 1H), 7.42–7.39 (m, 2H), 7.29–7.22 (m, 2H), 7.19 (t, J = 7.5 Hz, 1H), 7.06 (t, J = 7.4 Hz, 1H), 6.60 (s, 1H), 6.53 (d, J = 11.3 Hz, 1H), 4.88–4.83 (m, 1H), 3.91 (s, 3H), 3.89 (s, 3H), 3.71 (s, 3H), 3.03 (d, J = 5.2 Hz, 3H), 2.52–2,48 (m, 1H), 2.42–2.31 (m, 2H), 2.14–2.04 (m, 1H).

^{13}C NMR (126 MHz, CD$_2$Cl$_2$) δ 174.51, 165.99, 155.24, 153.11, 150.94, 150.51, 141.52, 139.19, 135.71, 134.71, 130.64, 130.43, 130.01, 129.60, 129.58, 126.83, 126.79, 123.26, 107.90, 107.46, 61.08, 61.07, 56.02, 52.86, 37.83, 30.11, 29.35.

Compound 15

Yellow solid, yield 23%.

ESI-MS for C$_{26}$H$_{27}$N$_3$O$_5$ (m/z): [M + H]$^+$ 462, [M + Na]$^+$ 484, [2M + H]$^+$ 923, [2M + Na]$^+$ 945, [M-H]$^-$ 460, [M + HCOO$^-$]$^-$ 506.

^{1}H NMR (500 MHz, CDCl$_3$) δ 9.35 (d, J = 7.0 Hz, 1H), 9.07 (d, J = 1.8 Hz, 1H), 8.48 (dd, J = 4.8, 1.5 Hz, 1H), 8.13–8.06 (m, 1H), 7.65 (s, 1H), 7.51 (d, J = 11.2 Hz, 1H), 7.31 (q, J = 5.1 Hz, 1H), 7.05 (dd, J = 7.9, 4.9 Hz, 1H), 6.61 (d, J = 11.4 Hz, 1H), 6.54 (s, 1H), 4.99–4.86 (m, 1H), 3.95 (s, 3H), 3.89 (s, 3H), 3.70 (s, 3H), 3.08 (d, J = 5.4 Hz, 3H), 2.51–2.45 (m, 1H), 2.40–2.34 (m, 1H), 2.33–2.27 (m, 1H), 2.17–2.09 (m, 1H).

^{13}C NMR (126 MHz, CDCl$_3$) δ 174.69, 165.09, 155.37, 153.01, 151.82, 151.42, 151.15, 148.87, 141.59, 139.62, 134.89, 134.61, 130.41, 129.34, 126.86, 123.08, 122.79, 108.49, 107.27, 61.53, 61.48, 56.15, 53.22, 36.83, 30.28, 29.58.

Compound 16

Yellow solid, yield 39%.

ESI-MS for C$_{26}$H$_{27}$N$_3$O$_5$ (m/z): [M + H]$^+$ 462, [M + Na]$^+$ 484, [2M + H]$^+$ 923, [2M + Na]$^+$ 945, [M-H]$^-$ 460, [M + HCOO$^-$]$^-$ 506.

^{1}H NMR (500 MHz, CDCl$_3$) δ 9.71 (d, J = 6.6 Hz, 1H), 8.37 (d, J = 5.8 Hz, 2H), 7.69 (s, 1H), 7.64 (d, J = 5.8 Hz, 2H), 7.54 (d, J = 11.2 Hz, 1H), 7.32–7.28 (m, 1H), 6.65 (d, J = 11.4 Hz, 1H), 6.53 (s, 1H), 4.98–4.81 (m, 1H), 3.95 (s, 3H), 3.87 (s, 3H), 3.71 (s, 3H), 3.10 (d, J = 5.4 Hz, 3H), 2.50–2.41 (m, 1H), 2.41–2.25 (m, 2H), 2.16–2.11 (m, 1H).

^{13}C NMR (126 MHz, CDCl$_3$) δ 174.51, 164.91, 155.37, 153.05, 151.64, 151.17, 150.18, 141.59, 140.46, 139.81, 134.59, 130.64, 126.78, 122.68, 120.99, 108.68, 107.27, 61.55, 61.47, 56.14, 53.46, 36.50, 30.29, 29.60.

Compound 18

Yellow solid, yield 38%.

ESI-MS for C$_{22}$H$_{29}$N$_3$O$_6$S (m/z): [M + H]$^+$ 464, [M + Na]$^+$ 486, [2M + H]$^+$ 927, [2M + Na]$^+$ 949, [M-H]$^-$ 462.

^{1}H NMR (500 MHz, CDCl$_3$) δ 7.85 (s, 1H), 7.45–7.41 (m, 2H), 6.58 (d, J = 11.3 Hz, 1H), 6.54 (s, 1H), 6.49–6.46 (m, 1H), 4.33–4.19 (m, 1H), 3.93–3.89 (m, 6H), 3.57 (s, 3H), 3.10 (d, J = 5.1 Hz, 3H), 2.58 (s, 6H), 2.49–2.39 (m, 2H), 2.35–2.26 (m, 1H), 2.01–1.90 (m, 1H).

^{13}C NMR (126 MHz, CDCl$_3$) δ 174.73, 155.46, 153.08, 150.77, 150.08, 141.39, 139.41, 134.59, 129.64, 126.34, 124.53, 108.22, 107.43, 61.34, 60.80, 56.48, 56.05, 39.91, 37.95, 30.50, 29.57.

Compound 21

Yellow solid, yield 83%.

ESI-MS for C$_{27}$H$_{27}$F$_3$N$_2$O$_6$S (m/z): [M + H]$^+$ 565, [M + Na]$^+$ 587, [2M + H]$^+$ 1129, [2M + Na]$^+$ 1151, [M-H]$^-$ 563.

^{1}H NMR (500 MHz, CDCl$_3$) δ 8.72 (d, J = 7.5 Hz, 1H), 8.07 (s, 1H), 7.92 (s, 1H), 7.84 (d, J = 8.2 Hz, 2H), 7.53 (d, J = 8.3 Hz, 2H), 7.48 (d, J = 11.5 Hz, 1H), 6.66 (d, J = 11.8 Hz, 1H), 6.46 (s, 1H), 4.16 (q, J = 8.8 Hz, 1H), 3.91 (s, 3H), 3.86 (s, 3H), 3.58 (s, 3H), 3.08 (d, J = 5.2 Hz, 3H), 2.45–2.31 (m, 1H), 2.31–2.18 (m, 2H), 2.16–2.10 (m, 1H).

^{13}C NMR (126 MHz, CDCl$_3$) δ 170.13, 155.43, 153.53, 150.65, 150.15, 144.53, 141.35, 134.75, 133.34, 131.89, 127.57, 125.82, 125.79, 125.49, 124.38, 123.51, 122.21, 111.26, 107.42, 61.29, 60.95, 56.63, 56.04, 38.98, 30.26, 29.78.

3.3.4. General Procedure for the Synthesis of Colchicine Derivatives **5–7, 9–12** and **14**

Compounds **5–7, 9–12** and **14** were obtained directly from compound **3**. To a solution of compound **3** (1.0 equiv.) in DCM corresponding carboxylic acid (1.1 equiv.) and 1-(3-dimethylaminopropyl)-3-ethylcarbodiimide hydrochloride (EDCI, 1.1 equiv.) were added. Reaction progress was monitored by LC-MS. Then the reaction mixture was diluted with EtOAc, washed with H$_2$O, 1M K$_2$CO$_3$, brine and dried over Na$_2$SO$_4$. The residue was purified using column flash chromatography (silica gel; DCM/MeOH) and next lyophilized from dioxane to give respective compound.

Compound **5**

Yellow solid, yield 93%.

ESI-MS for C$_{24}$H$_{30}$N$_2$O$_5$ (*m/z*): [M + H]$^+$ 427, [M + Na]$^+$ 449, [2M + H]$^+$ 853, [2M + Na]$^+$ 875, [M-H]$^-$ 425, [M + HCOO$^-$]$^-$ 471.

^{1}H NMR (500 MHz, CDCl$_3$) δ 7.88 (s, 1H), 7.51 (s, 1H), 7.45 (d, *J* = 11.1 Hz, 1H), 7.27–7.25 (m, 1H), 6.56 (d, *J* = 11.3 Hz, 1H), 6.51 (s, 1H), 4.76–4.68 (m, 1H), 3.92 (s, 3H), 3.87 (s, 3H), 3.61 (s, 3H), 3.08 (d, *J* = 5.4 Hz, 3H), 2.45–2.41 (m, 1H), 2.35–2.27 (m, 1H), 2.25–2.17 (m, 3H), 1.91 –1.85 (m, 1H), 1.65–1.55 (m, 2H), 0.87 (t, *J* = 7.4 Hz, 3H).

^{13}C NMR (126 MHz, CDCl$_3$) δ 175.10, 172.96, 155.22, 152.87, 151.43, 151.13, 141.52, 139.20, 134.61, 130.31, 126.94, 123.10, 108.13, 107.22, 61.45, 56.13, 52.21, 38.22, 37.45, 30.18, 29.54, 19.09, 13.93.

Compound **6**

Yellow solid, yield 73%.

ESI-MS for C$_{25}$H$_{32}$N$_2$O$_5$ (*m/z*): [M + H]$^+$ 441, [M + Na]$^+$ 463, [2M + H]$^+$ 881, [2M + Na]$^+$ 903, [M-H]$^-$ 439, [M + HCOO$^-$]$^-$ 485.

^{1}H NMR (500 MHz, CDCl$_3$) δ 7.86 (s, 1H), 7.50 (s, 1H), 7.44 (d, *J* = 11.1 Hz, 1H), 7.26–7.21 (m, 1H), 6.55 (d, *J* = 11.3 Hz, 1H), 6.51 (s, 1H), 4.76–4.68 (m, 1H), 3.93 (s, 3H), 3.88 (s, 3H), 3.61 (s, 3H), 3.08 (d, *J* = 5.4 Hz, 3H), 2.45–2.41 (m, 1H), 2.36–2.30 (m, 1H), 2.25–2.18 (m, 3H), 1.93–1.84 (m, 1H), 1.58–1.51 (m, 2H), 1.30–1.22 (m, 2H), 0.81 (t, *J* = 7.3 Hz, 3H).

^{13}C NMR (126 MHz, CDCl$_3$) δ 175.19, 173.02, 155.19, 152.85, 151.32, 151.15, 141.54, 139.11, 134.59, 130.19, 126.98, 123.13, 107.97, 107.20, 61.44, 56.13, 52.20, 37.46, 36.05, 30.19, 29.53, 27.70, 22.46, 13.76.

Compound **7**

Yellow solid, yield 24%.

ESI-MS for C$_{36}$H$_{54}$N$_2$O$_5$ (*m/z*): [M + H]$^+$ 595, [2M + H]$^+$ 1189, [M-H]$^-$ 593, [M + HCOO$^-$]$^-$ 639.

^{1}H NMR (500 MHz, CDCl$_3$) δ 8.18–7.90 (m, 2H), 7.73–7.53 (m, 2H), 6.88 (d, *J* = 10.1 Hz, 1H), 6.55 (s, 1H), 4.74 (s, 1H), 3.93 (s, 3H), 3.89 (s, 3H), 3.62 (s, 3H), 3.19 (s, 3H), 2.47 (d, *J* = 7.4 Hz, 1H), 2.39–2.08 (m, 5H), 1.54–1.49 (m, 2H), 1.28–1.16 (m, 26H), 0.86 (t, *J* = 7.0 Hz, 3H).

^{13}C NMR (126 MHz, CDCl$_3$) δ 175.09, 173.07, 155.23, 152.89, 151.32, 151.14, 141.55, 139.25, 134.58, 130.35, 126.91, 123.12, 108.24, 107.23, 61.45, 56.12, 52.16, 37.56, 36.39, 31.95, 30.18, 29.73, 29.69, 29.54, 29.53, 29.43, 29.39, 25.64, 22.72, 14.16.

Compound **9**

Yellow solid, yield 83%.

ESI-MS for C$_{22}$H$_{25}$ClN$_2$O$_5$ (*m/z*): [M + H]$^+$ 433/435, [M + Na]$^+$ 455/457, [2M + H]$^+$ 865, [2M + Na]$^+$ 887, [M-H]$^-$ 431.

^{1}H NMR (500 MHz, CDCl$_3$) δ 8.60–8.38 (m, 1H), 7.48–7.39 (m, 2H), 7.29 (q, J = 5.2 Hz, 1H), 6.56 (d, J = 11.4 Hz, 1H), 6.52 (s, 1H), 4.75–4.63 (m, 1H), 4.08–3.95 (m, 2H), 3.92 (s, 3H), 3.87 (s, 3H), 3.60 (s, 3H), 3.07 (d, J = 5.3 Hz, 3H), 2.50–2.43 (m, 1H), 2.40–2.31 (m, 1H), 2.28–2.21 (m, 1H), 2.04–1.93 (m, 1H).

^{13}C NMR (126 MHz, CDCl$_3$) δ 175.04, 166.12, 155.33, 152.97, 151.10, 150.18,141.57, 139.37, 134.41, 129.97, 126.80, 122.73, 108.18, 107.27, 61.45, 61.33, 56.14, 52.91, 42.63, 37.17, 30.02, 29.55.

Compound 10

Yellow solid, yield 46%.

ESI-MS for C$_{22}$H$_{24}$Cl$_2$N$_2$O$_5$ (*m/z*): [M + H]$^+$ 467/469, [M + Na]$^+$ 489/491, [2M + H]$^+$ 933/935, [2M + Na]$^+$ 957/959, [M-H]$^-$ 465/467.

^{1}H NMR (500 MHz, CDCl$_3$) δ 9.53 (d, J = 7.2 Hz, 1H), 7.56 (s, 1H), 7.53 (d, J = 11.2 Hz, 1H), 7.34 (q, J = 5.2 Hz, 1H), 6.64 (d, J = 11.4 Hz, 1H), 6.52 (s, 1H), 6.20 (s, 1H), 4.77–4.69 (m, 1H), 3.94 (s, 3H), 3.89 (s, 3H), 3.63 (s, 3H), 3.12 (d, J = 5.4 Hz, 3H), 2.46–2.44 (m, 1H), 2.38–2.23 (m, 2H), 1.97–1.91 (m, 1H).

^{13}C NMR (126 MHz, CDCl$_3$) δ 174.73, 164.19, 155.51, 153.12, 151.17, 150.51, 141.69, 139.81, 134.31, 130.45, 126.66, 122.71, 108.80, 107.36, 66.56, 61.52, 61.48, 56.17, 53.28, 37.17, 30.06, 29.66.

Compound 11

Yellow solid, yield 89%.

ESI-MS for C$_{24}$H$_{27}$F$_3$N$_2$O$_5$ (*m/z*): [M + H]$^+$ 481, [M + Na]$^+$ 503, [2M + H]$^+$ 961, [2M + Na]$^+$ 983, [M-H]$^-$ 479, [M + HCOO$^-$]$^-$ 525.

^{1}H NMR (500 MHz, CDCl$_3$) δ 8.77–8.65 (m, 1H), 7.56 (s, 1H), 7.49 (d, J = 11.2 Hz, 1H), 7.35–7.28 (m, 1H), 6.61 (d, J = 11.4 Hz, 1H), 6.51 (s, 1H), 4.75–4.70 (m, 1H), 3.94 (s, 3H), 3.88 (s, 3H), 3.62 (s, 3H), 3.10 (d, J = 5.4 Hz, 3H), 2.56–2.46 (m, 2H), 2.45–2.27 (m, 4H), 2.25–2.20 (m, 1H), 1.90–1.84 (m, 1H).

^{13}C NMR (126 MHz, CDCl$_3$) δ 174.99, 169.79, 155.36, 152.97, 151.33, 151.12, 141.57, 139.53, 134.54, 130.36, 127.98, 126.81, 122.89, 108.41, 107.25, 61.46, 61.34, 56.13, 52.52, 37.37, 30.16, 29.56, 29.33, 28.17.

Compound 12

Yellow solid, yield 89%.

ESI-MS for C$_{27}$H$_{28}$N$_2$O$_5$ (*m/z*): [M + H]$^+$ 461, [M + Na]$^+$ 483, [2M + H]$^+$ 921, [2M + Na]$^+$ 943, [M-H]$^-$ 459, [M + HCOO$^-$]$^-$ 505.

^{1}H NMR (500 MHz, CDCl$_3$) δ 8.36 (d, J = 7.3 Hz, 1H), 7.81 (d, J = 7.2 Hz, 2H), 7.68 (s, 1H), 7.49 (d, J = 11.2 Hz, 1H), 7.29–7.23 (m, 2H), 7.16 (t, J = 7.7 Hz, 2H), 6.57 (d, J = 11.4 Hz, 1H), 6.53 (s, 1H), 4.99–4.93 (m, 1H), 3.96 (s, 3H), 3.89 (s, 3H), 3.70 (s, 3H), 3.06 (d, J = 5.4 Hz, 3H), 2.50–2.45 (m, 1H), 2.41–2.37 (m, 1H), 2.34–2.26 (m, 1H), 2.11–2.06 (m, 1H).

^{13}C NMR (126 MHz, CDCl$_3$) δ 175.02, 167.10, 155.26, 152.91, 151.30, 151.20, 141.57, 139.18, 134.65, 133.84, 131.31, 130.17, 128.28, 127.17, 127.01, 123.23, 108.01, 107.28, 61.53, 61.49, 56.14, 52.85, 37.19, 30.30, 29.53.

Compound 14

Yellow solid, yield 57%.

ESI-MS for C$_{27}$H$_{27}$FN$_2$O$_5$ (*m/z*): [M + H]$^+$ 479, [M + Na]$^+$ 501, [2M + H]$^+$ 957, [2M + Na]$^+$ 979, [M-H]$^-$ 477, [M + HCOO$^-$]$^-$ 523.

^{1}H NMR (500 MHz, CDCl$_3$) δ 8.75 (s, 1H), 7.68 (s, 1H), 7.59 (d, J = 7.5 Hz, 1H), 7.53–7.47 (m, 2H), 7.31–7.26 (m, 1H), 7.10–7.05 (m, 1H), 6.97–6.92 (m, 1H), 6.61 (d, J = 11.4 Hz, 1H), 6.55 (s, 1H), 4.99–4.90 (m, 1H), 3.96 (s, 3H), 3.90 (s, 3H), 3.70 (s, 3H), 3.09 (d, J = 5.4 Hz, 3H), 2.53–2.47 (m, 1H), 2.43–2.37 (m, 1H), 2.35–2.27 (m, 1H), 2.18–2.10 (m, 1H).

^{13}C NMR (126 MHz, CDCl$_3$) δ 174.84, 165.56, 155.31, 152.98, 151.38, 151.20, 141.59, 139.42, 134.63, 130.36, 129.84, 126.92, 123.06, 122.53, 118.29, 118.12, 114.70, 114.52, 108.29, 107.27, 61.52, 61.50, 56.15, 53.09, 37.00, 30.31, 29.56.

3.3.5. Synthesis of 17

To a solution of compound 3 (1.0 equiv.) in DCM, N-(*tert*-Butoxycarbonyl)-N-[4-(dimethylazaniumylidene)-1,4-dihydropyridin-1-ylsulfonyl]azanide (4.0 equiv.) was added and the mixture was stirred at RT. Reaction progress was monitored by LC-MS. Then the reaction mixture was diluted with EtOAc, washed with H_2O, 10% citric acid, 1M K_2CO_3, brine and dried over Na_2SO_4. The residue was purified using column flash chromatography (silica gel; EtOAc/hexanes). To the obtained compound, 4M HCl/EtOAc was added and the reaction mixture was stirred at RT overnight. Next the solvent was removed under reduced pressure and the residue was purified using preparative HPLC (MeCN/H_2O) and lyophilized from dioxane to give the pure hydrochloride product 17 as a yellow solid with a yield of 21%.

ESI-MS for $C_{20}H_{25}N_3O_6S$ (*m/z*): $[M + H]^+$ 436, $[M + Na]^+$ 458, $[2M + H]^+$ 871, $[2M + Na]^+$ 893, $[M-H]^-$ 434.

^{1}H NMR (500 MHz, CDCl$_3$) δ 8.19 (s, 2H), 7.50–7.39 (m, 2H), 6.66 (s, 1H), 6.57 (s, 1H), 4.41–4.32 (m, 1H), 3.94 (m, 6H), 3.56 (s, 3H), 3.11 (s, 3H), 2.59–2.46 (m, 2H), 2.56–2.49 (s, 1H), 2.21 (s, 1H).

3.3.6. Synthesis of 19

To a solution of compound 3 (1.0 equiv.) and Et_3N (3.0 equiv.) in DCM in an ice bath, 2-chloroethanesulfonyl chloride (1.2 equiv.) diluted with DCM was slowly added. Next, the ice bath was removed and the reaction mixture was stirred at RT. Reaction progress was monitored by LC-MS. Then the reaction mixture was diluted with EtOAc, washed with 1M K_2CO_3, brine and dried over Na_2SO_4. The residue was purified using column flash chromatography (silica gel; EtOAc/MeOH) and lyophilized from dioxane to give the pure product 19 as a yellow solid with a yield of 64%.

ESI-MS for $C_{22}H_{26}N_2O_6S$ (*m/z*): $[M + H]^+$ 447, $[2M + H]^+$ 893, $[2M + Na]^+$ 915, $[M-H]^-$ 445.

^{1}H NMR (500 MHz, (CD$_3$)$_2$SO) δ 8.26 (d, *J* = 7.5 Hz, 1H), 8.04 (s, 1H), 7.41 (s, 1H), 7.23 (d, *J* = 11.2 Hz, 1H), 6.71 (s, 1H), 6.64 (d, *J* = 11.5 Hz, 1H), 6.48 (dd, *J* = 16.4, 9.9 Hz, 1H), 5.71 (dd, *J* = 21.1, 13.1 Hz, 2H), 3.84–3.76 (m, 4H), 3.73 (s, 3H), 3.37 (s, 3H), 2.95 (s, 3H), 2.49 (s, 1H), 2.11–2.01 (m, 2H), 1.88–1.82 (m, 1H).

^{13}C NMR (126 MHz, (CD$_3$)$_2$SO) δ 173.10, 155.58, 153.04, 150.65, 149.28, 141.12, 139.36, 137.66, 134.78, 128.80, 126.48, 125.64, 123.98, 108.88, 108.07, 61.19, 60.73, 56.26, 55.99, 38.70, 29.82.

3.3.7. Synthesis of 20

Compound 20 was obtained directly from compound 19. To 19 in DCM, morpholine was added in excess. Reaction progress was monitored by LC-MS. Then the mixture was diluted with EtOAc, washed with H_2O, brine and dried over Na_2SO_4. The residue was purified using column flash chromatography (silica gel; DCM/MeOH) and subsequently lyophilized from dioxane to give the pure product 20 as a yellow solid with a yield of 63%.

ESI-MS for $C_{26}H_{35}N_3O_7S$ (*m/z*): $[M + H]^+$ 534, $[2M + H]^+$ 1067, $[M-H]^-$ 532.

^{1}H NMR (500 MHz, CDCl$_3$) δ 7.72 (s, 1H), 7.43 (d, *J* = 11.2 Hz, 1H), 7.40–7.38 (m, 1H), 6.84–6.50 (m, 1H), 6.56 (d, *J* = 11.3 Hz, 1H), 6.53 (s, 1H), 4.48–4.35 (m, 1H), 3.93 (s, 3H), 3.90 (s, 3H), 3.63 (t, *J* = 4.5 Hz, 4H), 3.58 (s, 3H), 3.17–3.11 (m, 1H), 3.10 (d, *J* = 5.4 Hz, 3H), 3.07–2.99 (m, 1H), 2.83–2.76 (m, 1H), 2.75–2.69 (m, 1H), 2.51–2.33 (m, 7H), 1.99–1.91 (m, 1H).

^{13}C NMR (126 MHz, CDCl$_3$) δ 175.05, 155.45, 153.09, 150.89, 149.61, 141.54, 139.38, 134.35, 129.35, 129.06, 128.25, 126.38, 124.07, 108.00, 107.38, 61.37, 61.02, 56.09, 55.65, 53.37, 52.68, 51.08, 39.95, 30.38, 29.56.

3.4. Single Crystal X-ray Measurement

The single crystals of colchicine derivatives (6, 11, 12, 14, 15, 16, 18 and 19) were used for data collection on a four-circle KUMA KM4 diffractometer equipped with two-dimensional CCD area detector at room (295(1) K) and low temperature (100(1) K). The graphite monochromatized Mo-Kα radiation (λ = 0.71073 Å) and the ω-scan technique (Δω = 1°) were used for data collection. Lattice parameters were refined by the least-squares methods at all reflection positions. One image was monitored as a standard after every 40 images for a control of the crystal stability. Data collection and reduction along with absorption correction were performed using the CrysAlis software package [60]. The structures were solved by direct methods using SHELXT [61] giving positions of almost all non-hydrogen atoms. The structures were refined using SHELXL–2018 [62] with the anisotropic thermal displacement parameters. Hydrogen atoms were refined as rigid. Visualizations of the structures were made with the Diamond 3.0 program [63]. Details of the data collection parameters, crystallographic data and final agreement parameters are collected in Supplementary Table S1. The structures have been deposited with the Cambridge Crystallographic Data Center in the CIF format, no. CCDC 1980349–1980354 for **6**, **11**, **12**, CCDC 1980341–1980344 for **14** and **15**, CCDC 1980339–1980340 for **16** and CCDC 1980345–1980348 for **18** and **19** at 100 K and RT, respectively. Copies of this information can be obtained free of charge from The Director, CCDC, 12 Union Road, Cambridge, CB2 1EZ, UK (fax: +44 1223 336 033); email: deposit@ccdc.cam.ac.uk or www:http://www.ccdc.cam.ac.uk).

3.5. DFT Molecular Modeling

Molecular orbital calculations with full geometry optimization of colchicine derivatives (**6**, **11**, **12**, **14**, **15**, **16**, **18** and **19**) were performed with the Gaussian09 program package [52]. All calculations were carried out with the DFT level using the Becke3-Lee–Yang–Parr correlation functional (B3LYP) [53–56] with the 6–31+G basis set assuming the geometry resulting from the X-ray diffraction study as the starting structure. As convergence criteria, the threshold limits of 0.00025 and 0.0012 a.u. were applied for the maximum force and the displacement, respectively. The three-dimensional molecular electrostatic potential (3D MESP) maps are obtained on the basis of the DFT (B3LYP/6–31G) optimized. The calculated 3D MESP is mapped onto the total electron density isosurface ($0.008\ e\text{Å}^{-3}$) for each molecule. The color code of MESP maps is in the range of $-0.05\ e\text{Å}^{-1}$ (red) to $+0.05\ e\text{Å}^{-1}$ (blue).

3.6. In Vitro Antiproliferative Activity

3.6.1. Cell Lines and Culturing Conditions

Four human cancer cell lines and one murine normal cell line were used to evaluate antiproliferative activity of colchicine and its derivatives **1–21**: human lung adenocarcinoma (A549), human breast adenocarcinoma (MCF-7), human colon adenocarcinoma cell lines sensitive and resistant to doxorubicin (LoVo) and (LoVo/DX) respectively, and normal murine embryonic fibroblast cell line (BALB/3T3). The A549 cell line was purchased from the European Collection of Authenticated Cell Cultures (ECACC, Salisbury, UK). The MCF-7, LoVo and LoVo/DX cell lines was purchased from American Type Culture Collection (ATCC, Manassas, VA, USA). All the cell lines are maintained in the Institute of Immunology and Experimental Therapy (IIET), Wroclaw, Poland.

Human lung adenocarcinoma cell line was cultured in a mixture of OptiMEM and RPMI 1640 (1:1) medium (IIET, Wroclaw, Poland), supplemented with 5% fetal bovine serum HyClone (GE Healthcare, USA) and 2 mM L-glutamine (Sigma-Aldrich, Germany). Human breast adenocarcinoma cell line was cultured in a mixture of Eagle medium (IIET, Wroclaw, Poland), supplemented with 10% fetal bovine serum, 2 mM L-glutamine, 8 μg/mL insulin and 1% amino acids (Sigma-Aldrich, Germany). Human colon adenocarcinoma cell lines were cultured in a mixture of OptiMEM and RPMI 1640 (1:1) medium (IIET, Wroclaw, Poland), supplemented with 5% fetal bovine serum HyClone (GE Healthcare, USA), 2 mM L-glutamine, 1 mM sodium pyruvate (Sigma-Aldrich, Germany) and 10 μg/100 mL doxorubicin (Accord) for LoVo/DX. Murine embryonic fibroblast cells were cultured in Dulbecco medium (Gibco), supplemented with 10% fetal bovine serum (GE Healthcare, USA) and 2 mM L-glutamine (Sigma-Aldrich, Germany). All culture media contained antibiotics: 100 U/mL penicillin (Polfa-Tarchomin, Poland) and 0.1 mg/mL streptomycin (Sigma Aldrich, Germany). All cell lines were cultured during entire experiment in humid atmosphere at 37 °C and 5% CO_2.

3.6.2. Cell Viability Assays

Twenty-four hours before adding the tested compounds, all cell lines were seeded in 96-well plates (Sarstedt, Germany) in appropriate media with 0.5×10^4 cells per well for A549 cell line, 0.75×10^4 cells per well for MCF-7 cell line and 1.0×10^4 cells per well for LoVo, LoVo/DX and BALB/3T3 cell lines. All cell lines were exposed to each tested agent at different concentrations in the range 100–0.001 µg/mL for 72 h. The cells were also exposed to the reference drug cisplatin (Teva Pharmaceuticals, Poland) and doxorubicin (Accord Healthcare Limited, UK). Additionally, all cell lines were exposed to DMSO (solvent used for tested compounds) (POCh, Poland) at concentrations corresponding to those present in dilutions of tested agents. After 72 h sulforhodamine B assay (SRB) was performed [64].

SRB

After 72 h of incubation with the tested compounds, the cells were fixed in situ by gently adding of 50 µL per well of cold 50% trichloroacetic acid TCA (POCh, Poland) and were incubated at room temperature for one hour. Then the wells were washed four times with water and air dried. Next, 50 µL of 0.1% solution of sulforhodamine B (Sigma-Aldrich, Germany) in 1% acetic acid (POCh, Poland) were added to each well and were incubated at room temperature for 0.5 h. After incubation time, unbound dye was removed by washing plates four times with 1% acetic acid, whereas the stain bound to cells was solubilized with 150 µL of 10 mM Tris base (Sigma-Aldrich, Germany). Absorbance of each solution was read from a Synergy H4 Hybrid Multi-Mode Microplate Reader (BioTek Instruments, USA) at the 540 nm wavelength.

Results are presented as mean IC_{50} (concentration of the tested compound that inhibits cell proliferation by 50%) ± standard deviation. IC_{50} values were calculated in Cheburator 0.4, Dmitry Nevozhay software (version 1.2.0 software by Dmitry Nevozhay, 2004–2014, http://www.cheburator.nevozhay.com, freely available for each experiment [65]. Compounds at each concentration were tested in triplicates in a single experiment and each experiment was repeated at least three times independently. Results are summarized in Table 2.

3.7. Molecular Docking Studies

3.7.1. Ligand Preparation

The ligand structures were prepared using Ligprep from the Schrödinger suite [66]. Conformations and tautomeric states were assigned to the ligands by following the ligand preparation protocol implemented in Schrödinger suite with default settings. LigPrep generates variants of the same ligand with different tautomeric, stereochemical, and ionization properties.

3.7.2. Tubulin Model

The tubulin crystal structures available in the PDB are those for bovine protein. The bovine tubulin structure of tubulin (PDB ID: 1SA0) [67] was used as a template to construct the homology model of human αβ-tubulin isotypes (βI (UniProtKb: P07437), which is the most abundant isotype in most tumors using the Molecular Operating Environment (MOE) software package [68]. The sequence corresponding to the gene TUBA1A (UniProt ID: Q71U36) was chosen as a reference sequence for human tubulin, whereas gene TUBB associated to I isoform (UniProt ID: P07437) was chosen for human tubulin. Homology modeling was performed using MOE by setting the number of generated models to 10 and by selecting the final model based on MOE's generalized Born/volume integral (GB/VI) scoring function. The models used in the simulations performed for the present study were developed earlier and described in our previous publications [69]. These earlier investigations can also be considered to be validations of the computational model employed here since they were directly compared to the corresponding experimental data.

3.7.3. Molecular Dynamics Simulations

The missing hydrogens for heavy atoms were added using the tLEAP module of AMBER 14 with the AMBER14SB force field [70]. The protonation states of all ionizable residues were determined at pH = 7 using the MOE program [68]. Each protein model was solvated in a 12 Å box of TIP3P water. In order to bring the salt concentration to the physiological value of 0.15 M, 93 Na$^+$ ions and 57 Cl$^-$ ions were added. Minimization of the structure was carried out in two steps, using the steepest descent and conjugate gradient methods successively. At first, minimization was made in 2 ps on solvent atoms only, by restraining the protein-ligand complex. Next, minimization was run without the restraint in 10 ps. After minimization, the molecular dynamics (MD) simulations were carried out in three steps: heating, density equilibration, and production. At first, each solvated system was heated to 298 K for 50 ps, with weak restraints on all backbone atoms. Next, density equilibration was carried out for 50 ps of constant pressure equilibration at 298 K, with weak restraints. Finally, MD production runs were performed for all systems for 70 ns. The root-mean-square deviation (RMSD) of both the entire tubulin structure and the colchicine binding site were found to reach a plateau after 40 ns. Clustering analysis of the last 30 ns of the generated MD trajectory was carried out using the Amber's CPPTRAJ program [71] to identify representative conformations of the tubulin dimer. Clustering was made via the hierarchical agglomerative approach using the RMSD of atoms in the colchicine binding site as a metric. An RMSD cutoff of 1.0 Å was set to differentiate the clusters. On the basis of the clustering analysis, three representative structures of the tubulin dimer were found. The docking was performed on all the three representative structures and the one with the highest docking score was selected, which was the largest cluster (about 70% of the simulation) conformation of the tubulin structure. During the modeling, the cofactors including GTP, GDP, colchicine, and the magnesium ion located at the interface between α–and β–monomers were kept as part of the environment and included in the refinement step.

3.7.4. Docking Simulations

We used the AutoDock Vina [72] program to predict the binding pose of the ligands under flexible ligand and rigid receptor conditions. Dockbox package was used to facilitate preparing docking inputs and post-processing of the docking results [73]. Docking simulations performed with a cubic box (size 30.0 Å) were centered at the center of binding pockets and the docking was run separately on tubulin structure. Every generated pose was energy-minimized using Amber14 by keeping the protein fixed and was re-scored using the MOE's GBVI/WSA dG scoring function [68]. No constraints were applied in the docking studies. For each compound/protein-structure pair, the pose with the best score was identified and used as an initial configuration for molecular mechanics Gibbs–Boltzmann surface area MM/GBSA computations.

3.7.5. Binding Energy and Pairwise Per-Residue Free Energy Decomposition Calculations Using MM/GBSA Method

The MM/GBSA technique is used to calculate the free energy associated with the binding of double modified colchicine amides and sulfonamides [74]. This method combines molecular mechanics with continuum solvation models. We performed MM-GBSA integrated in Amber. The binding free energy is estimated as:

$$\Delta G_{bind} = \overline{G}_{complex} - \left[\overline{G}_{protein} + \overline{G}_{ligand}\right] \tag{1}$$

where G is the average free energy of the complex, protein, and ligand, are calculated according to the equation:

$$\overline{G} = \overline{E}_{M+}\overline{G}_{solvation} - T\overline{S} \tag{2}$$

where EMM are determined with the SANDER program and represent the internal energy (bond, angle, and dihedral), van der Waals and electrostatic interactions (see Equation (3)). TS is the entropy contribution estimated using normal mode (nmode) analysis.

$$\overline{E}_M = \overline{E}_{int} + \overline{E}_{elec} + \overline{E}_{vdW} \tag{3}$$

The solvation free energy can be calculated as the sum of polar and nonpolar contributions. The polar parts are obtained by using the generalized-born (GB) model—resulting in the MM/GBSA method, whereas the nonpolar terms are estimated from a linear relation (Equation (4)) to the solvent accessible surface area (SASA).

$$\overline{G}_{non-polar} = \gamma\, SASA + b \tag{4}$$

In the present study, a 2 ns-duration MD trajectory was run in TIP3P water using Amber14, for every top pose generated at the end of the docking step. It is worth noting that to assess the performance of MM/GBSA methodology [75], we evaluated the prediction accuracy of this method by various simulation protocols including 1 ns MD production calculations using PDBbind data set. Too long an MD simulation could be prejudicious for the overall success of the MM/GBSA method. According to this study and the common practice to calculate binding energies using MM/GBSA, we have decided to run MD production simulation for 2 ns. The MM/GBSA calculations were performed on a subset of 200 frames collected at regular time intervals from the trajectory. For PB calculations, an ionic strength of 0.0 nM (istrng = 0.0) and a solvent probe radius of 1.6 Å (prbrad = 1.6) were used. For GB calculations, the igb parameter was set to 5 that corresponds to a modified GB model equivalent to model II in reference. Pairwise free energy decomposition analysis was performed using the MM/GBSA decomposition process by the MM/GBSA program in AMBER 14 to compute the interaction between the inhibitors and each residue. For each of the tested compounds, the active residues estimated from MM/GBSA decomposition process and the best GB score out of the trajectories associated with the representative structures of the tubulin dimer were collected and are reported in Table 3 and Figure 4.

3.8. Calculation clogP

We used the Molinspiration online database (http://www.molinspiration.com, free of charge) to predict the clogP values for all synthesized compounds and collected them in Table 3 [76].

4. Conclusions

In an attempt to discover novel potent inhibitors of microtubule dynamics, eighteen novel double modified colchicine analogs comprising methylamine substituent at position C10 of ring C and amide or sulfonamide substituents at position C7 of ring B were successfully synthesized, purified and their structures were confirmed by spectroscopic analyses as well as X-ray measurements. Four human cancer cell lines (A549, MCF-7, LoVo, LoVo/DX) were used to evaluate the anticancer potency of all synthesized compounds.

Compared with unmodified colchicine, the majority of its studied derivatives exhibited excellent potency against A549, MCF-7, and LoVo cell lines. The antiproliferative activity of colchicine derivatives was in the nanomolar range and they also were characterized by lower IC_{50} values also than doxorubicin and cisplatin, commonly used as antitumor agents in cancer chemotherapy. The preliminary SAR revealed that the type of substituent at position C7 in ring B and the presence of $-NHCH_3$ group at position C10 in ring C of colchicine **1** were of cardinal importance to the compounds' cytotoxicity.

The calculated values of the selectivity index (SI) clearly show that it is possible to design more selective compounds than colchicine **1**. The most active double-modified colchicine derivatives were the compounds that included chloroacetamide and dichloroacetamide (**9**, **10**) and 2–chlorobenzamide (**13**) moiety (Table 2). However, in vitro tests showed that they did not have high SI values (except towards the LoVo cells) and *in vivo* testing should be carried out to determine their therapeutic potential.

But of all tested compounds, 4,4,4-trifluorobutyric amide of 10-*N*-methylaminocolchicine **11** was the most prominent. Compound **11** showed high activity towards A549, MCF7 and LoVo cell lines, with antiproliferative IC$_{50}$ values ranging between 10.4 and 14.6 nM as well as SI values higher than 5 for these three cell lines. The most selective towards MCF-7 cell line was compound **17** (SI was almost 10) and towards LoVo cell line the most selective were compounds **7**, **9**, **10**, and **13** (SI were over 6). So we conclude that the appropriate modification of colchicine molecule and synthesis of its analogs might overcome the toxicity, which is a major challenge in designing a potential colchicine-based drug candidate.

Compound **11** was subsequently identified as the that with potentially the best therapeutic index and therefore the most promising candidate for further development, as it showed strong in vitro anticancer activities with high SI against three human cancer cell lines. However, further in vivo studies should be conducted for the successful development of this compound.

Molecular docking study showed the ability of the obtained colchicine derivatives to bind into the active sites of βI-tubulin isotype with the well-defined binding modes. It is worthy to mention that 10-*N*-methylaminocolchicine based compounds serve as useful templates for the further development of the anticancer and antimitotic agents. Further evaluation should help to find more detailed structure-activity relationships of microtubule-targeting drugs and CBS inhibitors, which can help in rational drug design in future.

Supplementary Materials: Table S1: Details of the data collection parameters, crystallographic data and the final agreement parameters. (for compounds **6**, **11**, **12**, **14**, **15**, **16**, **18** and **19**); Table S2: Optimized parameters for colchicine derivatives (**6**, **11**, **12**, **14**, **15**, **16**, **18** and **19**), Figure S1: The LC-MS chromatogram and mass spectra of **2**; Figure S2: The ^{1}H NMR spectrum of **2** in CDCl$_3$; Figure S3: The ^{13}C NMR spectrum of **2** in CDCl$_3$; Figure S4: The LC-MS chromatogram and mass spectra of **3**; Figure S5: The ^{1}H NMR spectrum of **3** in CDCl$_3$; Figure S6: The ^{13}C NMR spectrum of **3** in CDCl$_3$; Figure S7: The LC-MS chromatogram and mass spectra of **4**; Figure S8: The ^{1}H NMR spectrum of **4** in CDCl$_3$, Figure S9: The ^{13}C NMR spectrum of **4** in CDCl$_3$, Figure S10: The LC-MS chromatogram and mass spectra of **5**; Figure S11: The ^{1}H NMR spectrum of **5** in CDCl$_3$, Figure S12: The ^{13}C NMR spectrum of **5** in CDCl$_3$; Figure S13: The LC-MS chromatogram and mass spectra of **6**; Figure S14: The ^{1}H NMR spectrum of **6** in CDCl$_3$; Figure S15: The ^{13}C NMR spectrum of **6** in CDCl$_3$; Figure S16: The LC-MS chromatogram and mass spectra of **7**; Figure S17: The ^{1}H NMR spectrum of **7** in CDCl$_3$; Figure S18: The ^{13}C NMR spectrum of **7** in CDCl$_3$; Figure S19: The LC-MS chromatogram and mass spectra of **8**; Figure S20: The ^{1}H NMR spectrum of **8** in CDCl$_3$; Figure S21:. The ^{13}C NMR spectrum of **8** in CDCl$_3$; Figure S22: The LC-MS chromatogram and mass spectra of **9**; Figure S23: The ^{1}H NMR spectrum of **9** in CDCl$_3$; Figure S24: The ^{13}C NMR spectrum of **9** in CDCl$_3$; Figure S25: The LC-MS chromatogram and mass spectra of **10**; Figure S26: The ^{1}H NMR spectrum of **10** in CDCl$_3$; Figure S27: The ^{13}C NMR spectrum of **10** in CDCl$_3$; Figure S28. The LC-MS chromatogram and mass spectra of **11**; Figure S29. The ^{1}H NMR spectrum of **11** in CDCl$_3$; Figure S30: The ^{13}C NMR spectrum of **11** in CDCl$_3$; Figure S31. The LC-MS chromatogram and mass spectra of **12**; Figure S32: The ^{1}H NMR spectrum of **12** in CDCl$_3$; Figure S33: The ^{13}C NMR spectrum of **12** in CDCl$_3$; Figure S34: The LC-MS chromatogram and mass spectra of **13**; Figure S35: The ^{1}H NMR spectrum of **13** in CD$_2$Cl$_2$; Figure S36: The ^{13}C NMR spectrum of **13** in CD$_2$Cl$_2$. Figure S37: The LC-MS chromatogram and mass spectra of **14**; Figure S38: The ^{1}H NMR spectrum of **14** in CDCl$_3$; Figure S39: The ^{13}C NMR spectrum of **14** in CDCl$_3$; Figure S40: The LC-MS chromatogram and mass spectra of **15**; Figure S41: The ^{1}H NMR spectrum of **15** in CDCl$_3$; Figure S42: The ^{13}C NMR spectrum of **15** in CDCl$_3$; Figure S43: The LC-MS chromatogram and mass spectra of **16**; Figure S44: The ^{1}H NMR spectrum of **16** in CDCl$_3$. Figure S45: The ^{13}C NMR spectrum of **16** in CDCl$_3$; Figure S46: The LC-MS chromatogram and mass spectra of **17**; Figure S47: The ^{1}H NMR spectrum of **17** in CDCl$_3$; Figure S48: The LC-MS chromatogram and mass spectra of **18**;Figure S49: The ^{1}H NMR spectrum of **18** in CDCl$_3$; Figure S50: The ^{13}C NMR spectrum of **18** in CDCl$_3$; Figure S51: The LC-MS chromatogram and mass spectra of **19**; Figure S52: The ^{1}H NMR spectrum of **19** in (CD$_3$)$_2$SO; Figure S53: The ^{13}C NMR spectrum of **19** in (CD$_3$)$_2$SO; Figure S54: The LC-MS chromatogram and mass spectra of **20**; Figure S55: The ^{1}H NMR spectrum of **20** in CDCl$_3$. Figure S56: The ^{13}C NMR spectrum of **20** in CDCl$_3$; Figure S57: The LC-MS chromatogram and mass spectra of **21**; Figure S58: The ^{1}H NMR spectrum of **21** in CDCl$_3$. Figure S59: The ^{13}C NMR spectrum of **21** in CDCl$_3$; Figure S60: Molecular structure of colchicine derivatives (**6**, **11**, **12**, **14**, **15**, **16**, **18** and **19**) at 295 K and 100 K.

Author Contributions: Conceptualization, J.K., and A.H.; methodology, J.K., A.H., J.J., J.W. and J.A.T.; software, J.J.; M.A.; validation, A.H., J.A.T. and J.J.; formal analysis, A.H. and J.K.; investigation, J.K., E.M., J.J. and M.A; resources, A.H.; J.K. and W.M.; data curation, J.K., M.A. and E.M.; writing—original draft preparation, J.K., J.J. and M.A.; writing—review and editing, W.M., A.H. J.W. and J.A.T.; visualization, J.K., J.J. and M.A.; supervision,

A.H.; project administration, A.H.; funding acquisition, A.H. and W.M. All authors have read and agreed to the published version of the manuscript.

Acknowledgments: Financial support by a grant No. 2016/21/B/ST5/00111 of the Polish National Science Centre (NCN) –is gratefully acknowledged. JAT gratefully acknowledges research support from NSERC and the Allard Foundation for his research.

References

1.   Amos, L.A. Microtubule structure and its stabilisation. *Org. Biomol. Chem.* **2004**, *2*, 2153–2160. [CrossRef] [PubMed]
2.   Wade, R.H. On and around microtubules: An overview. *Mol. Biotechnol.* **2009**, *43*, 177–191. [CrossRef] [PubMed]
3.   Hawkins, T.; Mirigian, M.; Selcuk Yasar, M.; Ross, J.L. Mechanics of microtubules. *J. Biomech.* **2010**, *43*, 23–30. [CrossRef] [PubMed]
4.   Wittmann, T.; Hyman, A.; Desai, A. The spindle: A dynamic assembly of microtubules and motors. *Nat. Cell Biol.* **2001**, *3*. [CrossRef]
5.   Jordan, M.A.; Wilson, L. Microtubules and actin filaments: Dynamic targets for cancer chemotherapy. *Curr. Opin. Cell Biol.* **1998**, *10*, 123–130. [CrossRef]
6.   Pellegrini, F.; Budman, D.R. Review: Tubulin function, action of antitubulin drugs, and new drug development. *Cancer Invest.* **2005**, *23*, 264–273. [CrossRef]
7.   Kumar, B.; Kumar, R.; Skvortsova, I.; Kumar, V. Mechanisms of Tubulin Binding Ligands to Target Cancer Cells: Updates on their Therapeutic Potential and Clinical Trials. *Curr. Cancer Drug Targets* **2016**, *17*, 357–375. [CrossRef]
8.   Capraro, H.G.; Brossi, A. Chapter 1 Tropolonic Colchicum Alkaloids. *Alkaloids Chem. Pharmacol.* **1984**, *23*, 1–70.
9.   Boyé, O.; Brossi, A. Tropolonic Colchicum Alkaloids and Allo Congeners. *Alkaloids Chem. Pharmacol.* **1992**, *41*, 125–176.
10. Hastie, S.B. Interactions of colchicine with tubulin. *Pharmacol. Ther.* **1991**, *51*, 377–401. [CrossRef]
11. Sapra, S.; Bhalla, Y.; Nandani Sharma, S.; Singh, G.; Nepali, K.; Budhiraja, A.; Dhar, K.L. Colchicine and its various physicochemical and biological aspects. *Med. Chem. Res.* **2013**, *22*, 531–547. [CrossRef]
12. Skoufias, D.A.; Wilson, L. Mechanism of Inhibition of Microtubule Polymerization by Colchicine: Inhibitory Potencies of Unliganded Colchicine and Tubulin-Colchicine Complexes. *Biochemistry* **1992**, *31*, 738–746. [CrossRef] [PubMed]
13. Bhattacharyya, B.; Panda, D.; Gupta, S.; Banerjee, M. Anti-mitotic activity of colchicine and the structural basis for its interaction with tubulin. *Med. Res. Rev.* **2008**, *28*, 155–183. [CrossRef] [PubMed]
14. Ravelli, R.B.G.; Gigant, B.; Curmi, P.A.; Jourdain, I.; Lachkar, S.; Sobel, A.; Knossow, M. Insight into tubulin regulation from a complex with colchicine and a stathmin-like domain. *Nature* **2004**, *428*, 198–202. [CrossRef]
15. Wiesenfeld, P.L.; Garthoff, L.H.; Sobotka, T.J.; Suagee, J.K.; Barton, C.N. Acute oral toxicity of colchicine in rats: Effects of gender, vehicle matrix and pre-exposure to lipopolysaccharide. *J. Appl. Toxicol.* **2007**, *27*, 421–433. [CrossRef]
16. Spiller, H.A. Colchicine. In *Encyclopedia of Toxicology*, 3rd ed.; Wexler, P., Ed.; Elsevier Inc.: London, UK, 2014; pp. 1007–1008.
17. Roubille, F.; Kritikou, E.; Busseuil, D.; Barrere-Lemaire, S.; Tardif, J.-C. Colchicine: An Old Wine in a New Bottle? *Antiinflamm. Antiallergy. Agents Med. Chem.* **2013**, *12*, 14–23. [CrossRef]
18. Mendis, S. Colchicine cardiotoxicity following ingestion of Gloriosa superba tubers. *Postgrad. Med. J.* **1989**, *65*, 752–755. [CrossRef] [PubMed]
19. Margolis, R.L.; Wilson, L. Addition of colchicine tubulin complex to microtubule ends: The mechanism of substoichiometric colchicine poisoning. *Proc. Natl. Acad. Sci. USA* **1977**, *74*, 3466–3470. [CrossRef]
20. Kuncl, R.W.; Duncan, G.; Watson, D.; Alderson, K.; Rogawski, M.A.; Peper, M. Colchicine Myopathy and Neuropathy. *N. Engl. J. Med.* **1987**, *316*, 1562–1568. [CrossRef]
21. Finkelstein, Y.; Aks, S.E.; Hutson, J.R.; Juurlink, D.N.; Nguyen, P.; Dubnov-Raz, G.; Pollak, U.; Koren, G.; Bentur, Y. Colchicine poisoning: The dark side of an ancient drug. *Clin. Toxicol.* **2010**, *48*, 407–414. [CrossRef]
22. Cocco, G.; Chu, D.C.C.; Pandolfi, S. Colchicine in clinical medicine. A guide for internists. *Eur. J. Intern. Med.* **2010**, *21*, 503–508. [CrossRef] [PubMed]
23. Zemer, D.; Revach, M.; Pras, M.; Modan, B.; Schor, S.; Sohar, E.; Gafni, J. A Controlled Trial of Colchicine in Preventing Attacks of Familial Mediterranean Fever. *N. Engl. J. Med.* **1974**, *291*, 932–934. [CrossRef] [PubMed]

24. Cerquaglia, C.; Diaco, M.; Nucera, G.; La Regina, M.; Montalto, M.; Manna, R. Pharmacological and clinical basis of treatment of Familial Mediterranean Fever (FMF) with colchicine or analogues: An update. *Curr. Drug Targets Inflamm. Allergy* **2005**, *4*, 117–124. [CrossRef] [PubMed]

25. Masuda, K.; Urayama, A.; Kogure, M.; Nakajima, A.; Nakae, K.; Inaba, G. Double-masked trial of cyclosporin versus colchicine and long-term open study of cyclosporin in Behçet's disease. *Lancet* **1989**, *333*, 1093–1096. [CrossRef]

26. Keith, M.P.; Gilliland, W.R. Updates in the Management of Gout. *Am. J. Med.* **2007**, *120*, 221–224. [CrossRef]

27. Hitzeman, N.; Stephens, R. Colchicine for acute gout. *Am. Fam. Physician* **2015**, *91*, 759–760. [PubMed]

28. Kerekes, P.; Sharma, P.N.; Brossi, A.; Chignell, C.F.; Quinn, F.R. Synthesis and Biological Effects of Novel Thiocolchicines. 3. Evaluation of *N*-Acyldeacetylthiocolchicines, *N*-(Alkoxycarbonyl)deacetylthiocolchicines, and O-Ethyldemethylthiocolchicines. New Synthesis of Thiodemecolcine and Antileukemic Effects of 2-Demeth. *J. Med. Chem.* **1985**, *28*, 1204–1208. [CrossRef]

29. Sun, L.; Hamel, E.; Lin, C.M.; Hastie, S.B.; Pyluck, A.; Lee, K.H. Antitumor Agents. 141. Synthesis and Biological Evaluation of Novel Thiocolchicine Analogs: *N*-Acyl-, *N*-Aroyl-, and *N*-(Substituted benzyl)deacetylthiocolchicines as Potent Cytotoxic and Antimitotic Compounds. *J. Med. Chem.* **1993**, *36*, 1474–1479. [CrossRef]

30. Majcher, U.; Urbaniak, A.; Maj, E.; Moshari, M.; Delgado, M.; Wietrzyk, J.; Bartl, F.; Chambers, T.C.; Tuszynski, J.A.; Huczyński, A. Synthesis, antiproliferative activity and molecular docking of thiocolchicine urethanes. *Bioorg. Chem.* **2018**, *81*, 553–566. [CrossRef]

31. Marzo-Mas, A.; Falomir, E.; Murga, J.; Carda, M.; Marco, J.A. Effects on tubulin polymerization and down-regulation of c-Myc, hTERT and VEGF genes by colchicine haloacetyl and haloaroyl derivatives. *Eur. J. Med. Chem.* **2018**, *150*, 591–600. [CrossRef]

32. Shen, L.H.; Li, H.Y.; Shang, H.X.; Tian, S.T.; Lai, Y.S.; Liu, L.J. Synthesis and cytotoxic evaluation of new colchicine derivatives bearing 1,3,4-thiadiazole moieties. *Chinese Chem. Lett.* **2013**, *24*, 299–302. [CrossRef]

33. Shen, L.H.; Li, Y.; Zhang, D.H.; Lai, Y.S.; Liu, L.J. Synthesis and evaluation of nitrate derivatives of colchicine as anticancer agents. *Chinese Chem. Lett.* **2011**, *22*, 768–770. [CrossRef]

34. Shen, L.H.; Wang, S.L.; Li, H.Y.; Lai, Y.S.; Liu, L.J. Synthesis and bioactivity of furoxan-based nitric oxide-releasing colchicine derivatives as anticancer agents. *Asian, J. Chem.* **2013**, *25*, 3294–3296. [CrossRef]

35. Kim, S.K.; Cho, S.M.; Kim, H.; Seok, H.; Kim, S.O.; Kwon, T.K.; Chang, J.S. The colchicine derivative CT20126 shows a novel microtubule-modulating activity with apoptosis. *Exp. Mol. Med.* **2013**, *45*, e19-e7. [CrossRef]

36. Lee, S.H.; Park, S.K.; Kim, J.M.; Kim, M.H.; Kim, K.H.; Chun, K.W.; Cho, K.H.; Youn, J.Y.; Namgoong, S.K. New synthetic thiocolchicine derivatives as low-toxic anticancer agents. *Arch. Pharm. (Weinheim)* **2005**, *338*, 582–589. [CrossRef]

37. Saeedi, M.; Goli, F.; Mahdavi, M.; Dehghan, G.; Faramarzi, M.A.; Foroumadi, A.; Shafiee, A. Synthesis and biological investigation of some novel sulfonamide and amide derivatives containing coumarin moieties. *Iran. J. Pharm. Res.* **2014**, *13*, 881–892.

38. Ashraf, Z.; Mahmood, T.; Hassan, M.; Afzal, S.; Rafique, H.; Afzal, K.; Latip, J. Dexibuprofen amide derivatives as potential anticancer agents: Synthesis, in silico docking, bioevaluation, and molecular dynamic simulation. *Drug Des. Devel. Ther.* **2019**, *13*, 1643–1657. [CrossRef]

39. Ragha Suma, V.; Sreenivasulu, R.; Subramanyam, M.; Rao, K.R.M. Design, Synthesis, and Anticancer Activity of Amide Derivatives of Structurally Modified Combretastatin-A4. *Russ. J. Gen. Chem.* **2019**, *89*, 499–504. [CrossRef]

40. Kachaeva, M.V.; Hodyna, D.M.; Semenyuta, I.V.; Pilyo, S.G.; Prokopenko, V.M.; Kovalishyn, V.V.; Metelytsia, L.O.; Brovarets, V.S. Design, synthesis and evaluation of novel sulfonamides as potential anticancer agents. *Comput. Biol. Chem.* **2018**, *74*, 294–303. [CrossRef]

41. Gul, H.I.; Yamali, C.; Sakagami, H.; Angeli, A.; Leitans, J.; Kazaks, A.; Tars, K.; Ozgun, D.O.; Supuran, C.T. New anticancer drug candidates sulfonamides as selective hCA IX or hCA XII inhibitors. *Bioorg. Chem.* **2018**, *77*, 411–419. [CrossRef]

42. Kiyoshi, A. N-methyldeacetylcolchiceinamide. Patent EP0607647(A1), 27 July 1994.

43. Winum, J.Y.; Toupet, L.; Barragan, V.; Dewynter, G.; Montero, J.L. N-(tert-Butoxycarbonyl)-N-[4-(dimethylazaniumylidene)-1,4-dihydropyridin-1-ylsulfonyl]azanide: A new sulfamoylating agent. Structure and reactivity toward amines. *Org. Lett.* **2001**, *3*, 2241–2243. [CrossRef] [PubMed]

44. Al-Riyami, L.; Pineda, M.A.; Rzepecka, J.; Huggan, J.K.; Khalaf, A.I.; Suckling, C.J.; Scott, F.J.; Rodgers, D.T.; Harnett, M.M.; Harnett, W. Designing anti-inflammatory drugs from parasitic worms: A synthetic small molecule analogue of the acanthocheilonema viteae product ES-62 prevents development of collagen-induced arthritis. *J. Med. Chem.* **2013**, *56*, 9982–10002. [CrossRef] [PubMed]

45. Cruz, C.M.; Ortega-Muñoz, M.; López-Jaramillo, F.J.; Hernández-Mateo, F.; Blanco, V.; Santoyo-González, F. Vinyl Sulfonates: A Click Function for Coupling-and-Decoupling Chemistry and their Applications. *Adv. Synth. Catal.* **2016**, *358*, 3394–3413. [CrossRef]

46. Lessinger, L.; Margulis, T.N. The crystal structure of colchicine. A new application of magic integers to multiple-solution direct methods. *Acta Crystallogr. Sect. B Struct. Crystallogr. Cryst. Chem.* **1978**, *34*, 578–584. [CrossRef]

47. McClure, W.O.; Paulson, J.C. The interaction of colchicine and some related alkaloids with rat brain tubulin. *Mol. Pharmacol.* **1977**, *13*, 560–575. [PubMed]

48. Hastie, S.B.; Williams, R.C.; Puett, D.; Macdonald, T.L. The binding of isocolchicine to tubulin. Mechanisms of ligand association with tubulin. *J. Biol. Chem.* **1989**, *264*, 6682–6688.

49. Politzer, P.; Laurence, P.R.; Jayasuriya, K. Molecular electrostatic potentials: An effective tool for the elucidation of biochemical phenomena. *Environ. Health Perspect.* **1985**, *61*, 191–202. [CrossRef]

50. Chemical Applications of Atomic and Molecular Electrostatic Potentials. Available online: https://www.springer.com/gp/book/9780306406577 (accessed on 13 April 2020).

51. Murray, J.S.; Politzer, P. The electrostatic potential: An overview. *Wiley Interdiscip. Rev. Comput. Mol. Sci.* **2011**, *1*, 153–163. [CrossRef]

52. Frisch, M.J.; Trucks, G.W.; Schlegel, H.B.; Scuseria, G.E.; Robb, M.A.; Cheeseman, J.R.; Scalmani, G.; Barone, V.; Mennucci, B.; Petersson, G.A.; et al. *Gaussian 09, Revision E.01.*; Gaussian, Inc: Wallingford, CT, USA, 2013.

53. Becke, A.D. Density-functional thermochemistry. IV. A new dynamical correlation functional and implications for exact-exchange mixing. *J. Chem. Phys.* **1996**, *104*, 1040–1046. [CrossRef]

54. Lee, C.; Yang, W.; Parr, R.G. Development of the Colle-Salvetti correlation-energy formula into a functional of the electron density. *Phys. Rev. B* **1988**, *37*, 785–789. [CrossRef]

55. Patterson, J.D. Density-functional theory of atoms and molecules. *Ann. Nucl. Energy* **1989**, *16*, 611. [CrossRef]

56. Bai, R.; Pei, X.F.; Boyé, O.; Getahun, Z.; Grover, S.; Bekisz, J.; Nguyen, N.Y.; Brossi, A.; Hamel, E. Identification of cysteine 354 of β-tubulin as part of the binding site for the a ring of colchicine. *J. Biol. Chem.* **1996**, *271*, 12639–12645. [CrossRef] [PubMed]

57. Chaudhuri, A.R.; Seetharamalu, P.; Schwarz, P.M.; Hausheer, F.H.; Ludueña, R.F. The interaction of the B-ring of colchicine with α-Tubulin: A novel footprinting approach. *J. Mol. Biol.* **2000**, *303*, 679–692. [CrossRef] [PubMed]

58. Cheung, C.H.A.; Wu, S.Y.; Lee, T.R.; Chang, C.Y.; Wu, J.S.; Hsieh, H.P.; Chang, J.Y. Cancer cells acquire mitotic drug resistance properties through beta i-tubulin mutations and alterations in the expression of beta-tubulin isotypes. *PLoS ONE* **2010**, *5*, 1–11. [CrossRef]

59. Ravanbakhsh, S.; Gajewski, M.; Greiner, R.; Tuszynski, J.A. Determination of the optimal tubulin isotype target as a method for the development of individualized cancer chemotherapy. *Theor. Biol. Med. Model.* **2013**. [CrossRef] [PubMed]

60. *CrysAlis CCD and CrysAlis RED, version 1171.32.15*; Oxford Diffraction Ltd: Abingdon, Oxford, UK, 2009.

61. Sheldrick, G.M. SHELXT-Integrated space-group and crystal-structure determination. *Acta Crystallogr. Sect. A Found. Crystallogr.* **2015**, *71*, 3–8. [CrossRef]

62. Sheldrick, G.M. Crystal structure refinement with SHELXL. *Acta Crystallogr. Sect. C Struct. Chem.* **2015**, *71*, 3–8. [CrossRef]

63. Brandenburg, K.; Putz, H. *DIAMOND*; Crystal Impact GbR: Bonn, Germany, 2006.

64. Skehan, P.; Storeng, R.; Scudiero, D.; Monks, A.; Mcmahon, J.; Vistica, D.; Warren, J.T.; Bokesch, H.; Kenney, S.; Boyd, M.R. New colorimetric cytotoxity assay for anticancer-drug screening. *J. Natl. Cancer Inst.* **1990**, *82*, 1107–1112. [CrossRef]

65. Nevozhay, D. Cheburator software for automatically calculating drug inhibitory concentrations from in vitroscreening assays. *PLoS ONE* **2014**, *9*, e106186. [CrossRef]

66. Schrödinger Schrödinger Release 2019–4: LigPrep. 2019. Available online: https://www.schrodinger.com/ligprep (accessed on 13 April 2020).

67. Löwe, J.; Li, H.; Downing, K.H.; Nogales, E. Refined structure of αβ-tubulin at 3.5 Å resolution. *J. Mol. Biol.* **2001**, *313*, 1045–1057. [CrossRef]

68. *Molecular Operating Environment (MOE)*; Chemical Computing Group Inc: Montreal, QC, Canada, 2012.

69. Klejborowska, G.; Urbaniak, A.; Maj, E.; Preto, J.; Moshari, M.; Wietrzyk, J.; Tuszynski, J.A.; Chambers, T.C.; Huczyński, A. Synthesis, biological evaluation and molecular docking studies of new amides of 4-chlorothiocolchicine as anticancer agents. *Bioorg. Chem.* **2020**, *97*. [CrossRef]

70. Case, D.; Babin, V.; Berryman, J.; Betz, R.; Cai, Q.; Cerutti, D.; Cheatham, T., III; Darden, T.; Duke, R.; Gohlke, H.; et al. *Amber 14*; University of California: San Francisco, CA, USA, 2014.

71. Roe, D.R.; Cheatham, T.E. PTRAJ and CPPTRAJ: Software for processing and analysis of molecular dynamics trajectory data. *J. Chem. Theory Comput.* **2013**, *9*, 3084–3095. [CrossRef] [PubMed]

72. Trott, O.; Olson, A.J. Software news and update AutoDock Vina: Improving the speed and accuracy of docking with a new scoring function, efficient optimization, and multithreading. *J. Comput. Chem.* **2010**, *31*, 455–461.

73. Preto, J.; Gentile, F. Assessing and improving the performance of consensus docking strategies using the DockBox package. *J. Comput. Aided. Mol. Des.* **2019**, *33*, 817–829. [CrossRef] [PubMed]

74. Hou, T.; Wang, J.; Li, Y.; Wang, W. Assessing the performance of the MM/PBSA and MM/GBSA methods. 1. The accuracy of binding free energy calculations based on molecular dynamics simulations. *J. Chem. Inf. Model.* **2011**, *51*, 69–82. [CrossRef] [PubMed]

75. Sun, H.; Duan, L.; Chen, F.; Liu, H.; Wang, Z.; Pan, P.; Zhu, F.; Zhang, J.Z.H.; Hou, T. Assessing the performance of MM/PBSA and MM/GBSA methods. 7. Entropy effects on the performance of end-point binding free energy calculation approaches. *Phys. Chem. Chem. Phys.* **2018**, *20*, 14450–14460. [CrossRef]

76. Molinspiration Property Calculation Service. Available online: http://www.molinspiration.com (accessed on 3 April 2020).

Permissions

List of Contributors

Sami A. Makharza
Leibniz Institute of Solid State and Material Research Dresden, 01069 Dresden, Germany
College of Pharmacy and Medical Sciences, Hebron University, Hebron 00970, Palestine

Giuseppe Cirillo
Leibniz Institute of Solid State and Material Research Dresden, 01069 Dresden, Germany
Department of Pharmacy, Health and Nutritional Sciences, University of Calabria, Rende (CS), 87036 Rende, Italy

Orazio Vittorio
Children's Cancer Institute, Lowy Cancer Research Centre, UNSW Sydney, Sydney 2031, Australia
ARC Centre of Excellence for Convergent Bio Nano Science and Technology, Australian Centre for Nano Medicine, UNSW Sydney, Sydney 2052, Australia
School of Women's and Children's Health, Faculty of Medicine, UNSW Sydney, Sydney 2052, Australia

Emanuele Valli
Children's Cancer Institute, Lowy Cancer Research Centre, UNSW Sydney, Sydney 2031, Australia
School of Women's and Children's Health, Faculty of Medicine, UNSW Sydney, Sydney 2052, Australia

Florida Voli
Children's Cancer Institute, Lowy Cancer Research Centre, UNSW Sydney, Sydney 2031, Australia

Annafranca Farfalla, Manuela Curcio, Francesca Iemma and Fiore Pasquale Nicoletta
Department of Pharmacy, Health and Nutritional Sciences, University of Calabria, Rende (CS), 87036 Rende, Italy

Ahmed A. El-Gendy
Department of Physics, University of Texas at El Paso, El Paso, TX 79968, USA

Gerardo F. Goya
Institute of Nanoscience of Aragon (INA) & Department of Condensed Matter Physics, University of Zaragoza, 50018 Zaragoza, Spain

Silke Hampel
Leibniz Institute of Solid State and Material Research Dresden, 01069 Dresden, Germany

Ayesha Jabeen, Ishita Gupta and Ala-Eddin Al Moustafa
College of Medicine, QU Health, Qatar University, Doha, Qatar
Biomedical Research Centre, Qatar University, Doha, Qatar

Anju Sharma, Semir Vranic and Halema F. Al Farsi
College of Medicine, QU Health, Qatar University, Doha, Qatar

Hadeel Kheraldine
College of Medicine, QU Health, Qatar University, Doha, Qatar
Biomedical Research Centre, Qatar University, Doha, Qatar
College of Pharmacy, Qatar University, Doha, Qatar

Krystal M. Butler-Fernández, Zulma Ramos, Joseph Bloom and Eliud Hernández
Department of Pharmaceutical Sciences, University of Puerto Rico, School of Pharmacy, San Juan 00936, Puerto Rico

Adela M. Francis-Malavé
Department of Biology, College of Natural Sciences, University of Puerto Rico, San Juan 00931, Puerto Rico

Suranganie Dharmawardhane
Department of Biochemistry, University of Puerto Rico, School of Medicine, San Juan 00936, Puerto Rico

Marcos Vilariño, Josune García-Sanmartín, Laura Ochoa-Callejero and Alfredo Martínez
Oncology Area, Center for Biomedical Research of La Rioja (CIBIR), 26006 Logroño, Spain

Alberto López-Rodríguez and Jaime Blanco-Urgoiti
CsFlowchem, Campus Universidad San Pablo CEU, Boadilla del Monte, 28668 Madrid, Spain

Shu Wang, Thomas F. Greene, Niamh M. O'Boyle, Niall O. Keely and Mary J. Meegan
School of Pharmacy and Pharmaceutical Sciences, Trinity College Dublin, Trinity Biomedical Sciences Institute, 152-160 Pearse Street, Dublin 2 DO2R590, Ireland

Azizah M. Malebari
Department of Pharmaceutical Chemistry, College of Pharmacy, King Abdulaziz University, Jeddah 21589, Saudi Arabia

Darren Fayne, Seema M. Nathwani and Daniela M. Zisterer
School of Biochemistry and Immunology, Trinity College Dublin, Trinity Biomedical Sciences Institute, 152-160 Pearse Street, Dublin 2 DO2R590, Ireland

Brendan Twamley and Thomas McCabe
School of Chemistry, Trinity College Dublin, Dublin 2 DO2R590, Ireland

Hazel O'Neill, John V Reynolds and Jacintha O'Sullivan
Trinity Translational Medicine Institute, Department of Surgery, Trinity College Dublin, D08W9RT Dublin, Ireland

Vinod Malik and Ciaran Johnston
Department of Radiology, St. James's Hospital, D08 X4RX Dublin, Ireland

Amira A. El-Sayed and Ahmed K. EL-Ziaty
Laboratory of Synthetic Organic Chemistry, Chemistry Department, Faculty of Science, Ain Shams University, Abbassia, Cairo 11566, Egypt

Abd El-Galil E. Amr
Pharmaceutical Chemistry Department, Drug Exploration & Development Chair (DEDC), College of Pharmacy, King Saud University, Riyadh 11451, Saudi Arabia
Applied Organic Chemistry Department, National Research Center, Cairo, Dokki 12622, Egypt

Elsayed A. Elsayed
Zoology Department, Bioproducts Research Chair, Faculty of Science, King Saud University, Riyadh 11451, Saudi Arabia
Chemistry of Natural and Microbial Products Department, National Research Centre, Dokki 12622, Cairo, Egypt

Kasipandi Muniyandi
Laser Research Centre, Faculty of Health Sciences, University of Johannesburg, 17011, Doornfontein 2028, South Africa
Bioprospecting Laboratory, Department of Botany, School of Life Sciences, Bharathiar University, Coimbatore, Tamil Nadu 641046, India

Blassan George and Heidi Abrahamse
Laser Research Centre, Faculty of Health Sciences, University of Johannesburg, 17011, Doornfontein 2028, South Africa

Thangaraj Parimelazhagan
Bioprospecting Laboratory, Department of Botany, School of Life Sciences, Bharathiar University, Coimbatore, Tamil Nadu 641046, India

Marcin Michalak
Department of Radiation Therapy and Gynecologic Oncology, Greater Poland Cancer Centre, Garbary 15, 61–866 Poznań, Poland

Michał Stefan Lach
Radiobiology Lab, Greater Poland Cancer Centre, Garbary 15, 61–866 Poznań, Poland
The Postgraduate School of Molecular Medicine, Medical University of Warsaw, Księcia Trojdena 2a, 02–109 Warsaw, Poland
Department of Electroradiology, Poznań University of Medical Sciences, Garbary 15, 61–866 Poznań, Poland

Michał Antoszczak and Adam Huczyński
Department of Medical Chemistry, Faculty of Chemistry, Adam Mickiewicz University, Uniwersytetu Poznańskiego 8, 61–614 Poznań, Poland

Wiktoria Maria Suchorska
Radiobiology Lab, Greater Poland Cancer Centre, Garbary 15, 61–866 Poznań, Poland
Department of Electroradiology, Poznań University of Medical Sciences, Garbary 15, 61–866 Poznań, Poland

Alhussein A. Ibrahimd
Applied Organic Chemistry Department, National Research Center, Cairo, Dokki 12622, Egypt

Mohamed F. El-Shehry
Pesticide Chemistry Department, National Research Center, Dokki 12622, Cairo, Egypt
Chemistry Department, Al-Zahrawy University College, Karbala 56001, Iraq

Hanaa M. Hosni
Pesticide Chemistry Department, National Research Center, Dokki 12622, Cairo, Egypt

Ahmed A. Fayed
Applied Organic Chemistry Department, National Research Center, Cairo, Dokki 12622, Egypt
Respiratory Therapy Department, College of Medical Rehabilitation Sciences, Taibah University, Madinah Munawara, 22624, Saudi Arabia

Julia Krzywik
Department of Medical Chemistry, Faculty of Chemistry, Adam Mickiewicz University, Uniwersytetu Poznańskiego 8, 61–614 Poznań, Poland
TriMen Chemicals, Piłsudskiego 141, 92–318 Łódź, Poland

Witold Mozga
TriMen Chemicals, Piłsudskiego 141, 92–318 Łódź, Poland

Maral Aminpour
Department of Oncology, University of Alberta, Edmonton, AB T6G 1Z2, Canada

Jan Janczak
Institute of Low Temperature and Structure Research, Polish Academy of Sciences, 50–950 Wrocław, Poland

Ewa Maj and Joanna Wietrzyk
Hirszfeld Institute of Immunology and Experimental Therapy, Polish Academy of Sciences, Rudolfa Weigla 12, 53–114 Wrocław, Poland

Jack A. Tuszyński
Department of Oncology, University of Alberta, Edmonton, AB T6G 1Z2, Canada
DIMEAS, Politecnico di Torino, Corso Duca degli Abruzzi, 24, 10129 Torino, Italy

Index

A

Actin Cytoskeleton, 33-35, 39, 49, 51-52, 56-59, 61

Actin Polymerization, 33-35, 39, 48-49

Adenocarcinoma, 52, 59, 62, 67, 108, 111, 116, 125, 127, 152, 156, 215

Alkaloids, 52, 62, 65, 143-144, 149, 153-154, 159, 220, 222

Angiogenesis, 17, 23-24, 28, 78, 114, 117-119, 122-123, 125, 127, 153, 161

Anthraquinones, 143-144, 149, 154, 159, 162-163

Anti-migratory Effect, 38, 49

Anticancer Agents, 2, 109-111, 129, 142, 148, 161, 169-170, 172, 191, 193, 221, 223

Antimitotic Agents, 65, 108, 110-112, 219

Apoptotic Cell Death, 104, 148

B

Biocompatibility, 2-4, 6, 13

Blood Brain Barrier, 2, 4, 78

C

Cell Culture, 25, 48, 51, 103, 139, 173-174

Cell Invasion, 16-18, 21, 23-24, 26-28, 30, 33

Cell Proliferation, 16-18, 23-24, 26, 29, 36, 51, 144, 153, 155, 160, 174, 184, 216

Cell Viability, 17, 26, 35-37, 39, 48, 79-80, 103, 140, 174, 182, 216

Chemotherapy, 1-2, 14, 16, 125, 127, 143-144, 164-165, 172, 176-177, 193, 201, 218, 220, 222

Cisplatin, 1, 11-15, 64, 162, 164, 166-167, 169-175, 177-178, 182, 189, 193, 201, 216, 218

Colchicine Amides, 193, 207, 217

Colchicine Binding Site, 76, 84-85, 87, 109, 193-195, 207-208, 217

Colorectal Cancer, 17, 63, 118, 125, 128, 158, 178

Column Flash Chromatography, 209-210, 212, 214

Combination Index, 170, 174-175

Confocal Microscopy, 57, 60, 84, 105, 107

Coumarins, 17, 24

Crystal Structure, 67, 69, 85, 106, 111, 113, 193, 222

Curcumins, 143-144, 149, 153

Cytotoxicity, 2, 15, 38, 59, 65, 78-80, 87, 103-104, 111, 113, 133, 135, 139, 142-143, 150, 152, 154, 156, 161, 177, 193, 201, 206-207, 218, 222

E

Elaeagnus Angustifolia, 16-18, 26, 28-29

Electron Impact, 88, 185

Electrospray Ionization, 41, 49, 88, 209

Endothelial Cells, 15, 63, 84, 108

Epithelial-mesenchymal Transition, 16, 30, 172, 175, 178

Extracellular Matrix, 33-34, 49

F

Fetal Bovine Serum, 11, 25-26, 59, 103, 140, 174-175, 215

Flavonoids, 17, 23-24, 30

Flow Cytometry, 18-19, 26, 80-82, 87, 104

Furanocoumarins, 143-144, 149-150

G

Gemcitabine, 164, 167-168, 170, 172, 175, 178

Gene Expression, 28, 57, 61, 119, 156, 159, 174, 177

Glioblastoma, 1-2, 6, 11-12, 14, 162

Glycolysis, 114, 116-118, 120

Graphite Oxide, 3, 9

H

Hepatocellular Carcinoma, 29, 66, 108, 119, 126, 133, 139, 172, 178

Heterocycles, 66, 140-142, 161

Heterogeneity, 116, 123

High-performance Liquid Chromatography, 88, 105, 107, 160

Hypoxia, 114, 116-120, 122-123, 125-128

I

Immunofluorescence, 35, 65, 84-85, 87, 105

Invadopodia, 33, 35, 39

L

Leukemia, 17, 31, 62, 78, 172, 175, 177, 191

M

Macrocybe Titans, 52, 54, 58, 63

Macrocybin, 52, 54-61

Maghemite, 1-4, 10, 14-15

Magnetic Vectorization, 8, 11

Mass Spectrometry, 41, 49-50, 52, 54, 88, 107

Microtubules, 66, 83-84, 104, 193, 207, 220

Molecular Dynamics, 207, 217, 223

Molecular Electrostatic Potential Map, 198, 200-201

Molecular Operating Environment, 106, 112-113, 216, 222

N

Nanographene Oxide, 1-2, 9, 14

Nanohybrids, 2-3, 13-14

Non-essential Amino Acids, 48, 103, 174, 176

Non-small Cell Lung Cancer, 63, 84, 112, 122, 127-128, 152, 177

Nuclear Magnetic Resonance, 40, 52, 60, 88, 107

O
Oesophageal Cancer, 121, 127

P
Phosphate Buffered Saline, 26, 174
Photodynamic Therapy, 13, 143-146, 154-159, 161-163
Photosensitizer, 155, 157-159
Pim Kinases, 184, 191
Polyacetylenes, 143-144, 149, 152
Polyvinylidene Difluoride, 175-176
Positron Emission Tomography, 114, 124-128
Pyrazolopyridine, 129, 132, 140

R
Reactive Oxygen Species, 2, 144-145, 155, 162
Resistance Index, 169, 174, 201

S
Salinomycin, 164-166, 168-171, 173, 176-178
Selectivity Index, 169, 174, 206, 218

Stratification, 120, 124, 127
Structure-activity Relationship, 33-34, 40, 107, 110, 135, 161, 167, 176, 195
Sulfonamides, 193, 201, 205-207, 209, 217, 221

T
Thermogravimetric Analysis, 1, 5
Thiazolidinone, 179, 181, 186
Thienopyrimidinone, 179-180, 189
Thin Layer Chromatography, 88, 107
Thiophenes, 143-144, 149, 152, 158, 160-161
Triethylamine, 70, 90, 95, 107, 188, 195
Triglycerides, 52, 54-55, 58
Tubulin Polymerization, 65-66, 82-84, 87, 104, 111-112, 207, 221

W
Western Blot Analysis, 27, 170, 172-175

X
Xenografts, 2, 125, 189

www.ingramcontent.com/pod-product-compliance
Lightning Source LLC
Chambersburg PA
CBHW080530200326
41458CB00012B/4394